GRS

Geriatrics Review Syllabus:
A Core Curriculum in Geriatric Medicine

Seventh Edition

Syllabus/Book 3

Editors-In-Chief

James T. Pacala, MD, MS, AGSF
Gail M. Sullivan, MD, MPH, AGSF

The Chief Editors were James T. Pacala, MD, MS and Gail M. Sullivan, MD, MPH; Syllabus Editors were Colleen Christmas, MD, G. Paul Eleazer, MD, Anne R. Fabiny, MD, Melinda S. Lantz, MD, and Annette Medina-Walpole, MD; Question Editors were John D. Gazewood, MD, MSPH, C. Bree Johnston, MD, MPH, and Gary J. Kennedy, MD; Consulting Editor on Ethnogeriatrics was Carmel Bitondo Dyer, MD; Consulting Editor on Pharmacotherapy was Judith L. Beizer, PharmD; Special Advisors were Samuel C. Durso, MD, MBA, and Michelle Eslami, MD; Medical Writers were Susan E. Aiello, DVM, ELS and Dalia Ritter; Indexer was L. Pilar Wyman; and Managing Editor was Andrea N. Sherman, MS.

Many thanks to Fry Communications for assistance in organizing the *Geriatrics Review Syllabus* material onto an editorial content management Web site and all production work including typesetting, graphic design, CD-ROM development, and printing. With more than 60 years in the information industry, Fry offers printing and ancillary services to publishers and other content providers.

Citation: Pacala JT, Sullivan GM, eds. *Geriatrics Review Syllabus: A Core Curriculum in Geriatric Medicine.* 7th ed. New York: American Geriatrics Society; 2010.

Geriatrics Review Syllabus: A Core Curriculum in Geriatric Medicine, 7th Edition. Cataloging in publication data is available from the Library of Congress.

Library of Congress Control Number: 2009906527

ISBN Number Book 3: 978-1-886775-52-7

10   9   8   7   6   5   4   3   2   1

INTRODUCTION

The core mission of the American Geriatrics Society (AGS) is to improve the health, independence, and quality of life of all older adults. Since the AGS published the first *Geriatrics Review Syllabus (GRS)* in 1989, the *GRS* has become recognized as the premier geriatric medicine resource supporting clinicians to stay current and to provide evidence-based, high quality care to older adults. To keep pace with advances in geriatric medicine, the AGS is proud to publish this seventh edition *(GRS7)*. Over 100 AGS members, leaders in the field of geriatric medicine, contributed to the *GRS7* as authors and question writers.

Contents

The *GRS7* is available as a 3-volume set of books and in CD-ROM format. Book 1 contains the *Syllabus* of 62 chapters and annotated references that allow the interested reader to pursue topics in greater depth. Book 2 contains 290 case-oriented, multiple-choice questions and is accompanied by an answer sheet for those participating in the continuing education program. Book 3 repeats the questions and contains answers, supporting critiques, and references to aid learner self-assessment. The CD-ROM format comprises the entire program.

The *Syllabus* is divided into six sections—Principles of Aging, Approach to the Patient, Care Systems, Syndromes, Psychiatry, and Diseases and Disorders. *GRS7* particularly highlights developments in geriatric medicine since publication of the sixth edition. When discussing specific drugs, the authors and editors verified that the information provided was up to date at the time of publication. Any mention of uses not specifically approved by the U.S. Food and Drug Administration (so called "off-label" uses) are tagged as OL.

New Features

New features in the seventh edition include added emphases on evidence-based medicine and on quality assessment and improvement. Authors were encouraged to include strength-of-evidence (SOE) ratings for key diagnostic, prognostic, and therapeutic information. Authors and editors also have endeavored to present measures of association (between risk factors or therapies and conditions) in terms of absolute risk as well as relative risk. The Assessing Care of Vulnerable Elders-3 (ACOVE-3) quality indicators have been appended to applicable chapters in *GRS7*. The 392 ACOVE-3 indicators, published in 2007 in the *Journal of the American Geriatrics Society*, can be used by practitioners to measure and improve the quality of care they provide to older adults. Please see the inside cover for further explanation of the SOE rating system and of the ACOVE-3 indicators.

Multiple Choice Questions

The question editors, using questions drafted by question writers, have developed an entirely new set of 290 case-oriented, multiple-choice self-study questions. These questions are designed to complement material in the *Syllabus* chapters. The questions draw on the entire knowledge base of geriatric medicine, rather than just material from the *Syllabus* text. We recommend that participants prepare for answering these questions by first reading through the *Syllabus* chapters. Material addressed in the questions that is not discussed in the chapters is discussed in the critiques. The questions have been developed independently of any specialty board and will not be a part of any secure board certification examination.

CME and MOC Credits

The *GRS* self-assessment program provides participants with the option of applying for 85 Continuing Medical Education (CME) credits through the American Medical Association, American Academy of Family Physicians, and American Osteopathic Association. For information on self-scoring or submitting answer sheets for CME credit, please see the Program Guidelines (p xxix). In addition, the American Board of Internal Medicine (ABIM) has approved the CD-ROM version of the *GRS7* self-assessment program for 110 lifelong learning points for ABIM diplomates who are enrolled in the Maintenance of Certification (MOC) program. See Program Guidelines for further instructions.

We hope the *GRS7* will meet our goal of enhancing participants' knowledge base and practice patterns when caring for older adults by providing a self-study tool that is current, concise, scholarly, and clinically relevant. We encourage your comments and suggestions, as the AGS continually strives to better serve its members and the older adults they treat.

Learning Objectives

The learning objectives for this activity have been designed to address participant knowledge, competence, performance, and patient outcomes. At the conclusion of this program, participants should be able to:

- Describe the general principles of aging and the biomedical and psychosocial issues of aging (knowledge);

- Discuss legal and ethical issues related to geriatric medicine (knowledge/competence);

- Evaluate the financing of health care for older adults (knowledge/competence);

- Identify the basic principles of geriatric medicine, including assessment, geriatric pharmacotherapy, prevention, exercise, palliative care, rehabilitation, and sensory deficits (knowledge/competence);

- Use state-of-the-art approaches to geriatric care while providing care in hospital, office-practice, nursing-home, and home-care settings (performance);

- Diagnose and manage geriatric syndromes, including dementia, delirium, urinary incontinence, malnutrition, osteoporosis, falls, pressure ulcers, sleep disorders, pain, dysphagia, and dizziness (performance);

- Apply relevant information from the fields of internal medicine, neurology, psychiatry, dermatology, and gynecology to the care of older patients (performance);

- Adjust patient care in the light of evidence-based data regarding the particular risks and needs of ethnic, racial, and sexual patient groups (patient outcomes);

- Use quality indicators to assess and improve the care of older adults in their own practices (performance/patient outcomes); and

- Employ evidence-based data to increase the effectiveness of teaching geriatrics to all health professionals (performance).

Other Resources

The intent of the *GRS* is to provide an up-to-date resource that covers the broad scope of geriatric medicine. Other AGS products are designed to complement the GRS7 in caring for older adults. The practice handbook *Geriatrics At Your Fingertips*, published annually, provides practical, up-to-date information for clinicians. The AGS publication *Doorway Thoughts: Cross-Cultural Health Care for Older Adults* is designed to raise awareness of differences between various ethnic groups and to heighten sensitivity to cultural issues in the care of older adults. Another supplemental product is the *GRS Teaching Slides*, available as a subscription through the AGS Web site (http://www.frycomm.com/ags/teachingslides/.) The slide presentations in Microsoft® Power Point® are based on each of the *GRS* chapters and suitable for faculty, fellows, residents, and students. Each presentation is designed for approximately a 1-hour seminar and may be used as a stand-alone lecture or as a complement to one's own personal teaching materials. These and other publications, including resources and clinical practice guidelines, are available at www.americangeriatrics.org.

PROGRAM GUIDELINES

PRE-ACTIVITY ASSESSMENT

To assess changes in participant knowledge and competence, the *GRS7* contains both a pre-activity assessment and a Continuing Medical Education (CME) exam (post-test). The pre-activity assessment is designed to test participant knowledge before reading the *GRS7 Syllabus*. These data will be used to help the American Geriatrics Society (AGS) measure the effectiveness of this CME activity.

Before reading the *GRS7 Syllabus*, please complete the first 10 questions of Book 2 and record your answers on either the enclosed bubble sheet form or online at www.MyCECenter.com. Click on the home page icon button for the *GRS7* exam.

CONTINUING EDUCATION CREDITS

Accreditation

The AGS is accredited by the Accreditation Council for Continuing Medical Education (ACCME) to provide CME for physicians.

CME Credit Hours

American Medical Association (AMA) ■ The AGS designates this educational activity for a maximum of **85 AMA PRA Category 1 Credit(s)**™. Physicians should only claim credit commensurate with the extent of their participation in the activity. The credit is available from May 1, 2010 through April 30, 2013.

American Academy of Family Physicians (AAFP) ■ This activity has been reviewed and is acceptable for up **to 85 Prescribed credit(s) by the AAFP.** AAFP accreditation begins May 1, 2010. Term of approval is for 2 year(s) from this date, with option for yearly renewal. The AGS will apply for renewal of Prescribed credits for the period April 30, 2012 to April 30, 2013, following the review of the *GRS7* for currency of content in mid-2011.

American Osteopathic Association (AOA) ■ The **AOA** has determined that the *GRS7* is eligible for up to **85 hours in Category 2-B of AOA CME** from May 1, 2010 through April 30, 2013.

Method of Participation

Based on pilot tests, this activity should take approximately 85 hours to complete. To receive CME credit, participants must complete the pre-activity assessment, read the *GRS7 Syllabus*, select the type of CME requested, and complete and submit the CME exam (post-test) with at least 70% of the questions answered correctly.

Methods of Submission and Notification of CME Examination Performance

For those using the *GRS7* Question Book, the CME exam (post-test) answers may be submitted either online or by completing the enclosed bubble sheet answer form and mailing it to Program Management Services, Inc. (PMSI) with the enclosed envelope. All score results are considered confidential. The type of CME credit requested must be indicated online or on the bubble sheet.

To complete and submit your CME exam (post-test) answers using the *GRS7* Question Book, please choose one of the following methods:

1 ■ Go online to www.MyCEcenter.com to complete the CME exam (post-test). Please click the *GRS7* icon button, which appears on the home page, and follow all instructions carefully. You do not have to complete the entire exam at one time. You may save your answers, revise, and complete the exam at your own pace. Once your answers are successfully submitted, your exam results will be **immediately** available and you will be able to download and/or print your CME certificate of completion, check credits earned, and reprint your CME certificate and Personal Performance Results.

2 ■ Complete the CME exam (post-test) manually with the enclosed bubble sheet form and mail it to PMSI for scoring in the enclosed envelope. PMSI will grade your exam and mail your Personal Performance Results to you. For those who successfully complete the program, a CME certificate, based on your CME selection, will be enclosed with the report. For those who do not successfully complete the program, another answer sheet will be enclosed with an offer to take the exam again. Please allow a minimum of 3-4 weeks for processing if you mail your exam results.

If you lose the return envelope, mail your bubble sheet form to: PMSI, P.O. Box 490, East Islip, NY 11730. Only regular U.S. mail is accepted. Mail that requires a signature will be returned to the sender.

CD-ROM Program Submission: If you are using the *GRS7* CD-ROM program, on completion of all of the questions, answers may be uploaded directly to PMSI for processing of CME. For those who successfully complete the program, participants may log onto www.MyCEcenter.com to download and/or print their CME certificate along with their Personal Performance Report.

American Board of Internal Medicine (ABIM) Maintenance of Certification (MOC)

Diplomates of the ABIM who are recertifying may also obtain 110 MOC lifelong learning points through the *GRS7* CD-ROM self-assessment program. This is in addition to Category 1 credit. ABIM MOC lifelong learning points are *not* available through the online or bubble sheet exam formats, *only* through the *GRS7* CD-ROM program. For those eligible to apply for the ABIM MOC lifelong learning points, complete the required section during the program registration and your answers will be forwarded to ABIM for processing.

Submission and Notification Questions

Questions about submissions and CME certificates should be directed to PMSI at **1-800-232-4422 or 631-563-1604.**

User Eligibility for CME Credits

Each copy of the *GRS7* program is valid for CME credits for only one participant.

QUESTION ANALYSIS

AGS will post an analysis of participant performance on the *Syllabus* questions to the AGS Web site (http://www.americangeriatrics.org) once 250 answer sheets have been scored.

USER EVALUATION

The AGS would appreciate participants' comments about the *GRS7* program through the user evaluation enclosed with the program. Comments and suggestions will be taken into consideration by those planning the next edition.

Congruity of Content between *Syllabus* and Questions

Because the *Syllabus* chapters and the questions with critiques are written by different authors, questions may not always correlate directly with the *Syllabus*. In the event that a question's content is not addressed in the correlating chapter, its answer is fully supported in the question critique.

UPDATES AND ERRATA

Important updates, such as medication alerts, will be posted as necessary on the AGS Web site: http://www.americangeriatrics.org.

Please report any errata to: info.amger@americangeriatrics.org, Attention: *GRS* Managing Editor. Identified errata will be posted on the AGS Web site: http://www.americangeriatrics.org.

AGS GERIATRICS RECOGNITION AWARD

The Geriatrics Recognition Award (GRA) was developed by the AGS to encourage health care professionals to acquire special knowledge and keep abreast of the latest developments in geriatrics through continuing education programs. The GRA demonstrates a health care professional's commitment to providing quality care to patients by participating in continuing education programs in geriatrics. It provides professional recognition of a health care professional's special knowledge in geriatrics sought by many employers.

CME credits earned from successfully completing the *GRS7* may be applied toward the GRA. To receive more information and an application, please provide your mailing address to the American Geriatrics Society, CME Department, Empire State Building, Suite 801, 350 Fifth Avenue, New York, NY 10118, telephone (212) 308-1414, fax (212) 832-8646.

GRS7 Online (Web version)

The *GRS7* will soon be available via the Web through institutional subscriptions. Subscribers can purchase yearly access to the full *GRS7 Syllabus* along with the questions and critiques for all of their students and faculty to use through their institutional intranets. For more information on this great teaching resource, please contact Elvy Ickowicz at 212-308-1414 or eickowicz@americangeriatrics.org.

QUESTIONS, ANSWERS, SUPPORTING CRITIQUES, AND REFERENCES

Note: The table of Normal Laboratory Values on the inside back cover may be consulted for any of the questions in this book.

1. A 72-yr-old woman comes to the office for preoperative evaluation before left total-knee replacement. Despite the worsening pain in her left knee, she remains active, and gardens and plays golf 4 days a week. She has no known allergies and has never smoked. Both her parents lived into their nineties. History includes mild hypertension, for which she takes atenolol 25 mg/d.

   On physical examination, blood pressure is 121/82 mmHg and resting heart rate is 70 beats per minute. Other than osteoarthritic changes in both knees, left worse than right, her examination is unremarkable. Serum chemistries and CBC are within normal limits. ECG shows no conduction delays and no ischemic changes.

   Which of the following is most appropriate for perioperative management of this patient?

   (A) Increase atenolol dosage to 50 mg/d; continue perioperatively.
   (B) Discontinue atenolol immediately before surgery; restart 48 hours after surgery.
   (C) Continue atenolol at the current dosage.
   (D) Discontinue atenolol; begin an ACE inhibitor plus a statin.

   ANSWER: C

   This patient has a Revised Cardiac Risk Index of 0 (normal creatinine level; no heart failure, ischemic heart disease, or diabetes; and no history of cerebrovascular disease). For patients at low cardiac risk (index of 0 or 1) who are already on a β-blocker for hypertension, angina, arrhythmias, or other cardiac problems, β-blocker treatment should be continued perioperatively (SOE=C).

   Perioperative β-blockers should not be started in patients at low cardiac risk (index of 0 or 1) who do not already take a β-blocker; in these patients, β-blockers offer no benefit and may be harmful (SOE=B). The available evidence suggests that benefit from β-blockers is primarily limited to patients with a Revised Cardiac Risk Index >2 who are undergoing major noncardiac surgery.

   Increasing the dosage of β-blocker in a low-risk patient affords no benefit and may precipitate perioperative hypotension or bradycardia. Abrupt discontinuation of the β-blocker could result in rebound hypertension and tachycardia. In this patient, there is no indication for starting an ACE inhibitor.

   References
   1. Fleisher LA, Beckman JA, Brown KA, et al. ACC/AHA 2007 Guidelines on Perioperative Cardiovascular Evaluation and Care of Noncardiac Surgery: A report of the American College of Cardiology/American Heart Association Task Force on Practice Guidelines. *J Am Coll Cardiol.* 2007;50(17):159–241.
   2. Lindenauer PK, Pekow P, Wang K, et al. Perioperative beta-blocker therapy and mortality after major noncardiac surgery. *N Engl J Med.* 2005;353(4):349–361.
   3. Salerno SM, Carlson DW, Soh EK, et al. Impact of perioperative cardiac assessment guidelines on management of orthopedic surgery patients. *Am J Med.* 2007;120(11):181–185.

2. A 70-yr-old man comes to the office because he is bothered by increasing urinary urgency over the last few months. He has had lower urinary tract symptoms associated with benign prostatic hyperplasia; these have been well controlled with tamsulosin over the past year. He now describes the sudden need to go to the bathroom, occasionally associated with losing "a few drops" of urine before he gets to the toilet. His usual symptoms of frequency and urgency have also become more troublesome. He has no dysuria, hematuria, chills, fever, or symptoms related to sexual activity. History includes dyslipidemia and hypertension. In addition to tamsulosin, he takes atorvastatin and lisinopril.

On examination, blood pressure is 110/70 mmHg and heart rate is 60 beats per minute. Digital rectal examination is unchanged from previous years: he has a well-defined, nontender prostate about 20 mL in size, with no asymmetry, nodules, or induration.

The patient's levels of prostate-specific antigen have slowly increased over the past few years, from 2.5 to 3.25 at his last evaluation 2 mo ago. A urine sample analyzed in the office is normal. Postvoid residual volume is 80 mL on ultrasonography.

Which of the following is the most appropriate next step?

(A)   Urine culture after prostate massage
(B)   Transrectal ultrasonography
(C)   Treatment with tolterodine
(D)   Treatment with finasteride

ANSWER: C

This patient has overactive bladder syndrome associated with benign prostatic hyperplasia and a relatively small prostate. Overactive bladder syndrome is increasingly recognized as an important cause of lower urinary tract symptoms in men with benign prostatic hyperplasia. This patient's symptoms of increasing urinary frequency, urgency, and urge incontinence are classic for this syndrome. In a randomized trial of men with benign prostatic hyperplasia and symptoms of overactive bladder, adding an antimuscarinic agent (extended-release tolterodine) to an α-blocker was associated with greater clinical improvement than treatment with an α-blocker alone (SOE=A), at least in men with a postvoid residual urine volume of <200 mL (mean, 53 mL). Urinary retention was rare in this trial.

   Treatment with finasteride is unlikely to improve symptoms of urgency; finasteride also tends to be more effective in men with large prostates. Chronic bacterial or nonbacterial prostatitis is unlikely, given the normal urinalysis and absence of pelvic pain or irritation. Transrectal ultrasonography is appropriate only when biopsy is indicated for possible prostate cancer.

References

1. Kaplan SA, Roehrborn C, Rovner ES, et al. Tolterodine and tamsulosin for treatment of men with lower urinary tract symptoms of overactive bladder: a randomized clinical control trial. *JAMA*. 2006;296(19):2319–2328.

2. Roehrborn CG. Current medical therapies for men with lower urinary tract symptoms and benign prostatic hyperplasia: achievements and limitations. *Rev Urol*. 2008;10(1):14–25.

3.   An 88-yr-old man comes to the office because he has been feeling more tired than usual, and yesterday he fell in his bedroom. He was hospitalized with pneumonia 2 mo ago; he received daily physical and occupational therapy in a nursing facility for 4 wk and was then discharged home at maximal function. He has a history of Parkinson's disease, hypertension, and osteoarthritis. Medications include carbidopa/levodopa, hydrochlorothiazide, metoprolol, and acetaminophen.

Which of the following is most likely to yield additional information useful for reducing his risk of falling?

(A)   Serum electrolytes
(B)   Vitamin D level
(C)   Postural blood pressure
(D)   Timed Up and Go test

ANSWER: C

Up to 70% of patients with Parkinson's disease fall in a given year. This patient's recent fall and his fatigue may be related to the orthostasis associated both with Parkinson's disease and with carbidopa/levodopa (SOE=A). He should be evaluated for postural hypotension. Furthermore, he has had several recent transitions—from the hospital to a nursing facility to home. Changes in medication regimen are a common cause of complications in transition of care, raising the possibility that the patient's hypertension is being overtreated. Both hydrochlorothiazide and metoprolol may be lowering his blood pressure excessively.

   Serum electrolytes should be checked because of the patient's fatigue and because he takes hydrochlorothiazide. Low sodium or potassium concentrations could cause the patient's symptoms, but orthostasis remains the primary consideration in this case. Inadequate levels of vitamin D are common in older adults, and supplementation with vitamin D_3 can decrease fall risk. Checking the vitamin D level is appropriate in the overall management of fall risk but is a secondary consideration in this situation. The Timed Up and Go test is a good screen for functional balance, strength, and gait but would not yield specific useful information in this situation. Because the patient has recently undergone intensive rehabilitation, results of the Timed Up and Go test are not likely to lead to further interventions to improve his physical function.

References

1. Dennison AC, Noorigian JV, Robinson KM, et al. Falling in Parkinson disease: identifying and prioritizing risk factors in recurrent fallers. *Am J Phys Med Rehab.* 2007;86(8):621–631.
2. Jackson C, Gaugris S, Sen SS, et al. The effect of cholecalciferol (vitamin D$_3$) on the risk of fall and fracture: a meta-analysis. *QJM.* 2007;100(4):185–192.

4. A 78-yr-old woman comes to the office because she has recurrent syncope and falls that do not correlate to time of day or activity. The episodes are not preceded by symptoms and have not been accompanied by incontinence or major injury. She reports no chest pain, palpitations, or acute illnesses. She had percutaneous angioplasty and a bare-metal stent inserted 10 yr ago for single-vessel right coronary artery disease. Medications include a diuretic, aspirin, amlopidine, clopidogrel, and a statin.

On examination, blood pressure is 148/84 mmHg supine and 152/86 mmHg standing. Pulse is 70 beats per minute in supine and standing positions. Lungs are clear, and heart sounds are normal. There is a 1/6 diamond-shaped murmur at the left sternal border. Distant pulses are intact, and there is no ankle edema. A recent echocardiogram showed a left ventricular ejection fraction of 55% without segmental wall motion abnormalities and aortic sclerosis.

As the patient is dressing, she complains of lightheadedness; the office staff obtains a rhythm strip that shows third-degree heart block with a 4-sec pause.

Which of the following therapies is indicated for this diagnosis?

(A) Discontinue amlodipine.
(B) Warfarin therapy
(C) Permanent pacemaker implantation
(D) Internal cardiac defibrillator implantation
(E) Scopolamine patch

ANSWER: C

This patient has intermittent third-degree heart block and recurrent syncope. Permanent pacemaker implantation is indicated (SOE=C). Indications for pacing are complex because they depend on both the disease process and the patient. Indications for pacing are based on the presence of symptoms, the magnitude of the bradycardia, and the reversibility or natural history of the disease. The more strongly a bradyarrhythmia can be correlated with symptoms, the stronger the recommendation for pacing. Likewise, the more extreme the bradycardia or atrioventricular (AV) block, the stronger the recommendation for pacing. Reversibility of a disease process would typically lead against recommendations for pacing (eg, bradycardia due to a drug that can be stopped). Conversely, a natural history that predicts worsening progression of bradycardia or block (eg, myotonic muscular dystrophy) increases the recommendation for pacing.

Amlodipine is a dihydropyridine calcium channel blocker, a class of calcium channel blocker that does not cause AV conduction block or sinus node depression in people. Warfarin therapy is inappropriate because the patient does not have an indication for anticoagulation. Implantable defibrillators are used for ventricular rhythm disorders, such as ventricular fibrillation or refractory ventricular tachycardia, or are implanted in patients with coronary artery disease, prior myocardial infarction, and low ejection fraction to prolong life. None of these indications is present in this patient. Scopolamine patches do not affect AV conduction in vivo.

Reference

1. Epstein AE, DiMarco JP, Ellenbogen KA, et al. ACC/AHA/HRS 2008 Guidelines for Device Based Therapy of Cardiac Rhythm Abnormalities. *J Am Coll Cardiol.* 2008;51(21):e1–62.

5. In a four-physician practice, approximately 60% of patients are ≥65 yr old and enrolled in traditional fee-for-service Medicare. The physicians accept Medicare assignment and are participating ("PAR") Medicare providers. At the beginning of the next fiscal year, CMS will cut all Medicare reimbursement rates by 10%. Because the practice income is derived primarily from reimbursement from CMS, a significant reduction in practice income is anticipated and raises unattractive options (eg, cutting expenses by letting staff go, or less income for the same amount of work).

Which of the following strategies would increase the reimbursement that the clinic receives *directly* from CMS?

(A) Perform and bill for more services.
(B) Charge higher fees for services.
(C) Become a nonparticipating provider.
(D) Become a concierge physician.
(E) Become a Medicare Advantage provider.

ANSWER: A

Traditional Medicare operates under a standard fee-for-service reimbursement system, in which the amount of reimbursement is based on the volume and intensity of services performed and billed. If the Medicare fee schedule is reduced, reimbursement can be increased by performing and billing for greater volume and higher-intensity services. Participating Medicare providers are not allowed by law to charge higher fees. Theoretically, total reimbursement could be increased by no longer participating as a Medicare provider, but then reimbursement must be obtained directly from patients. By law, concierge physicians are not allowed to obtain reimbursement directly from CMS; they must sign an agreement not to receive payments from CMS for 2 yr. Becoming a Medicare Advantage provider could also theoretically increase total reimbursement, depending on the nature of the negotiated contract. However, the provider would then receive reimbursement directly from the Medicare Advantage plan, rather than from CMS.

References

1. American Medical Association. *Medicare Participation Options for Physicians.* http://www.ama-assn.org/ama1/pub/upload/mm/399/medicarepayment08.pdf (accessed Nov 2009).
2. Centers for Medicare & Medicaid Services. *Medicare & You 2008.* http://www.medicare.gov/Publications/Pubs/pdf/10050.pdf, p. 13 (accessed Nov 2009).

6. A 78-yr-old woman comes to the office because she has had mid- to low-back pain for approximately 2 mo. The pain was initially mild, but it has become more severe and persistent over the past several weeks. She now has pain in virtually all positions; it decreases when she lies down but does not completely resolve.

On examination, there is mild limitation in range of motion of the lumbar spine. There is full mobility of both hips without pain. The straight-leg raise test is normal bilaterally. Strength is normal in the proximal and distal muscles of the lower legs. Both toes are upgoing. MRI of the lumbar spine demonstrates significant stenosis most prevalent at the L3-L4 and L4-L5 areas.

Which of the following is the most appropriate next step?

(A) Epidural steroid injection
(B) Intensive physical therapy
(C) MRI of the thoracic spine
(D) Surgical consultation
(E) Trial of a lumbar sacral corset with metal stays

ANSWER: C

The presence of bilateral upgoing toes is of great concern in this patient and demands evaluation of the thoracic spine (SOE=D). Upgoing toes is an upper motor neuron sign and should not be present with disease of the lumbar spine, because the spinal cord ends at L1 and any abnormalities of the cauda equina would result in lower-motor neuron signs. The presence of gradually progressive, nonpositional pain suggests an underlying tumor as the cause of this patient's back pain.

In older adults, diagnostic imaging tests of the lumbar spine have high false-positive rates. One study found a 21% incidence of lumbar spinal stenosis in adults ≥60 yr old with no history of low-back pain or sciatica. The presence of an anatomic abnormality on diagnostic imaging tests should never lead to a diagnosis unless that abnormality is consistent with the clinical presentation.

This patient's gradually progressing pain over 2 mo, with no significant changes with position, is not consistent with a diagnosis of lumbar spinal stenosis. The classic feature of lumbar spinal stenosis is pain with standing and walking, which is relieved with sitting. The stenosis usually produces intermittent positional pain; it is not severe and persistent, and it should not bother the patient throughout the day. Therefore, epidermal injection, intensive physical therapy, surgical consultation, and trial of a lumbar sacral corset are not indicated for this patient.

References

1. Katz JN, Harris MB. Lumbar spinal stenosis. *N Engl J Med.* 2008;358(8):818–825.
2. Siemionow K, McLain R. When back pain is not benign. A concise guide to differential diagnosis. *Postgrad Med.* 2006;119(2):62–69.
3. Winters ME, Kluetz P, Zilberstein J. Back pain emergencies. *Med Clin North Am.* 2006;90(3):505–523.

7. An 85-yr-old woman with significant osteoporosis is brought to the office by her daughter, who wants to know whether once-yearly infusion of zoledronic acid may be started for her mother. The patient has moderate dementia and osteoporosis, and drug adherence is a major problem, according to her daughter.

The patient and daughter are cautioned that osteonecrosis of the jaw has been reported. Dental consultation is recommended to confirm that the patient has no active oral infection and to manage sites at high risk of infection. Additionally, the patient is advised to have biannual dental care for cleaning, minimizing periodontal inflammation, addressing caries, and performing endodontic therapy for nonrestorable teeth.

Which of the following is the basis for these preventive strategies?

(A) Good-quality patient-oriented evidence
(B) Limited-quality patient-oriented evidence
(C) Consensus guidelines
(D) No evidence

ANSWER: C

Being aware of the evidence on which clinical guidelines are based can help clinicians weigh the risks and benefits of various treatment strategies as applied to particular patients.

Osteonecrosis of the jaw has received widespread attention and continues to be of concern to many patients and clinicians, yet the actual incidence appears to be extremely low. It has been most commonly reported with intravenous bisphosphonate treatment among patients with malignancy (eg, multiple myeloma and metastatic carcinoma to the skeleton). Approximately 60% of cases develop after dentoalveolar surgery (such as tooth extraction) to treat infections, and the remaining 40% are probably related to infection, denture trauma, or other physical trauma. Recommended preventive strategies include removing all foci of dental infection before starting bisphosphonate therapy, but these guidelines are not based on high-quality clinical evidence (SOE=C).

The most widely cited trial of intravenous bisphosphonate therapy (zoledronic acid 5 mg annually) for osteoporosis included over 2,000 participants; no cases of osteonecrosis of the jaw were reported. It is unknown what, if any, dental prophylaxis was provided in this trial.

The absolute magnitude of the risk of osteonecrosis with intravenous bisphosphonate therapy is uncertain. The optimal approach to preventing this complication is still under investigation.

References

1. Black DM, Delmas PD, Eastell R, et al. Once-yearly zoledronic acid for treatment of postmenopausal osteoporosis. *N Engl J Med.* 2007;356(18):1809–1822.
2. Johnson B. A once-yearly IV infusion of zoledronic acid prevented fractures in postmenopausal women with osteoporosis. *ACP J Club.* 2007;147(2):31.
3. Woo S, Hellstein J, Kalmar J. Narrative review: bisphosphonates and osteonecrosis of the jaws. *Ann Intern Med.* 2006;144(10):753–761.

8. A 70-yr-old Chinese-American man comes to the office because he has a widespread maculopapular eruption with formation of flaccid bullae and erosions. For 2 days before the rash, he had fever, odynophagia, and eye pain. Over the next few days, the rash evolved to extensive sloughing and peeling of the skin. History includes hypertension, diabetes, and peripheral neuropathy. Two weeks ago, he began carbamazepine at 200 mg q12h for peripheral neuropathy. Other medications include glipizide, felodipine, simvastatin, and enteric-coated aspirin.

On examination, the sloughing and peeling involve 40% of the patient's body surface. His oral mucosa has erosions and exudates. He also has bilateral conjunctivitis.

The patient is admitted to a burn unit.

Which of the following is the most likely diagnosis?

(A) Bullous pemphigoid
(B) Staphylococcal scalded skin syndrome
(C) Disseminated herpes zoster
(D) Toxic epidermal necrolysis

ANSWER: D

Stevens-Johnson syndrome (SJS) and toxic epidermal necrolysis (TEN) are severity variants of the same disease, characterized by epidermal detachment. In SJS, skin detachment affects <10% of the body surface; in TEN, detachment affects >30% of the body. When skin detachment is between 10% and 30%, the syndrome is considered overlap SJS/TEN. The mortality for SJS is between 1% and 3%; mortality is 30% for TEN. Often, fever and mucosal involvement develop days before the rash appears. Initial lesions are macular and can form target lesions with purpuric centers. The lesions can coalesce and progress to superficial flaccid bullae. Usually at least two mucous surfaces are involved. Epidermal necrosis is pathognomonic for SJS and TEN.

SJS and TEN are rare reactions to medications. More than 200 medications have been implicated, but the most common are antibiotics, NSAIDs, and anticonvulsants. The risk of SJS or TEN from carbamazepine is significantly increased in patients who have the HLA-B*1502 allele, which is found in individuals with ancestry from across broad areas of Asia, including South Asian Indians. In 2007, the FDA alerted healthcare professionals of changes to the prescribing information, including a new boxed warning for carbamazepine: "Patients with ancestry in at-risk populations should be screened for the HLA-B*1502 allele prior to starting carbamazepine. Patients who test positive for HLA-B*1502 should not be treated with carbamazepine unless the expected benefit clearly outweighs the increased risk of SJS/TEN." Given the Chinese ancestry of this patient, he should not have been given carbamazepine without genetic testing.

Bullous pemphigoid is a bullous disorder mainly found in older adults. The bullae are tense, not flaccid, because they are subepidermal. Oral involvement is seen in about 20% of cases and is rare in drug-induced pemphigoid.

Staphylococcal scalded skin syndrome is caused by exfoliative exotoxins released by group 2 staphylococci. It presents as a generalized, superficial exfoliative dermatitis without mucosal involvement. Because the exotoxins are cleared renally, it usually affects neonates and infants, due to their immature renal clearance, and adults with renal insufficiency or immunodeficiency.

Pemphigus vulgaris also presents with flaccid, easily ruptured bullae. Oral involvement is present in 60%, but is less common in drug-induced pemphigus. Histopathologic examination is essential for definitive diagnosis of bullous disorders.

The lesions of herpes zoster are small vesicles, or blisters, on an erythematous base. They appear in clusters and in various stages of healing, and distributed along a single dermatome. New lesions appear every few days and heal with crusting over 1–2 wk. Although there can be mucosal involvement, the lesions are clearly different from those of TEN on appearance.

References
1. Carr DR, Houshmand E, Heffernan, MP. Approach to the acute, generalized, blistering patient. *Semin Cutan Med Surg*. 2007;26(3):139–146.
2. Cotliar J. Approach to the patient with a suspected drug eruption. *Semin Cutan Med Surg*. 2007;26(3):139–146.
3. Information on Carbamazepine (marketed as Carbatrol, Equetro, Tegretol, and generics). http://www.fda.gov/Drugs/DrugSafety/PostmarketDrugSafetyInformationforPatientsandProviders/ucm107834.htm (accessed Nov 2009).

9. A 74-yr-old man is brought to the office by his daughter because he has had several noninjurious falls in the past 3 mo.

On examination, blood pressure is 130/80 mmHg. He walks with a shuffling gait and a stooped posture. He has masked facies, increased arm rigidity, and a resting tremor.

What is the most appropriate initial treatment for this patient?

(A)   Amantadine
(B)   Levodopa
(C)   Ropinirole
(D)   Bromocriptine
(E)   Selegiline

ANSWER: B

This patient has Parkinson's disease. Parkinson's disease is seen in about 100 per 100,000 adults in the population. The most frequent presenting sign is a unilateral coarse resting tremor. Other signs are rigidity, bradykinesia, loss of postural reflexes, and gait disturbance. Variable features include autonomic dysfunction, masked facies, depression, fatigue, weight loss, and constipation. Parkinson's disease is characterized pathologically by loss of dopaminergic pigmented neurons in the substantia nigra. The remaining neurons contain abnormal inclusions consisting of protein aggregates (Lewy bodies).

Motor symptoms are most improved by levodopa/carbidopa, which is the most effective short-term treatment available (SOE=A). In long-term use, levodopa/carbidopa is associated with development of an "on-off" phenomenon and dyskinesias. Dopamine agonists such as ropinirole and bromocriptine are less effective than carbidopa/levodopa, more costly, and associated with increased risk of confusion in older adults. Selegiline is also a first-line agent for Parkinson's disease, but it is less effective than carbidopa/levodopa. The severity of this patient's symptoms warrant treatment with carbidopa/levodopa. Amantadine is useful for treatment of dyskinesias but not for treatment of bradykinesia and rigidity (SOE=A).

References

1. Rao G, Fisch L, Srinivasan S, et al. Does this patient have Parkinson disease? *JAMA*. 2003;289(3):347–353.
2. Stowe RL, Ives NJ, Clarke C, et al. Dopamine agonist therapy in early Parkinson's disease. *Cochrane Database Syst Rev*. 2008;(2):CD006564.
3. Suchowersky O, Reich S, Perlmutter J, et al. Practice Parameter: diagnosis and prognosis of new onset Parkinson disease (an evidence-based review): report of the Quality Standards Subcommittee of the American Academy of Neurology. *Neurology*. 2006;66(7):968–975.

10. A 76-yr-old woman comes to the office because over the past day she has had progressive painful swelling of the wrist, such that she is now unable to use her left hand. She has had similar episodes involving her knee and ankle over the past year. History includes hypertension, coronary artery disease, and osteoarthritis of the hands. Medications include aspirin 81 mg/d, hydrochlorothiazide 12.5 mg/d, and acetaminophen 1 gram q8h.

On examination, the patient has no fever. Her left hand is diffusely swollen, with wrist pain and tenderness; her right hand is tender over the second and third metacarpophalangeal joints. Her knees are warm to touch and hurt with movement. Uric acid level is 10.2 mg/dL, BUN is 30 mg/dL, and creatinine is 2.5 mg/dL.

In addition to discontinuing her hydrochlorothiazide, which of the following treatments is most appropriate?

(A) Intra-articular corticosteroid injection
(B) Oral corticosteroids
(C) Oral colchicine
(D) Oral probenecid
(E) Oral allopurinol

ANSWER: B

This patient has polyarticular gout. Flares are best managed with intramuscular or short-term oral corticosteroid therapy (prednisone 30 mg/d for 5 days). Joint aspiration and intra-articular corticosteroid therapy are appropriate for gout attacks of 1 or 2 accessible joints (knee, wrist, elbow, ankle) but not if there is concurrent involvement of small hand joints (SOE=C).

If corticosteroids and NSAIDs are contraindicated, analgesics alone are an acceptable alternative. Colchicine can alleviate

an acute attack, but at dosages associated with significant nausea, vomiting, and diarrhea. Urate-lowering therapy should not be started during an acute gouty attack.

The patient will continue to be susceptible to flares once this episode resolves. It is reasonable to consider urate-lowering therapy weeks after the current attack resolves. Initial intervention may include discontinuing diuretic therapy: 90% of cases of chronic hyperuricemia in older adults result from reduced renal excretion that is due to renal disease or medications, especially diuretics. Although aspirin at low dosages reduces uric acid clearance, it may be required for cardio-vascular prophylaxis. Probenecid, a uricosuric agent, is less effective in patients with renal insufficiency (creatinine clearance <40 mL/min). Allopurinol lowers serum urate concentration by blocking uric acid formation but should not be used during an acute flare.

References

1. Fox R. Management of recurrent gout. *BMJ*. 2008;336(7639):329.
2. Janssens HJ, Lucassen PL, Van de Laar FA, et al. Systemic corticosteroids for acute gout. *Cochrane Database Syst Rev*. 2008;(2):CD005521.
3. Keith MP, Gilliland WR. Updates in the management of gout. *Am J Med*. 2007;120(3): 221–224.
4. Pascual E, Sivera F. Therapeutic advances in gout. *Curr Opin Rheumatol*. 2007;19(2):122–127.
5. Singh H, Torralba KD. Therapeutic challenges in the management of gout in the elderly. *Geriatrics*. 2008;63(7):13–18, 20.

11. A 79-yr-old man is being discharged from the hospital after treatment for acute cholecystitis. History includes insulin-dependent diabetes mellitus, mild dementia, major depressive disorder, and recurrent falls (two in the past 6 mo). He has been hospitalized twice in the past year. He was delirious during the current hospitalization but is less confused at discharge. He lives with his daughter, who assists him with bathing and dressing. Arrangements are in place for a visiting nurse during the period immediately after discharge.

Medications during hospitalization included NPH and regular insulin, donepezil, acetaminophen, and a third-generation cephalosporin with metronidazole.

Which of the following is most likely to reduce this patient's risk of falls immediately after discharge?

(A) Supplemental vitamin D
(B) In-home occupational therapy
(C) Consultation with a podiatrist
(D) Consultation with an optometrist

ANSWER: B

The risk of a fall at home is greatest in the 2-wk period immediately after hospital discharge. Risk factors for falls during this period include impaired balance, new confusion or delirium, use of first-generation antidepressants, history of ≥2 falls in the past year, previous use of an assistive device for ambulation, prehospitalization dependency for ADLs, and greater number of hospitalizations in the prior year. This patient is at substantial risk.

Two studies on interventions designed to decrease falls in the period immediately after discharge both examined the value of home visits by an occupational therapist. In each study, the intervention included modification of environmental hazards, training in safe behaviors, and inclusion of mobility or functional aids. In both studies, patients who had home visits by an occupational therapist had fewer falls than patients who did not have occupational therapy at home (SOE=B).

A meta-analysis suggested that vitamin D supplements may reduce fall risk by about 20%, but a more recent study found that supplementation with cholecalciferol and calcium had a neutral effect on fall risk in men. There are no data on the use of vitamin D supplements to specifically reduce the risk of falls immediately after hospital discharge.

Podiatric or optometric consultation may theoretically reduce the risk of falls early after discharge, but these interventions in this setting have not been studied. However, in one randomized study of frail older outpatients, comprehensive vision and eye assessment with appropriate treatment did not reduce fall risk.

References

1. Bischoff-Ferrari HA, Orav EJ, Dawson-Hughes B. Effect of cholecalciferol plus calcium on falling in ambulatory older men and women: a 3-year randomized controlled trial. *Arch Intern Med.* 2006;166(4):424–430.
2. Burleigh E, McColl J, Potter J. Does vitamin D stop inpatients falling? A randomized controlled trial. *Age Ageing.* 2007;36(5):507–513.
3. Cumming RG, Ivers R, Clemson L, et al. Improving vision to prevent falls in frail older people: a randomized trial. *J Am Geriatr Soc.* 2007;55(2):175–181.
4. Cumming RG, Thomas M, Szonyi G, et al. Home visits by an occupational therapist for assessment and modification of environmental hazards: a randomized trial of falls prevention. *J Am Geriatr Soc.* 1999;47(12):1397–1402.
5. Nikolaus T, Bach M. Preventing falls in community-dwelling frail older people using a home intervention team (HIT): results from the randomized Falls-HIT trial. *J Am Geriatr Soc.* 2003;51:300–305.

12. Which of the following agents increases bone mass and reduces fracture risk by stimulating osteoblast activity and promoting bone formation?

(A) Oral bisphosphonates
(B) Estrogen
(C) Human parathyroid hormone
(D) Selective estrogen-receptor modulators
(E) Zoledronic acid

ANSWER: C

A number of medications are available for treatment of osteoporosis. At a mechanistic level, osteoporosis medications can be considered in terms of whether they act on bone resorption (antiresorptive agents) or on bone formation (anabolic agents). Most agents for osteoporosis are antiresorptive agents, including calcium, vitamin D, estrogen, selective estrogen-receptor modulators, bisphosphonates, and calcitonin.

Teriparatide, human parathyroid hormone, is the only anabolic therapy for osteoporosis approved by the FDA. Teriparatide increases bone mass and reduces fracture risk by stimulating osteoblast activity and promoting bone formation.

Teriparatide (20 mcg/d or 40 mcg/d) increases bone mineral density and decreases the risk of both vertebral and nonvertebral fractures in postmenopausal women with prior vertebral fractures or corticosteroid-induced osteoporosis (SOE=A). Teriparatide also increases bone mineral density at the lumbar spine and femoral neck in men with osteoporosis (SOE=A). Its effect on hip fractures has not been assessed.

Treatment with human parathyroid hormone is associated with usually transient increases in serum calcium. If the increases persist, they can be managed by decreasing calcium and vitamin D supplements. There is no clear consensus on how or when to use human parathyroid hormone in clinical practice. It is administered by daily subcutaneous injections and is substantially more expensive than bisphosphonates.

References

1. Bauer DC. Review: Human parathyroid hormone reduces fractures and increases bone mineral density in severe osteoporosis. *ACP J Club*. 2006;145(3):71.
2. Cranney A, Papaioannou A, Zytaruk N, et al. Parathyroid hormone for the treatment of osteoporosis: a systematic review. *CMAJ*. 2006;175(1):52–59.
3. Sambrook P, Cooper C. Osteoporosis. *Lancet*. 2007; 367(9527):2010–2018.

13. A 65-yr-old woman comes to the office because she has facial rash with stinging, burning, and tender pimples. The rash began recently and is causing increasing redness.

On examination, there is erythema underlying central facial papules and pustules with telangiectasias. The distribution is over the central region of her face and includes her cheeks and chin.

Which of the following is the most appropriate initial approach?

(A) Ketoconazole
(B) Tetracycline
(C) Biopsy
(D) Antinuclear antibody titer
(E) Review of exposure to skin irritants

ANSWER: B

This patient has stage III papulopustular rosacea, a vascular disorder with distinct, predictable symptoms. Correct diagnosis and early treatment are important because, untreated, rosacea can progress to irreversible disfigurement and even visual loss. Rosacea usually involves the cheeks, nose, chin, and forehead, with a predilection for the nose in men. There is no specific test for rosacea, but its characteristic appearance, distribution, discrete course, older age population, and response to various therapies allow accurate diagnosis. Although rosacea is incurable, its progress can be controlled and even halted through medical therapy and lifestyle modification. Besides avoiding triggers, management includes antibiotic therapy, such as tetracycline (SOE=A), especially for stage III lesions. Topical metronidazole can be used alone, or in combination with oral antibiotics, particularly for earlier stage disease.

The differential diagnosis of rosacea includes seborrheic dermatitis, which is treated with topical ketoconazole. Seborrheic dermatitis presents with a greasy scale and eczematous changes but no papules, pustules, or telangiectasias. Its pattern of distribution involves the paranasal area, the nasolabial grooves, and areas beyond the face, such as the scalp. Seborrheic dermatitis can coexist with rosacea.

Sarcoidosis can mimic rosacea clinically as well as histologically by producing red papules on the face, but biopsy of the lesion will reveal sarcoidal granulomas. This patient does not have the pigmentary changes, atrophy, scarring, and adherent scaling that are characteristic of systemic lupus erythematosus. Conversely, the pustules found in rosacea are not characteristic of lupus. However, a low antinuclear antibody titer can be present in rosacea. Contact dermatitis can resemble rosacea, but it is usually pruritic and has a cutaneous linear pattern, which follows the size and shape of contact by the external causal agent.

References

1. Conde JF. Managing rosacea: a review of the use of metronidazole alone and in combination with oral antibiotics. *J Drugs Dermatol*. 2007;6(5):495–498.
2. Fowler JF Jr. Combined effect of anti-inflammatory dose doxycycline (40-mg doxycycline, USP monohydrate controlled-release capsules) and metronidazole topical gel 1% in the treatment of rosacea. *J Drugs Dermatol*. 2007;6(6):641–645.
3. Powell FC. Clinical practice. Rosacea. *N Engl J Med*. 2005;352(8):793–803.

14. A 65-yr-old recently retired man comes to the office because he has recurring episodes of urinary frequency associated with perineal discomfort. He reports that he has had a "nervous bladder" for much of his life but had never seen a physician for this. Over the last year, however, he has had a mild to moderately uncomfortable sensation that initially seemed to come and go but now is present most days and uncomfortable enough to cause him distress. He has been married for 35 yr and has been sexually active and monogamous for that time. He reports no problems associated with sexual activity, and has no chills, fever, incontinence, or difficulty starting or stopping urinary stream. He has never sought counseling or medical care for anxiety. He has no chronic disorders and takes no medications.

On examination, blood pressure is 140/80 mmHg and pulse is 80 beats per minute. His prostate is estimated at 15 mL, with no asymmetry, nodule, or induration. He notes mild tenderness during palpation. Urinalysis done after digital rectal examination reveals 3 or 4 WBCs per high-power field and is otherwise unremarkable. Cultures from that urine sample (including for *Mycobacterium tuberculosis*) are unremarkable. Prostate-specific antigen level is 3.2 ng/mL, and urine cytologies are negative.

Which of the following is the most appropriate next step?

(A) Finasteride therapy
(B) α-Agonist therapy
(C) Transrectal ultrasonography
(D) CT of the pelvis
(E) Psychiatric evaluation

ANSWER: B

This patient has chronic pelvic pain syndrome. While this syndrome can present at any age, the risk increases with age; it has been reported in up to 13% of men ≥65 yr old. Chronic pelvic pain syndrome is a clinical diagnosis based on history of chronic pelvic pain and symptoms associated with voiding in the absence of inflammatory processes in the urinary tract. Urinary tract cancer and recurrent infection—including tuberculosis—must be excluded. There is no specific test for this syndrome. Administration of α-blockers for 3–6 mo had a beneficial effect in most published trials, although differences in study design and outcome measures limit the strength of the evidence (SOE=B).

Measurement of prostate-specific antigen is not helpful, and increased levels in the absence of active infection would warrant an evaluation independent of pelvic pain. Imaging of any kind is not useful unless other diagnoses are suspected. Finasteride has not been shown to be helpful in the treatment of chronic pelvic pain syndrome. While anxiety and psychologic diagnoses must be considered, this patient has no overt evidence of significant psychopathology; thus, psychiatric evaluation is not indicated at this time.

References

1. Mishra VC, Browne J, Emberton M. Role of alpha-blockers in type III prostatitis: a systematic review of the literature. *J Urol.* 2007;177(1):25–30.
2. Nadler RB, Collins MM, Propert KJ, et al. Prostate specific antigen test in diagnostic evaluation of chronic prostatitis/chronic pelvic pain syndrome. *Urology.* 2006;67(2):337–342.
3. Shaeffer AJ. Chronic prostatitis in the chronic pelvic pain syndrome. *N Engl J Med.* 2006;355(16):1690–1698.

15. An 82-yr-old man comes to the office because he has had severe pain in his left knee for 6 wk. He can no longer transfer independently. History includes rheumatoid arthritis. He takes an NSAID, hydroxychloroquine, methotrexate, and folate at maximal dosages for his arthritis. An injection to the joint has given no relief.

He is enrolled in traditional Medicare Parts A and B and has a stand-alone Part D policy through a private insurance company. The monthly premium for the Part D policy is $36, with an annual deductible of $295 (in 2009). Co-payment and co-insurance amounts vary by medication, and his policy includes a "doughnut hole" (coverage gap). His prescription medications currently cost him $180/mo. His income is $2,000/mo pension in addition to Social Security.

On examination, the left knee is swollen, warm, and exquisitely tender, with effusion. CBC is normal, serum rheumatoid factor is strongly positive, and erythrocyte sedimentation rate is 105 mm/h.

Etanercept, an antitissue necrosis factor medication, offers the best chance of improving function and avoiding nursing-home admission. However, the patient believes the price— $1,100/month—to be prohibitive. Etanercept, as well as other medications in the same class, is not available in a generic preparation.

Which of the following is accurate?

(A) He can enroll in hospice care, which offers complete Medicare coverage of all medications.
(B) He can enroll in Medicaid, which offers additional medication coverage.
(C) Some private plans provide payment within the coverage gap, which would likely reduce his total out-of-pocket expenses.
(D) Substituting generic preparations for his other medications would reduce costs and avoid the coverage gap.
(E) Coverage of medication costs resumes once expenses exceed the upper limit of the coverage gap.

ANSWER: E

This patient has exhausted less-expensive treatments for rheumatoid arthritis and now faces the prospect of financing more expensive treatment. His total medication costs will increase to about $15,000 per year. The vast majority of this will be covered by his current Part D plan: Once the "doughnut hole" is exceeded (corresponding to roughly $4,350 in total annual out-of-pocket expenses in 2009, which the patient may be able to afford), Medicare Part D covers 95% of additional drug costs. Many patients misunderstand the coverage gap and mistakenly believe that once a patient has reached it, all Medicare benefits are lost. Indeed, the new medicine would propel his medication costs through the coverage gap and beyond.

The history does not suggest that he has ≤6 mo to live, and therefore hospice care is inappropriate. His income is likely too high to qualify for medical assistance, so switching to Medicaid is not possible until his medical costs exceed his state's income and asset limits. Changing Part D plans is an option, but he would have to wait until the next enrollment period. In addition, if he chose a Part D plan with doughnut-hole coverage, he would have much higher premiums, and total out-of-pocket costs would likely be similar. In addition, the few Part D plans with doughnut-hole coverage usually provide generic drug coverage only. Substituting generic preparations for as many of his medications as possible may lower his total medication costs, but the cost of the etanercept will far overwhelm reductions through generic prescribing.

References
1. Hsu J, Fung V, Price M, et al. Medicare beneficiaries' knowledge of Part D prescription drug program benefits and responses to drug costs. *JAMA*. 2008;299(16):1929–1936.
2. Centers for Medicare & Medicaid Services. *Medicare Prescription Drug Coverage: Things to Consider*. http://www.medicare.gov/pdp-things-to-consider.asp (accessed Nov 2009).

16. An 84-yr-old-man comes to the office to get information on minimizing muscle loss. He is vigorous and healthy, with no chronic diseases. He has heard that muscle loss is a serious problem with aging and may contribute to frailty. He would like to take medication to delay or minimize muscle loss associated with aging.

Which of the following is most likely to minimize the patient's muscle loss?

(A) Testosterone
(B) Dehydroepiandrosterone
(C) Growth hormone
(D) Vitamin D
(E) No medication

ANSWER: E

No supplement or medication has been proved to increase function in older men with sarcopenia without significant adverse events. Studies of testosterone replacement have been inconclusive, although one trial showed improvement in function.

Dehydroepiandrosterone has not been shown to consistently improve strength or function in older men. Growth hormone can improve muscle strength, but the adverse events and cost prohibit its use. Vitamin D supplements are associated with fewer falls in frail older adults with vitamin D insufficiency, but its role in preventing sarcopenia is unknown. The therapy consistently shown to prevent sarcopenia is resistance training and exercise (SOE=A).

References
1. Borst SE. Interventions for sarcopenia and muscle weakness in older people. *Age Ageing*. 2004;33(6):548–555.
2. Chin A, Paw MJ, van Uffelen JG, et al. The functional effects of physical exercise training in frail older people: a systematic review. *Sports Med*. 2008;38(9):781–793.

17. A 70-yr-old woman with a relatively new diagnosis of type 2 diabetes mellitus and past history of hypertension comes to your office for evaluation. She is independent in ADLs and IADLs, walks daily, and has no exercise-induced symptoms. She does not smoke and drinks one glass of red wine daily. Although she states that she follows an American Heart Association low-fat diet, she has always had difficulty controlling her weight. She is on rosiglitazone 4 mg/d, lisinopril 20 mg/d, atorvastatin 20 mg/d, aspirin 325 mg/d, and calcium plus vitamin D q12h.

On examination, weight is 80 kg (176 lb, body mass index = 30 kg/m^2), sitting blood pressure is 130/80 mmHg without orthostatic changes, and heart rate is 60 beats per minute and regular. Cardiopulmonary examination is unremarkable except for 1+ pedal edema. Peripheral pulses are intact.

The ankle-brachial index is 0.8.

Laboratory results:

Hemoglobin A$_{1c}$	5.8%
Creatinine	1 mg/dL
Potassium	4.6 mEq/L
Low-density lipoprotein (LDL)	80 mg/dL
High-density lipoprotein	57 mg/dL
Triglycerides	140 mg/dL

Which of the following medication changes would you recommend?

(A)   Increase lisinopril to 40 mg.
(B)   Replace rosiglitazone with metformin.
(C)   Increase atorvastatin to 40 mg.
(D)   Add clopidogrel.
(E)   Advise patient to stop alcohol use.

ANSWER: B

This patient has diabetes mellitus, peripheral edema, and evidence of peripheral vascular disease. Studies suggest that use of thiazolidinediones is associated with increases in body weight, peripheral edema, and heart failure (SOE=A). Rosiglitazone has been associated with an increased risk of myocardial infarction, but the magnitude and significance of the risk continue to be debated (SOE=B). It would be appropriate in this patient to replace the rosiglitazone with metformin based on metformin's potential cardiovascular benefits and rosiglitazone's potential cardiovascular risks (SOE=B).

In the United Kingdom Prospective Diabetes Study (UKPDS) trial, initial treatment of overweight patients with type II diabetes with metformin was associated with less mortality than usual care. At 10 yr, initial intensive treatment of type II diabetes with metformin (in overweight patients) or sulfonylurea/insulin was associated with continued benefits (including a reduction in all diabetes-related end points, all-cause mortality, and myocardial infarction) over usual care with dietary restriction only (SOE=A).

The strength of diabetes mellitus as a cardiovascular risk factor has been increasingly recognized. Some experts consider the presence of diabetes to be equivalent in risk to that of coronary heart disease. Risk reduction strategies include controlling blood pressure to <135/80 mmHg and reducing lipids to a level similar to that recommended for patients with cardiovascular disease (LDL <100, based on 2004 National Cholesterol Education Project guidelines). More recent randomized trials suggest that patients with type II diabetes without evidence of cardiovascular disease benefit from statin therapy with a target LDL of <100 (SOE=A), but what the ideal LDL target should be, and whether it should be individualized based on risk factors, is still uncertain. This patient's blood pressure, LDL, and triglycerides are at target levels for diabetic patients, so there is no indication to increase her lisinopril or atorvastatin (SOE=A). Antiplatelet therapy with aspirin or clopidogrel can reduce the risk of cardiovascular events and slow progression of disease. However, there is no evidence that the addition of clopidogrel would be preferable to aspirin alone in this patient without documented cardiovascular disease (SOE=A).

References

1. Bhatt DL, Fox KA, Hacke W, et al. Clopidogrel and aspirin versus aspirin alone for the prevention of atherothrombotic events. *N Engl J Med.* 2006;354(16):1706–1717.
2. Grundy SM, Cleeman JI, Merz CN, et al; Coordinating Committee of the National Cholesterol Education Program. Implications of recent clinical trials for the National Cholesterol Education Program Adult Treatment Panel III Guidelines. *Circulation.* 2004;110(2):227–239.
3. Colhoun HM et al. Primary prevention of cardiovascular disease with atorvastatin in type 2 diabetes in the Collaborative Atorvastatin Diabetes Study (CARDS): multicentre randomised placebo-controlled trial. *Lancet.* 2004;364(9435):685–696.
4. Holman RR, Paul SK, Bethel MA, et al. 10-year follow up of intensive glucose control in type 2 diabetes. *N Engl J Med.* 2008;359(15):1577–1589.
5. Lipscombe LL, Gomes T, Levesque LE, et al. Thiazolidinediones and cardiovascular outcomes in older patients with diabetes. *JAMA.* 2007;298(22):2634–2643.

18.   A 65-yr-old woman with breast cancer metastatic to bone is evaluated in preparation for hospital discharge. She is on a continuous IV infusion of morphine 4 mg/h and she has received 3 breakthrough rescue doses of 4 mg each over the past 24 h. Her pain is generally well controlled on this regimen, and she is alert and talkative.

Which of the following oral regimens is most likely to provide appropriate pain relief?

(A) Oxycodone 20 mg q3h as needed
(B) Short-acting morphine 30 mg q3h
(C) Long-acting morphine 30 mg q12h, with short-acting morphine 15 mg q2h for breakthrough pain
(D) Long-acting morphine 150 mg q12h, with short-acting morphine 30 mg q2h for breakthrough pain

ANSWER: D

Practitioners should have a systematic approach to opioid conversion. Although many equianalgesic calculators are available, many conversion tables represent an oversimplification of pharmacologic principles that cannot substitute for clinical experience and caution.

Conversion from intravenous to oral morphine first requires calculation of the total intravenous dose of opioid that the patient has received over the past 24 hours, and then multiplication by 3. In this case, the patient has received 108 mg IV in the past 24 hours (4 mg/h × 24 hours plus 3 × 4 mg). The oral equivalent is 324 mg (108 mg × 3) over 24 hours.

Long-acting morphine comes in 30-mg capsules that cannot be split; they can be administered q8h or q12h. Therefore, the best oral standing dosage would be long-acting morphine 150 mg q12h (total dose 300 mg, close to the total of 324 mg above).

Breakthrough doses should usually be 10% of the daily equivalent of oral morphine. For this patient, 10% of the total oral dose is 30 mg. Her breakthrough dose should be 30 mg q2h as needed.

References

1. Mercadante S, Arcuri E. Pharmacological management of cancer pain in the elderly. *Drugs Aging*. 2007;24(9):761–776.
2. Patanwala AE, Duby J, Waters D, et al. Opioid conversions in acute care. *Ann Pharmacother*. 2007;41(2):255–266.

19. A 70-yr-old male smoker has a history of hypertension, dyslipidemia, diabetes mellitus, and nonvalvular atrial fibrillation.

Which of the following most increases his risk of stroke?

(A) Cigarette smoking
(B) Hypertension
(C) Dyslipidemia
(D) Atrial fibrillation

ANSWER: D

Among men, the incidence of stroke is 4.5 per 1,000 between the ages of 65 and 74 yr, and 9.3 per 1,000 between 75 and 84 yr. The contribution of factors to a person's stroke risk varies by age. For a 70-yr-old man, the relative risk from nonvalvular atrial fibrillation is 3.3; the relative risk from hypertension is 2; from cigarette smoking, 1.8; and from dyslipidemia, 2 (SOE=B).

The high prevalence of hypertension makes it the largest overall contributor to stroke risk in the population, with a population-attributable risk of 30%. This relationship is true in all age groups, except in adults >80 yr old, in whom the increased prevalence of nonvalvular atrial fibrillation results in a population-attributable risk of 23%, while that of hypertension is 20%.

Reference

1. Goldstein LB, Adams R, Alberts MJ, et al. Primary prevention of ischemic stroke: a guideline from the American Heart Association/American Stroke Association Stroke Council: cosponsored by the Atherosclerotic Peripheral Vascular Disease Interdisciplinary Working Group; Cardiovascular Nursing Council; Clinical Cardiology Council; Nutrition, Physical Activity and Metabolism Council; and the Quality of Care and Outcomes Research Interdisciplinary Working Group. *Circulation*. 2006:113(24):e873–e923.

20. A 76-yr-old woman is transferred from a rehabilitation facility to the hospital after she falls and fractures her right hip. She was recovering from a recent hospitalization for pneumonia and exacerbation of COPD that left her profoundly deconditioned. She uses a combined steroid and long-acting β-agonist inhaler and takes oral steroids for exacerbations. She is not oxygen dependent. She has no history of dementia but believes she has been more forgetful over the past year.

She is vigorously hydrated, her pain is controlled with narcotics, and surgery is planned for the next morning under general anesthesia.

Which of the following would be most likely to reduce her risk of postoperative delirium?

(A) Start low-dose intravenous haloperidol and continue for 48 hours after surgery.
(B) Start oral donepezil and continue indefinitely.
(C) Obtain preoperative consultation with a geriatrician for a multifactorial risk-reduction strategy.
(D) Provide stress doses of intravenous steroids perioperatively.
(E) Avoid opioid analgesia after surgery.

ANSWER: C

The prevalence of delirium in older hospitalized adults is as high as 60%. In-hospital development of delirium is associated with increased mortality, functional decline, longer hospital stay, and discharge to a long-term care facility. Risk factors associated with development of in-hospital delirium are older age, chronic cognitive impairment, immobility, sleep deprivation, compromised hearing or vision, dehydration or volume overload, malnutrition, polypharmacy, bladder catheterization, anemia, pain, electrolyte disturbances, hypoxemia, and infection. Proactive geriatrics consultation to address common risk factors reduced the occurrence of delirium by one-third in patients undergoing hip surgery (SOE=B).

The use of prophylactic haloperidol does not prevent delirium but can decrease the severity of the delirium and reduce the length of stay (SOE=B). However, in some studies, use of antipsychotics in patients with dementia has resulted in increased mortality; until there is further data about the safety of antipsychotics in patients with delirium, they should be used cautiously (SOE=D). The use of prophylactic noncompetitive cholinesterase inhibitors, such as donepezil, offers no benefit over placebo (SOE=B). Stress doses of intravenous steroids may have been necessary if this patient had used systemic steroids chronically before surgery. Because this patient uses oral steroids only for exacerbations, stress doses may add to the patient's confusion through adverse events affecting the CNS.

Withholding analgesics would not decrease the risk of delirium. In fact, poorly controlled pain is a risk factor for delirium (SOE=B).

References
1. Inouye SK, Bogardus ST, Charpentier PA, et al. A multicomponent intervention to prevent delirium in hospitalized older patients. *N Engl J Med.* 1999;340(9):669–676.
2. Kalisvaart KJ, de Jonghe JF, Bogaards MJ, et al. Haloperidol prophylaxis for elderly hip surgery patients at risk for delirium: a randomized placebo-controlled study. *J Am Geriatr Soc.* 2005;53(10):1658–1666.
3. Marcantonio ER, Flacker JM, Wright RJ, et al. Reducing delirium after hip fracture: a randomized trial. *J Am Geriatr Soc.* 2001;49(5):516–522.
4. Siddiqi N, Stockdale R, Britton AM, et al. Interventions for preventing delirium in hospitalized patients. *Cochrane Database System Rev.* 2007;(2):CD005563.
5. Vaurio LE, Sands LP, Wang Y, et al. Postoperative delirium: the importance of pain and pain management. *Anesth Analg.* 2006;102(4):1267–1273.

21. A 73-yr-old woman comes to the office for follow-up and medication refills. Her examination is unchanged since her last visit 3 mo ago, except that her weight has decreased from 99.8 kg (220 lb) to 92.5 kg (204 lb). She expresses surprise about the weight loss: "It's a miracle I didn't gain a ton. Since my daughter and grandchildren moved out, all I do is watch TV!"

Which one of the following is most appropriate?

(A) Set exercise and diet goals, and schedule follow-up in 2 mo.
(B) Discuss the weight loss and evaluate her for causes.
(C) Administer the Simplified Nutritional Assessment Questionnaire.
(D) Encourage her to continue to lose weight.
(E) Suggest a nutritional supplement to help her regain the lost weight.

ANSWER: B

This patient's unintentional weight loss is clinically significant (>5% in 3 mo) and requires attention even though she is overweight (SOE=A). Discussion of weight loss and evaluation for reversible causes are appropriate. Laboratory evaluation is part of a thorough evaluation for unintentional weight loss (SOE=C), as is age-appropriate screening for cancer. This patient may have provided an important clue to the cause of her weight loss: she may feel isolated (watching television most of the time and her family relocating to a different area). Screening for major depressive disorder may be warranted, because it is a common cause of weight loss and anorexia in older adults (SOE=B). If evaluation confirms that the patient is healthy, her goals for weight management (healthy, nonrestrictive diet and exercise) should be discussed.

Offering nutritional supplements to a patient with clinically significant unintentional weight loss without understanding the causes of the weight loss is inappropriate. Increasing caloric intake can lead to increased body fat and obese sarcopenia, because the patient is sedentary. This in turn can lead to functional decline (SOE=B).

The Simplified Nutritional Assessment Questionnaire is a validated risk-assessment instrument for community-dwelling and institutionalized adults. It is highly predictive for weight loss (SOE=B). In this case, however, significant weight loss is already present, and the questionnaire alone will not provide an evaluation of the causes of weight loss.

References

1. Chapman IM. Nutritional disorders in elderly. *Med Clin North Am.* 2006;90:887–907.
2. Rolland Y, Kim MJ, Gammack J, et al. Office management of weight loss in older persons. *Am J Med.* 2006;119(12):1019–1026.
3. Thompson Martin C, Kayser-Jones J, Stotts N, et al. Nutritional risk and low weight in community living older adults: a review of literature. *J Gerontol A Bio Sci Med Sci.* 2006;61(9):927–934.

22. A 75-yr-old woman with Alzheimer's disease is admitted to the hospital with a femoral neck fracture of the left hip and undergoes successful cemented hip arthroplasty within 24 h of admission. She resides in an assisted-living facility and walked independently before the fracture. Two weeks before the fracture, her score on the Mini–Mental State Examination was 15/30. Her daughter asks about rehabilitation options for her mother.

Which of the following is most appropriate for this patient?

(A) Arrange for immediate trial of rehabilitation.
(B) Do not recommend rehabilitation because of patient's dementia.
(C) Postpone rehabilitation because of patient's dementia.
(D) Postpone rehabilitation because of cemented prosthesis.

ANSWER: A

According to results of a randomized, controlled trial, patients with mild to moderate dementia who fracture a hip are likely to have better outcomes with rehabilitation than without. Patients with mild dementia are as successful as patients with normal cognitive function in returning to independent living. Further, after 1 yr, significantly fewer patients with moderate dementia who received rehabilitation are in institutional care (SOE=A).

There is no evidence that waiting to start rehabilitation is beneficial, and any delay in mobilization can lead to serious adverse outcomes, such as deconditioning, pressure sores, and pneumonia (SOE=A).

Mobilization is allowed on the second or third postoperative day with compression screws and uncemented or cemented prostheses. Adequate pain control is essential to promote full participation in rehabilitation (SOE=D).

In older adults with hip fracture, surgery within 24 hours is associated with reduced pain and length of hospital stay. Cemented prostheses are associated with less pain at 1 yr and later, and may be associated with better mobility. Rehabilitation after hip fracture improves outcome in terms of functional status. Home-based care can be as effective as care provided in a rehabilitation facility for patients with dementia.

References

1. Cameron I, Crotty M, Currie C, et al. Geriatric rehabilitation following fractures in older people: a systematic review. *Health Technology Assessment.* 2000;4(2):111.
2. Giusti A, Barone A, Pioli G. Rehabilitation after hip fracture in patients with dementia. *J Am Geriatr Soc.* 2007;55(8):1309–1310.
3. Huusko TM, Karppi P, Avikainen V, et al. Randomised, clinically controlled trial of intensive geriatric rehabilitation in patients with hip fracture: subgroup analysis of patients with dementia. *BMJ.* 2000;321(7269):1107–1111.
4. Khan F, Ng L, Gonzalez S, et al. Multidisciplinary rehabilitation programmes following joint replacement at the hip and knee in chronic arthropathy. *Cochrane Database Syst Rev.* 2008;(2):CD004957.
5. Parker MJ, Gurusamy K. Arthroplasties (with and without bone cement) for proximal femoral fractures in adults. *Cochrane Database Syst Rev.* 2006;(3):CD001706.

23. An 83-yr-old nursing home resident with advanced Alzheimer's disease has steadily lost nearly 8.2 kg (18 lb), or 11% of his weight, over 11 mo. His current weight is 66.2 kg (146 lb; body mass index, 22 kg/m^2). He gained about 8.2 kg (18 lb) 6 yr ago, after he entered the nursing home, and then maintained his weight until this year. He has not had any hospitalizations, acute infections, or other serious medical problems in the last 20 mo. Since his admission, he has had a slow, steady decline in cognitive function. He is fully ambulatory and attends most meals in the residents' dining hall; he needs minimal feeding assistance (set-up only). He is on a 2,600-kcal regular diet that was modified to include finger foods and nightly snacks. According to chart documentation, he only rarely consumes <75% of the food served, but a 2-day calorie count indicates that his consumption is closer to 40% of what he is served.

Besides a comprehensive evaluation for potentially reversible causes of the resident's weight loss, which of the following should be done?

(A) Prescribe 1 can (240 mL) of a polymeric oral supplement with each meal.
(B) Refer the resident for placement of a percutaneous endoscopic gastrostomy tube.
(C) Change the diet from regular to puréed.
(D) Implement a program of individualized feeding assistance.
(E) Start mirtazapine.

ANSWER: D

Of the choices provided, the best option is to work with the nursing staff to implement a program of individualized feeding assistance (SOE=B). Several recent controlled-intervention trials demonstrate that 90% of residents with inadequate nutrient intake increase food consumption by at least 15% in response to feeding assistance provided by appropriately trained staff. As part of this program, residents with low nutrient intake are monitored more closely and provided social stimulation, encouragement to eat, verbal cueing, and help in choosing menu items. Physical assistance is provided only as needed. Studies indicate that a 2-day trial of feeding assistance is a valid method of determining whether a given resident would respond. The intervention is offered both during and between meals.

The resident in this case is probably an ideal candidate for individualized feeding assistance. His progressive decline in cognitive function places him at increased risk of a continued decline in nutrient intake, as confirmed by the 2-day calorie counts. Nursing staff consider him a self-feeder; self-feeders often respond better than others to individualized feeding assistance.

One drawback of individualized feeding assistance is that it requires significantly more time than nursing home staff usually spend on feeding care. To address this issue, nursing homes can adopt alternative staffing models such as the "paid feeding assistant" program. A second issue is identifying residents in need of assistance. Chart documentation may not be accurate, and nursing staff tend to overestimate how much food residents consume, particularly when the resident is considered to be a self-feeder. A decline in a nursing home resident's intake can initially go unnoticed. For this reason, the nutrient intake of residents who are losing weight should be carefully assessed.

Although each of the other options has merit, none is optimal for the patient at this time. If nutrient intake remains low after implementing the feeding assistance program, a polymeric oral supplement can be added. However, supplements are generally most effective when offered between, rather than with, meals. Because there is no specific indication for a puréed diet, this option is not appropriate at this time. If the assessment provides evidence that the patient is depressed, a trial of an antidepressant would be appropriate. However, there is little evidence that mirtazapine is more effective than other types of antidepressants in improving nutrient intake (SOE=B).

References

1. Aoyama L, Weintraub N, Reuben DB. Is weight loss in the nursing home a reversible problem? *J Am Med Dir Assoc.* 2005;6(4):250–256.
2. Keller HH, Gibbs AJ, Boudreau LD, et al. Prevention of weight loss in dementia with comprehensive nutritional treatment. *J Am Geriatr Soc.* 2003;51(7):945–952.
3. Rigler SK, Webb MJ, Redford L, et al. Weight outcomes among antidepressant users in nursing facilities. *J Am Geriatr Soc.* 2001;49(1):49–55.
4. Simmons SF, Schnelle JF. Individualized feeding assistance care for nursing home residents: staffing requirements to implement two interventions. *J Gerontol A Biol Sci Med Sci.* 2004;59(9):966–973.

5. Simmons SF, Bertrand R, Shier V, et al. A preliminary evaluation of the paid feeding assistant regulation: impact on feeding assistance care process quality in nursing homes. *Gerontologist*. 2007;47(2):184–192.
6. Simmons SF. Quality improvement for feeding assistance care in nursing homes. *J Am Med Dir Assoc*. 2007;8(3 Suppl):S12–S17.

24. An 84-yr-old woman undergoes total hip replacement after falling and fracturing her hip. She lives at home with her 82-yr-old husband, who is confined to a wheelchair because of severe rheumatoid arthritis. The patient has diabetes mellitus, osteoporosis, and mild dementia. She has insurance coverage through standard fee-for-service Medicare Parts A and B.

On the third hospital day, she has no fever and her lungs are clear. She is taking adequate nourishment, and her weight is stable. Warfarin was begun after surgery; INR is 1.5. She requires a maximal assist of 1 to transfer and ambulate, and she has normal functioning of her arms. She tolerates physical therapy for 20 min before she is too fatigued to continue. Hospital discharge for the next day is discussed.

Which of the following is the most appropriate setting for now?

(A) Inpatient rehabilitation facility
(B) Nursing home with rehabilitation services
(C) Nursing home with dementia unit
(D) Her own home with home physical therapy
(E) She is not ready for discharge and should stay in the hospital.

ANSWER: B

This patient is medically stable and requires rehabilitation after hip replacement. Because she needs nursing services (eg, medication monitoring) and rehabilitation (ie, physical therapy and other rehabilitation services <3 hours/day), discharge to a nursing home with rehabilitation services is the most suitable option. The first 20 days of nursing-home care after hospitalization is fully covered through Medicare Part A.

The patient no longer requires hospitalization; she can continue to receive anticoagulation adjustments outside the hospital. According to Medicare rules, a patient must require hospital-level care—ie, a relatively intense, multidisciplinary team approach to rehabilitative care—to qualify for coverage in an inpatient rehabilitation facility.

Because this patient is medically stable, requires only physical therapy without other types of rehabilitation, and can tolerate only 20 min of physical therapy at a time, she is not a candidate for admission to an inpatient rehabilitation facility. Her dementia is mild and not the chief cause of her current disability, making admission to a nursing-home dementia unit less appropriate. Discharge to home is also inappropriate, because her husband is unable to assist her with transfers and other ADLs.

References
1. Centers for Medicare & Medicaid Services. *Medicare Benefit Policy Manual*. Chapter 1. Inpatient Hospital Services Covered Under Part A. http://www.cms.hhs.gov/manuals/Downloads/bp102c01.pdf, p. 24 (accessed Nov 2009).
2. Centers for Medicare & Medicaid Services. *Medicare & You 2008*. http://www.medicare.gov/Publications/Pubs/pdf/10050.pdf, p. 13 (accessed Nov 2009).

25. An 85-yr-old black man comes to the office because he wants to get a new pair of eyeglasses. He lives alone in a town 65 miles away and is accompanied by his nephew. When called to the examining room, he walks slowly with a cane, which he bumps into the wall several times. He pauses at the doorway of the examining room and waits for his nephew to assist him into the chair. The patient has not seen a doctor since his wife died 5 yr ago. He is withdrawn and answers questions curtly. He says he has "mild diabetes and arthritis in his hands," and takes no medications. The nephew is worried about his uncle's living conditions, describing the uncle's home as filthy. The nephew had hired a housekeeper, but the uncle kicked her out because she moved the chairs in his room. According to the nephew, the patient refuses to leave the house and spends all his time in one room. At this point, the patient states that he is ready to return home.

Which of the following is the most appropriate next step?

(A) Depression screen
(B) Vision assessment
(C) Cognition assessment
(D) Comprehensive assessment

ANSWER: B

The patient, who has come for a new pair of eyeglasses, appears to have problems with vision: he uses his cane and hands to guide him in an unknown environment, and at home he has adapted by living in one room and keeping his surroundings constant. The patient's behavior is likely related to impaired vision. How much of his functional decline is a result of poor vision cannot be judged until his vision needs are addressed. The best approach is to focus on the patient's main concern and examine his eyes, after which he may be referred to an ophthalmologist or optometrist.

Vision impairment is the most common treatable cause of disability in older adults; its prevalence reaches 50% after age 75. It can contribute to sensory deprivation (SOE=B), delirium (SOE=A), functional decline (SOE=A), motor vehicle collisions (SOE=B), and falls (SOE=A). Age-related bilateral cataracts are the leading cause of reversible blindness in the United States. Macular degeneration is the leading cause of blindness among white Americans. Age-related primary open-angle glaucoma is the leading cause of blindness in black Americans; diabetes, which this patient may have, is also a risk factor for glaucoma. Many older adults assume that vision problems are a normal part of aging and may not seek attention. Assessment of vision is a routine part of geriatric assessment. It is easy to do in almost any clinical setting as long as the patient is able to cooperate. Patients in whom vision impairment is suspected or who are not able to cooperate should be referred to a specialist.

Vision loss is a significant risk factor for major depressive disorder (SOE=A). Screening this patient for major depressive disorder would be appropriate after his vision problems have been addressed. While evaluation for cognitive impairment should be part of any comprehensive geriatric assessment, doing so during this visit may not be effective and may damage a future relationship with the patient, who is focused on improving his vision.

References
1. Jung S, Coleman A, Weintraub NT. Vision screening in the elderly. *J Am Med Dir Assoc.* 2007;8(6):355–362.
2. Sloan FA, Ostermann J, Brown DS, et al. Effects of changes in self-reported vision on cognitive, affective and functional status and living arrangements among the elderly. *Am J Ophthalmol.* 2005;140(4):618–627.
3. Sterns GK, McCormick GJ. Ophthalmologic disorders. In: Duthie EH, Katz PR, Malone ML, eds. *Practice of Geriatrics.* 4th ed. Philadelphia: Saunders; 2007:310–315.

26. A 71-yr-old man comes to the office because over the past 8 mo he has had violent movements during sleep. He kicks, punches, and at times yells, usually 2–3 hours after he falls asleep. On a few occasions, he remembers dreams in which he is running away or fighting with someone. According to his wife, he snores lightly a few nights per week and gets up once nightly to urinate. History includes Parkinson's disease and major depressive disorder without recurrence. His only medication is pramipexole. A sleep study reports increased motor activity during sleep and no clinically significant sleep apnea.

Which of the following should be prescribed?

(A) Clonazepam
(B) Venlafaxine
(C) Ropinirole
(D) Trazodone
(E) Gabapentin

ANSWER: A

Rapid eye movement (REM) sleep behavior disorder is characterized by complex, often violent motor behaviors associated with dream enactment. Most cases typically manifest themselves in adults ≥60 yr old (SOE=A). The dream enactment is associated with loss of muscle atonia during REM sleep. Polysomnography demonstrates increased muscle activity during sleep, including intermittent loss of REM sleep–associated muscle atonia. REM sleep behavior disorder has been seen in association with Parkinson's disease (SOE=B).

Management of REM sleep behavior disorder involves pharmacologic agents as well as interventions that address environmental safety. Clonazepam 0.5–1 mg at bedtime is effective in 90% of cases (SOE=B). There is little evidence of abuse, and only infrequent reports of tolerance in this group of patients. Use of clonazepam should be monitored carefully in older adults at risk of falls or respiratory disorders. The combination of drug therapy and implementation of safety precautions, including padding sharp edges and removing objects near the bed, offers safe and effective management.

Other medications that can be effective in REM sleep behavior disorder are levodopa, dopamine agonists, and melatonin (SOE=C). Melatonin, a food supplement, is not approved by the FDA, and its pharmacologic preparation is poorly regulated.

Venlafaxine is a selective serotonin- and norepinephrine-reuptake inhibitor that has been shown to either induce or increase motor activity in sleep, including REM sleep, and should be avoided in patients with REM sleep behavior disorder (SOE=B). Neither ropinirole nor gabapentin is indicated for treatment of REM sleep behavior disorder.

Trazodone is a sedative antidepressant with limited use because of its potential to lower blood pressure. Its use as a sleep hypnotic is off-label, and it would not be the best choice for this patient.

References

1. Gagnon JF, Postuma RB, Montplaisir J. Update on the pharmacology of REM sleep behavior disorder. *Neurology*. 2006;12;67(5):742–747.
2. Mahowald MW, Schenck CH, Bornemann MA. Pathophysiologic mechanisms in REM sleep behavior disorder. *Curr Neurol Neurosci Rep*. 2007;7(2):167–172.
3. Winkelman JW, James L. Serotonergic antidepressants are associated with REM sleep without atonia. *Sleep*. 2004;27(2):317–321.

27. An 85-yr-old man presents with jaundice associated with anorexia, weight loss, and pruritus. Abdominal CT reveals a pancreatic mass 2.3 cm in size, with multiple liver lesions, and right upper quadrant ultrasound reveals biliary dilatation with compression from surrounding tumor. Endoscopic ultrasound is performed with biopsy revealing pancreatic adenocarcinoma. The patient is otherwise healthy and very active, and independent on all IADLs and ADLs. The patient states that quality of life is more important to him than survival.

In reviewing the palliative care options with this patient, which of the following treatments are appropriate to discuss, given his symptoms and goals of care?

(A) Surgical resection
(B) Biliary stent placement and chemotherapy
(C) Chemotherapy
(D) Radiation

ANSWER: B

Pancreatic cancer is a devastating diagnosis and historically is associated with both poor prognosis and poor quality of life. Overall 5-yr survival rates are <6%. Most patients present with advanced or metastatic disease; the median life expectancy is 3–6 mo with metastatic disease.

The optimal treatment of metastatic pancreatic cancer is still uncertain, and all options provide limited benefit. A patient's particular circumstances in terms of symptoms, goals, and preferences need to be strongly considered when deciding on possible palliative treatment options.

Biliary decompression with biliary stenting can relieve jaundice, pruritus, and improve appetite, and would be an appropriate palliative option to discuss with the patient (SOE=A). Many chemotherapeutic agents have been used to treat advanced pancreatic cancer. Gemcitabine provides "clinical benefit" (improvement in pain, performance status, or weight) with fairly limited toxicity in about one-fourth of patients (SOE=A), so would be an appropriate option to discuss with this patient. 5-Fluorouracil-based chemotherapy modestly increased survival compared with best supportive care alone (SOE=A) but is associated with much more toxicity than gemcitabine, so it would be less appropriate for this patient. Benefits of any chemotherapeutic regimen must be weighed against burdens, which include the need for regular infusions, blood tests, and chemotherapy-related adverse events. Surgical resection would be potentially curative for an early pancreatic cancer (SOE=A) but not for a metastatic cancer. Radiation is not an appropriate treatment option for pancreatic cancer.

References

1. Jemal A, Siegel R, Ward E, et al. Cancer statistics, 2009. *CA Cancer J Clin*. 2009;59(4):225–249.
2. Nieto J, Grossbard ML, Kozuch P, et al. Metastatic pancreatic cancer 2008: is the glass less empty? *Oncologist*. 2008;13(5):562–576.
3. Neoptolemos JP, Stocken DD, Friess H, et al. A randomized trial of chemoradiotherapy and chemotherapy after resection of pancreatic cancer. *N Engl J Med*. 2004;350(12):1200–1210.
4. Sultana A, Smith CT, Cunningham D, et al. Meta-analyses of chemotherapy for locally advanced and metastatic pancreatic cancer. *J Clin Oncol*. 2007;25(18):2607–2615.

28. A resident of a nursing facility has fallen twice in the last month, without injury. He uses a rolling walker and participates in recreational programs. He has moderately severe Alzheimer's disease, major depressive disorder, osteoarthritis, and hypertension.

Which of the following should be undertaken *first* in evaluating his risk of future falls?

(A) Review the circumstances of his past falls.
(B) Evaluate his strength and balance.
(C) Review his medications.
(D) Check for postural hypotension.

ANSWER: A

The first step in evaluating a person who has had falls, whether in the community or in an institutional setting, is to review the circumstances of the fall(s) (SOE=C). Because older adults may be unable to recall circumstances of the fall because of cognitive impairment, a key question is whether the fall was observed and where it occurred. For residents of nursing facilities, a detailed incident report can help determine the most effective intervention for preventing future falls. If the person lost consciousness or was lightheaded, cardiovascular and neurologic evaluations are appropriate. If an environmental hazard (eg, a wet floor, clutter in the room, unstable furniture) contributed to the fall, the hazard should be eliminated. If the falls occurred at the same time of day (eg, at change of shift or while the patient tried to get to the bathroom after dinner), a change in staffing and supervision at vulnerable times may be effective.

Fall prevention in nursing facilities is best accomplished by a multidisciplinary approach (SOE=C). Once the circumstances of the falls are known, evaluation by a physical therapist could help in determining whether the resident needs to improve strength and balance, or whether he or she would benefit from an assistive device (or from retraining in safe use of the device). The physician should review medications and reduce the dosage or eliminate some, if possible. Postural hypotension is seen in ≥50% of residents in nursing facilities. Often it is due to medications, but it can also be caused by autonomic dysfunction. Some older adults may have postprandial hypotension that causes lightheadedness and falls; again, inquiring about the timing of falls may lead to this diagnosis.

References

1. American Geriatric Society and British Geriatrics Society. *Clinical Practice Guideline for the Prevention of Falls in Older Persons.* New York: American Geriatrics Society; 2009. http://www.americangeriatrics.org/
2. Gupta V, Lipsitz LA. Orthostatic hypotension in the elderly: diagnosis and treatment. *Am J Med.* 2007;120(10):841–847.

29. An 85-yr-old man with macular degeneration is evaluated because of a sudden change in behavior and weight loss. He is recently widowed and has moved into an assisted-living facility. When his family visits, they are stunned to find him withdrawn, quiet, and losing weight. Previously, he had lived in his home for 50 yr and had managed ADLs and IADLs with assistance from his wife. Several years ago, he received services from a local agency for the blind and visually impaired.

Physical examination is normal except for low vision. Results of the Mini–Mental State Examination and Geriatric Depression Scale are normal. Examination by his ophthalmologist shows no change in the macular degeneration.

Which of the following is the most appropriate next step?

(A) Start antidepressant medications.
(B) Encourage participation in group activities.
(C) Obtain a complete medical evaluation to assess the weight loss.
(D) Refer to a vision rehabilitation specialist.
(E) Refer to a geriatric psychiatrist.

ANSWER: D

The patient functioned well in his home. He knew where everything was located. He was able to get a cup of tea, dial the phone, go for a walk, and visit friends. Although he and his wife depended on each other for support, they could function independently at home. Thinking he could no longer live alone, his family did not take into account the benefits of a known home layout. In the new facility, his room layouts are unfamiliar. It is likely that he has difficulty accessing the dining room without assistance. A vision rehabilitation specialist can assess the new environment and ensure that the patient receives additional instruction in orientation and mobility so that he can navigate independently and safely. He may benefit from a talking watch to assist him to be on time for meals. The rehabilitation specialist can provide information on lighting to the staff, so that the patient can have sufficient light to eat his meals, and can instruct staff in creating plates that accentuate the color contrast of the food. With this assistance, he may obtain independence (and gain weight) in the new setting.

Loss of vision is associated with major depressive disorder in older adults. The prevalence of depression among patients with age-related macular degeneration is approximately 30%; depression is a major cause of excess disability (SOE=A). A return to independence may prevent major depressive disorder in this patient.

Encouraging participation in group activities may be beneficial but will be more successful once the patient has the tools for more independence. A complete medical evaluation is indicated if weight loss persists after the patient is oriented to the dining hall and his own room, and it is clear that he has access to meals.

References

1. American Academy of Ophthalmology Vision Rehabilitation Committee. *Preferred Practice Pattern Guidelines. Vision Rehabilitation for Adults.* San Francisco, CA: American Academy of Ophthalmology; 2007. Available at: http://one.aao.org/CE/PracticeGuidelines/PPP.aspx (accessed Nov 2009).
2. Brody BL, Gamst AC, Williams RA, et al. Depression, visual acuity, comorbidity, and disability associated with age-related macular degeneration. *Ophthalmology.* 2001;108(10):1893–1901.
3. Sloan FA, Ostermann J, Brown DS, et al. Effects of changes in self-reported vision on cognitive, affective, and functional status and living arrangements among the elderly. *Am J Ophthalmol.* 2005;140(4):618–627.

30. A 67-yr-old man comes to the office with his family to obtain a second medical opinion. He has lost 18 kg (40 lb) in the past 6 mo, is weak, spends most of his time in bed, no longer participates in family activities, and is no longer interested in watching sporting events on television. He tends to sit quietly and let his family answer questions, but when questioned directly, he indicates that he cannot swallow solids or liquids because his throat is blocked. His family reports that he eats and drinks small amounts. He believes he has undiagnosed cancer that the doctors have yet to find.

Physical examination and cognitive assessment reveal some mild difficulties in recall. According to the medical records he provides, radiography and CT of the chest are normal, and upper endoscopy is unremarkable. Physical examination and several sets of blood work have been obtained, none of which indicate dehydration, anemia, or hepatic or renal dysfunction.

Which of the following is the most likely explanation for these findings?

(A) Occult lung cancer
(B) Vascular dementia
(C) Alzheimer's disease
(D) Major depressive disorder with psychotic features
(E) Parkinson's disease with psychotic symptoms

ANSWER: D

In older adults, the presentation of major depressive disorder with psychotic features is often masked by concomitant physical symptoms. This patient has a sustained belief of a physical abnormality not supported by medical evidence. The belief alone, however, is not sufficient for diagnosis of major depressive disorder with psychotic features. The patient has other suggestive signs and symptoms: psychomotor retardation, loss of interest, loss of energy, social withdrawal, and increased time in bed. These symptoms likely reflect depressive disorder rather than physical impairment, with the normal test results. Patients with occult malignancy can present with weight loss and poorly articulated physical complaints. However, the preponderance of depressive symptoms and his loss of interest in activities (eg, watching sports on television) that are unaffected by his physical limitations make occult malignancy unlikely. A primary psychiatric concern is also suggested by his delusional belief that he cannot swallow. This is contradicted by his family, as well as by his previous examinations.

Major depressive disorder with psychotic features (in this case, somatic delusion) responds poorly to pharmacotherapy with an antidepressant alone, and usually requires the addition of an antipsychotic agent. However, the addition of an antipsychotic agent is not always effective and can also increase adverse events. Although its availability is limited and it can be less acceptable to patients, electroconvulsive therapy is the treatment of choice for older adults who have major depressive disorder with psychotic features.

Diagnosis of dementia requires the presence of memory impairment and at least one other deficit in another cognitive area such as language, executive function, or fine-motor coordination. Consequently, vascular dementia and Alzheimer's disease are unlikely. However, in a subgroup of older depressed adults with memory problems, dementia developed in subsequent years. The absence of symptoms of a movement disorder tends to exclude Parkinson's disease, although major depressive disorder can precede the onset of movement disorder in a subgroup of patients.

References

1. Ishihara L, Brayne C. A systematic review of depression and mental illness preceding Parkinson's disease. *Acta Neurol Scand.* 2006;113(4):211–220.

2. Koenig HG, Blazer DG, Steffens DC. Mood disorders. In: Blazer DG, Steffens DC, eds. *The American Psychiatric Publishing Textbook of Geriatric Psychiatry.* 4th ed. Washington, DC: American Psychiatric Publishing; 2009.

3. Manepalli JN, Gebretsadik M, Hook, J, et al. Differential diagnosis of the older patient with psychotic symptoms. *Primary Psychiatry.* 2007;14(8):55–62.

4. Murphy CF, Alexopoulos GS. Cognition and late-life depression. *Primary Psychiatry.* 2004;11(5):54–58.

31. An 80-yr-old man is brought to the emergency department because his cognition is rapidly deteriorating, his temperature is 39.4°C (103°F), and he has upper abdominal pain. His family reports that he has steroid-dependent COPD. He smokes one-half pack of cigarettes daily. He has not been eating well and has lost 4.5 kg (10 lb) over the last 4 mo. He uses a walker to ambulate short distances within the house and is dependent on his family for all IADLs.

Surgical evaluation and ultrasound study are highly suggestive of cholecystitis and possible abscess. Admission laboratory data show a WBC count of $19 \times 10^3/mm^3$ and a BUN of 32 mg/dL. He is vigorously rehydrated before undergoing emergent cholecystectomy under general anesthesia.

Which of the following is most likely to reduce his risk of postoperative pulmonary complications?

(A) Incentive spirometry
(B) Total parenteral hyperalimentation
(C) Postoperative epidural analgesia
(D) Routine nasogastric decompression

ANSWER: A

Risk factors for postoperative pneumonia include type of surgery (abdominal aortic aneurysm repair and thoracic and upper abdominal surgery carry the greatest risk), older age, diminished functional status, weight loss >10% over the previous 6 mo, history of COPD, use of general anesthesia, impaired sensorium, history of stroke, increased BUN, transfusion of >4 units of packed RBCs, emergent surgery, smoking, chronic steroid use, and consumption of >2 drinks containing alcohol daily. Risk reduction can be maximized by discontinuing tobacco smoking at least 6–8 wk before planned surgery (SOE=A), regrettably not an option for patients requiring emergency intervention.

This patient is at extremely high risk of postoperative pulmonary complications because of multiple risk factors. Aggressive interventions should be in place to minimize risk. Lung expansion therapy (such as incentive spirometry, continuous positive airway pressure, and deep breathing exercises) helps prevent decreased lung volumes and atelectasis associated with surgery and bed rest (SOE=A).

While nutrition support, including total parenteral nutrition in a patient unable to eat, is crucial to long-term management, such support provides no advantage in an acute situation (SOE=B).

Epidural analgesia does not appear to be more effective than patient-controlled intravenous analgesia in preventing postoperative pneumonia (SOE=B). However, intraoperative use of shorter-acting neuromuscular-blocking drugs may be superior to general anesthesia alone in minimizing postoperative pulmonary complications.

Routine nasogastric decompression until bowel function returns does not reduce the risk of postoperative pneumonia. Nasogastric decompression after surgery should be reserved for patients who have nausea, vomiting, or symptomatic abdominal distention, or for patients who cannot tolerate oral intake (SOE=B).

References

1. Arozullah AM, Khuri SF, Henderson WG, et al. Development and validation of a multifactorial risk index for predicting postoperative pneumonia after major non-cardiac surgery. *Ann Intern Med.* 2001;135(10):847–857.

2. Lawrence VA, Cornell JE, Smetana GW. Strategies to reduce postoperative pulmonary complications after noncardiothoracic surgery: systematic review for the American College of Physicians. *Ann Intern Med.* 2006;144(8):596–608.

3. Smetana GW, Lawrence VA, Cornell JE. Preoperative pulmonary risk stratification for noncardiothoracic surgery: systematic review for the American College of Physicians. *Ann Intern Med.* 2006;144(8):581–595.
4. Thompson DA, Makary MA, Dorman T, et al. Clinical and economic outcomes of hospital acquired pneumonia in intra-abdominal surgery patients. *Ann Surg.* 2006:243(4):547–552.

32. A 75-yr-old man comes to the office because he has an ulcer on his tongue that is not painful except when he eats acidic or spicy foods. He does not remember when he first noticed it. His last dental examination was 2 yr ago. He smoked 2 packs daily for 30 yr, but stopped smoking 20 yr ago. He has hypertension controlled with medication.

On examination, there is a 2 × 2–cm nonhealing, indurated ulcer on the left lateroventral border of the tongue next to a broken filling.

Which of the following is the next best step?

(A) Refer patient to dentist to have filling restored.
(B) Refer for immediate biopsy of the lesion.
(C) Instruct patient to use an OTC local anesthetic gel to relieve the pain.
(D) Explain to patient that this is a canker sore that will resolve on its own in 7–10 days.
(E) Recommend that the patient avoid acidic or spicy foods until the sore heals.

ANSWER: B

The clinical appearance of the ulcer—large and indurated, with rolled, firm edges—and its unknown duration make biopsy essential. Oral cancer claims approximately 8,000 lives in the United States each year. It is most common in people ≥40 yr old, especially in those with a history of smoking. Although head and neck cancer accounts for only 3% of all new cancer cases and 2% of all cancer deaths in the United States annually, it is the fifth most common malignancy worldwide. Tobacco and alcohol are the primary etiologic agents.

Squamous cell carcinoma, which accounts for 96% of all oral cancers, is usually preceded by dysplasia presenting as white epithelial lesions on the oral mucosa (leukoplakia), red and white lesions (erythroplakia), or a nonhealing ulcer. Early diagnosis and treatment markedly improve outcome and survival.

Although the defective tooth filling could have precipitated the ulcer, the duration and clinical appearance of the ulcer indicate a precancerous or cancerous lesion. An OTC local anesthetic gel may provide temporary pain relief, but it does not treat precancerous, cancerous, or any other oral lesions. Canker sore is unlikely: a canker sore has a short duration and is a shallow ulcer covered by a yellowish white, removable, fibrinous membrane and surrounded by an erythematous halo.

Avoiding spicy or acidic foods is not indicated; the patient needs immediate biopsy of the lesion (SOE=C).

References
1. Braakhuis BJ, Tabor MP, Leemans CR, et al. Second primary tumors and field cancerization in oral and oropharyngeal cancer: molecular techniques provide new insights and definitions. *Head Neck.* 2002;24(20):198–206.
2. Cinamon U, Hier MP, Black MJ. Age as a prognostic factor for head and neck squamous cell carcinoma: should older patients be treated differently? *J Otolaryngol.* 2006;35(1):8–12.
3. Jemal A, Clegg LX, Ward E, et al. Cancer Statistics, 2008. *CA Cancer J Clin.* 2008;58:71–96.
4. Rogers LQ, Courneya KS, Robbins KT, et al. Physical activity and quality of life in head and neck cancer survivors. *Support Care Cancer.* 2006;14(10):1012–1029.

33. An 85-yr-old woman is brought to the office by her family because she has visual hallucinations of children and small animals when she is alone in a room. At times she has been disturbed and agitated by these hallucinations. Her family also notes that she is having more difficulty walking, and at times has hand tremors when she sits quietly. She has a 9-mo history of short-term memory loss, word-finding difficulties, and difficulty paying bills and preparing meals. Examination is unremarkable except for cogwheel rigidity and resting tremors.

Which of the following is the most likely diagnosis?

(A) Parkinson's disease with dementia
(B) Alzheimer's disease
(C) Dementia with Lewy bodies
(D) Huntington's disease

ANSWER: C

This patient likely has Lewy body dementia, as suggested by the occurrence of dementia within 1 yr of onset of extrapyramidal symptoms (eg, lead-pipe or cogwheel rigidity, bradykinesia, resting tremor) with prominent, distinct visual hallucinations. Individuals typically have a dementia in which memory impairment in the earlier stages may not be as pronounced as deficits in attention, executive function, and visuospatial ability. An expert consortium agreed that in addition to dementia, criteria for diagnosis of Lewy body dementia should include 2 of the following: fluctuating cognition, parkinsonian features, and recurrent visual hallucinations that are typically well formed and detailed. Features that suggest Lewy body dementia include rapid-eye movement sleep behavior disorder, severe neuroleptic sensitivity, and reduced striatal dopamine transporter activity on functional neuroimaging (such as single photon emission computed tomography [SPECT] or positron emission tomography [PET]). Supportive features include unexplained falls, major depressive disorder, autonomic dysfunction (eg, orthostatic hypotension, urinary incontinence), transient loss of consciousness, and systematized delusions.

Although Parkinson's disease presents with extrapyramidal symptoms, initially these symptoms occur without memory loss or psychosis. Hallucinations can occur in patients with Alzheimer's disease (typically at mid-stage), but extrapyramidal symptoms usually occur later in the disease, and are generally not characterized by tremors but by bradykinesia and rigidity. Huntington's disease is characterized by cognitive impairment and choreiform movement.

References

1. Karim S, Byrne EJ. Treatment of psychosis in elderly people. *Advances in Psychiatric Treatment.* 2005;11:286–296.
2. Manepalli JN, Gebretsadik M, Hook J, et al. Differential diagnosis of the older patient with psychotic symptoms. *Primary Psychiatry.* 2007;14(8):55–62.
3. McKeith IG, Dickson DW, Lowe J, et al. Diagnosis and management of dementia with Lewy bodies: Third report of the DLB Consortium. *Neurology.* 2005;65(12):1863–1872.
4. Mintzer J, Targum SD. Psychosis in elderly patients: classification and pharmacotherapy. *J Geriatr Psychiatry Neurol.* 2003;16(4):199–206.

34. A 78-yr-old man comes to the office because he volunteers at the local hospital and is required to get a tuberculin skin test annually. A tuberculosis skin test (PPD) using 5 tuberculin units was done a year ago when he first started. At that time, the test was read as 4 mm of induration and interpreted as negative. On retesting now a year later, there is 16 mm of induration. He has no symptoms, and chest radiograph is negative. He is on coumadin for atrial fibrillation but has no other problems and no other medications.

What is the most appropriate next step in management?

(A) Observation only
(B) Annual chest radiography
(C) Repeat PPD testing in 6 mo
(D) Treatment with pyrazinamide plus rifampin for 2 mo
(E) Treatment with isoniazid for 9 mo

ANSWER: E

The proper interpretation of this PPD is that the patient is a recent converter (ie, induration enlarged from <10 mm to ≥15 mm within 2 yr). However, it is possible he has undergone a "booster" response in which the first PPD done a year ago "boosted" his T-cell memory so that a second PPD resulted in a greater reaction. This is why two-step testing is recommended for new long-term care residents and staff and for all healthcare personnel. In either case, a positive test warrants therapy. All patients with a positive PPD should have active disease excluded by a thorough examination and chest radiograph; if this evaluation is negative, 9 mo of INH is the appropriate treatment. This is true despite the drug interaction with warfarin; this patient will simply need his INR monitored closely. In this case, he also would qualify for INH therapy based only on the size of the PPD reaction (≥15 mm) which is always considered positive regardless of other factors, including age, underlying illness, prior administration of BCG vaccine, etc. In those with specific risk factors, which are quite common in older adults (eg, diabetes, gastrectomy/ achlorhydria, excessive weight loss, chronic renal disease, etc), a PPD ≥10 mm of induration is considered positive. In immunocompromised patients, in those with changes on chest radiographs typical of prior tuberculosis, and in those recently exposed to someone with active disease, a PPD ≥5 mm of induration is considered positive.

This patient has a 10% risk of developing active tuberculosis within 2 yr and works in a healthcare setting; thus, observation and annual chest radiography are not indicated. Repeat PPD testing will not change management options and is not needed. Treatment with pyrazinamide and rifampin has been shown effective in treating latent tuberculosis in patients with human immunodeficiency virus infection but is considered a second-line therapy to 9 mo of isoniazid treatment (SOE=A).

References

1. American Thoracic Society. Targeted tuberculin testing and treatment of latent infection. *Am J Resp Crit Care Med.* 2000;161(4 Pt 2):S221–S247.
2. American Thoracic Society. Diagnostic standards and classification of tuberculosis in adults and children. *Am J Resp Crit Care Med.* 2000;161(4 Pt 1):1376–1395.
3. Marion CR, High KP. Tuberculosis in older adults. In: Yoshikawa TT, Norma DC, eds. *Infectious Disease in the Aging: A Clinical Handbook.* New York: Humana Press; 2009:97–110.

35. A 69-yr-old patient comes to the office because she has vulvar burning and soreness. On examination, there is evidence of vulvar scarring, glassy erythematous erosions, white striae along the margins of the labia minora and vestibule, and vaginal involvement. A specimen is obtained for biopsy.

Which of the following is the most likely diagnosis?

(A) Lichen sclerosus
(B) Lichen planus
(C) Lichen simplex chronicus
(D) Vulvar atrophy
(E) Squamous hyperplasia

ANSWER: B

The skin of the vulva loses elasticity with aging. Underlying fat and connective tissue undergo degeneration with a loss of collagen and thinning of the epithelial layer. Vulvar skin changes are classified as either non-neoplastic lesions or vulvar intraepithelial neoplasias. Non-neoplastic lesions include lichen sclerosus, squamous hyperplasia, condylomata, lichen simplex chronicus, and lichen planus.

Vulvar lichen planus is considered uncommon. However, it can be difficult to diagnose and is frequently confused with candidiasis or vulvodynia. It can be isolated to the vulva or part of a generalized skin eruption. The cause of lichen planus is not known, although an autoimmune mechanism has been proposed. It can be drug-induced: β-blockers, NSAIDs, and ACE inhibitors have all been implicated. Lichen planus differs from lichen sclerosus in that the lesions of lichen sclerosus are typically shiny, white or pink, and parchment-like, and do not involve the vagina. Vaginal involvement has been reported in up to 70% of women with erosive lichen planus. Diagnosis of lichen planus is confirmed by biopsy of lesions. Treatment consists of very high-potency corticosteroids (clobetasol 0.5% or halbetasol) applied topically.

Lichen simplex chronicus is an eczematous disease characterized by itching and scratching. Lesions are usually small, round, itchy spots that thicken and become leathery from scratching. They are usually located over the labia majora. Lichen simplex chronicus is seen in women who are genetically atopic. Common triggers include psychologic distress, heat, sweating, and excessive dryness. Successful treatment depends on identification and elimination of aggravating factors. Oral or topical steroids and antihistamines may be necessary to reduce inflammation and relieve intense itching.

Vulvar atrophy results from estrogen deficiency and is characterized by itch, redness, or soreness of the vulva. Typically, there is pale, dry vaginal epithelium that is smooth and shiny. It is treated with low-dose topical estrogen cream.

Squamous cell hyperplasia can result from repetitive scratching or rubbing from irritants. It is often confused with lichen simplex chronicus. Squamous cell hyperplasia appears as ill-defined, single or scattered, whitish, thickened, and sometimes verrucous plaques. Itching is common. The clitoris, labia minora, and inner aspects of the labia majora are affected. It has malignant potential: 10% of cases progress to invasive carcinoma. All vulvar skin changes should be biopsied if they do not respond to standard therapies.

References

1. Bauer A, Rodiger C, Greif C, et al. Vulvar dematatoses—irritant and allergic contact dermatitis of the vulva. *Dermatology.* 2005;210(2):143–149.
2. Cooper SM, Wojnarowska F. Influence of treatment of erosive lichen planus of the vulva on its prognosis. *Arch Dermatol.* 2006;142(3):289–294.
3. Lynch PJ. Lichen simplex chronicus (atopic/neurodermatitis) of the anogenital region. *Dermatol Ther.* 2004;17(1):8–19.

4. Smith YR, Haefner HK. Vulvar lichen sclerosus: pathophysiology and treatment. *Am J Clin Dermatol.* 2004;5(2):105–125.

36. Which of the following is true regarding health literacy?

(A) Health literacy is the degree to which a person can obtain, process, and understand information to make appropriate health decisions.

(B) People with limited health literacy are more likely to ask questions about care during physician visits.

(C) Health status, rate of hospitalization, and healthcare costs of people with limited health literacy are similar to those of persons with adequate literacy.

(D) In the United States, 12% of the population lacks health literacy.

ANSWER: A

Health literacy is the degree to which a person can obtain, process, and understand health information to make appropriate health decisions. Literacy level appears to be an important determinant of a patient's participation in medical encounters: people with limited health literacy are less likely to ask questions about care during physician visits and more likely to make medication errors. Limited health literacy can affect a person's ability to learn about his or her medical conditions and treatments.

People with limited health literacy have less health knowledge, worse health status, more hospitalizations, higher healthcare costs, and poorer outcomes than people with adequate literacy (SOE=A). They are less likely to use preventive services and more likely to use hospitals and emergency departments. Inadequate knowledge about health, incorrect use of medication, poorer health status, and higher hospitalization rates related to limited health literacy increase healthcare costs by almost $100 billion each year.

According to the National Assessment of Adult Literacy survey conducted in 2003 by the U.S. Department of Education, only 12% of the adult population has sufficient skills to allow them to deal with complex and challenging tasks requiring health literacy. An additional 53% has intermediate skills, meaning they can deal with most tasks they encounter that require health literacy. The remainder of the population—36%, or nearly 90 million adults—has inadequate health literacy skills.

References

1. Katz MG, Jacobson TA, Veledar E, et al. Patient literacy and question-asking behavior during the medical encounter: a mixed-methods analysis. *J Gen Intern Med.* 2007;22(6):782–786.

2. Kutner M, Greenberg E, Jin Y, et al. The Health Literacy of America's Adults: Results from the 2003 National Assessment of Adult Literacy (NCES 2006-483). Washington, DC: National Center for Education Statistics, U.S. Department of Education; 2006.

3. Joint Commission on Accreditation of Healthcare Organizations. "*What Did the Doctor Say?" Improving Health Literacy to Protect Patient Safety*. Chicago, IL: Joint Commission on Accreditation of Healthcare Organizations; 2007.

37. A 72-yr-old man is evaluated because nurses are concerned about his agitation, which increases markedly in the evenings. He underwent emergency hip replacement 3 days ago after he fell and fractured his hip. He requires antipsychotic agents to control his agitation at night: he yells "help me" constantly and is determined to get out of bed alone and walk. In the year before his fall, he had stopped working and driving; the reasons are unclear. History includes hypertension, benign prostatic hyperplasia, and osteoarthritis. There is no history of dementia. On examination, he appears confused and is disoriented to place and time. He has some pain with hip movements. Neurologic findings are nonfocal.

Which of the following is most helpful in establishing the diagnosis of delirium?

(A) Order electrolytes, BUN, glucose, and thyrotropin.

(B) Determine why the patient stopped working and driving.

(C) Perform the digit-span memory test.

(D) Order CT of the brain.

(E) Review the patient's medication list.

ANSWER: C

The patient appears delirious, which is common in hip fracture patients. Delirium is diagnosed on the basis of change in cognitive function and attentional deficit. The digit-span memory test—asking the patient to repeat a series of numbers—is a useful assessment for attention. Cognitive assessment can include detailed orientation questions or formal cognitive screening tests, such as the Montreal Cognitive Assessment (MCCA) or Confusion Assessment Method (CAM). The sensitivity and specificity of CAM in acute medical patients are approximately 95% and 90%, respectively

(SOE=B). The Delirium Rating Scale–Revised 98 is another commonly used tool.

Because dementia is the strongest risk factor for developing delirium, establishing the baseline cognitive status of the patient is useful. The patient may have preexisting cognitive deficits: he recently stopped driving and working. Further history is required to determine whether these events were due to cognitive deficits. However, evaluation for risk factors would not substitute for tests for delirium.

CT of the brain may be performed to determine the cause of delirium, but it does not diagnose delirium. It is most useful in the presence of new focal neurologic symptoms or falls. Determining primary and contributing causes of the delirium requires reviewing all medications and conducting laboratory and other tests as indicated by the patient's history and findings on examination.

References

1. Inouye SK. Delirium in older persons. *N Engl J Med.* 2006;354(11):1157–1165.
2. Wei LA, Fearing MA, Sternberg EJ, et al. The Confusion Assessment Method: a systematic review of current usage. *J Am Geriatr Soc.* 2008;56(5):823–830.

38. An 86-yr-old woman with alcohol dependence comes to the office to establish care, accompanied by a geriatric care manager who has been hired by her children to look after her. The patient lives alone and has limited social support. Her family has often unsuccessfully attempted to help the patient with her alcohol dependence; they currently have little interaction with her. The patient describes periods of sobriety alternating with relapses, during which she can consume up to 1 liter of vodka in a day. Her most recent treatment experience included a psychiatric inpatient stay 4 mo ago. The patient left against medical advice after 2 days, vowing never to be hospitalized in a psychiatric facility again. She states that she has never had alcoholism-related pharmacologic treatment, alcohol withdrawal seizures, or severe reactions during prior detoxifications. She has tried and rejected Alcoholics Anonymous. She is unable to estimate the amount of alcohol she consumes daily. Her geriatric care manager is unsure of her level of consumption, and notes that the patient is able to have alcohol delivered to her home. The patient's history also includes major depressive disorder, gastroesophageal reflux disease, and osteoporosis. Medications include citalopram, omeprazole, and alendronate, although the patient reports taking no prescribed medications for the past several months. At the end of the visit, the patient asks for help with her alcohol problem.

Which of the following is the most appropriate first step?

(A) Instruct the patient to stop drinking.
(B) Prescribe disulfiram and a short-acting benzodiazepine.
(C) Recommend admission to psychiatric inpatient facility.
(D) Recommend hospital admission for alcohol detoxification.
(E) Prescribe naltrexone and refer her to the local Alcoholics Anonymous chapter.

ANSWER: D

The first step in treatment for this patient is alcohol detoxification. Outpatient detoxification can be considered for medically stable adults with good social support but is not appropriate for this patient. The decision to seek inpatient detoxification is also supported by preliminary research demonstrating that increasing age is associated with both increased severity and duration of withdrawal symptoms (SOE=B). Given the patient's negative reaction to a psychiatric inpatient stay, she is not likely to accept referral to another psychiatric inpatient facility. Thus, alcohol detoxification within a medical facility constitutes the most appropriate first step in management (SOE=C). The hospitalization will be covered by Medicare.

Disulfiram, an aldehyde dehydrogenase inhibitor, is an aversive therapy that works by causing an accumulation of acetaldehyde, which is responsible for the uncomfortable symptoms (eg, flushing, palpitations, nausea, vomiting) that occur when alcohol is consumed. Although the evidence is weak for use of disulfiram in relapse prevention, case reports suggest that it may have value for some patients. However, disulfiram is not recommended for use among older adults because of concerns related to cardiovascular effects. Research is sparse on the role of naltrexone, an opioid antagonist that reduces craving and emotional response to the pleasurable effects of alcohol, in preventing relapse in older adults. In a study of alcohol-dependent male veterans 50–70 yr old, naltrexone was well tolerated and was associated with less relapse to significant drinking when compared with placebo. Naltrexone cannot be given until a patient is abstinent from alcohol.

The patient's negative reaction to Alcoholics Anonymous should be explored after detoxification to determine whether this type of supportive therapy may have a role in helping her maintain abstinence.

Simply substituting a benzodiazepine for alcohol is neither safe nor effective.

References

1. Blow FC, Serra AM, Barry KL. Late-life depression and alcoholism. *Current Psychatry Rep.* 2007;9:14–19.
2. McKeon A, Frye MA, Delanty N. The alcohol withdrawal syndrome. *J Neurol Neurosurg Psychiatry.* 2007;79(8):854–862.
3. Oslin DW. Evidenced-based treatment of geriatric substance. *Psychiatr Clin North Am.* 2005;28(4):897–911.

39. A 75-yr-old woman with established osteoporosis wishes to discuss advertisements she has seen for ibandronate and risedronate. She currently takes alendronate and wonders whether she would benefit more from a different agent. She has not had a fracture.

Which of the following is the best agent for preventing fracture?

(A) Alendronate
(B) Ibandronate
(C) Pamidronate
(D) Risedronate
(E) Data are not available to answer her question.

ANSWER: E

Bisphosphonates are effective in reducing fracture risk among postmenopausal women with osteoporosis. When compared with placebo, these agents prevent vertebral, nonvertebral, and hip fractures (SOE=A). Patients are exposed to considerable advertising about the benefits of these agents, different dosing regimens, and convenience. Studies have not been identified that demonstrate the superiority of one agent over another in preventing fractures (SOE=A). A systematic review of studies of agents used to treat osteoporosis identified the following design issues: 1) few studies compared different agents within the same class; 2) most head-to-head comparisons of agents from different classes reported intermediate outcomes (eg, changes in bone mineral density or in markers of bone turnover) rather than differences in fracture incidence; and 3) no

trial with head-to-head comparisons of ≥2 agents had a sufficient sample size to detect even large differences in fracture risk.

Only 2 head-to-head trials were designed to compare fracture outcomes. In one, no difference was found between risedronate and etidronate for the prevention of vertebral fractures. In the other, which compared raloxifene and alendronate, not enough participants were recruited to test differences in fracture outcomes. The authors of the above-mentioned systematic review concluded that "1) within the bisphosphonate class, superiority for prevention of fractures has not been shown for any agent; 2) superiority for the prevention of vertebral fractures has not been demonstrated for bisphosphonates compared with calcitonin, calcium, or raloxifene; and 3) on the basis of 6 inadequately powered randomized trials, fracture prevention did not differ between bisphosphonates and estrogen."

References

1. Kushida K, Fukunaga M, Kishimoto H, et al. A comparison of incidences of vertebral fracture in Japanese patients with involutional osteoporosis treated with risedronate and etidronate: a randomized, double-masked trial. *J Bone Miner Metab.* 2004;22(5):469–478.
2. MacLean C, Newberry S, Maglione M, et al. Systematic review: comparative effectiveness of treatments to prevent fractures in men and women with low bone density or osteoporosis. *Ann Intern Med.* 2008;148(3):197–213.
3. Recker RR, Kendler D, Recknor CP, et al. Comparative effects of raloxifene and alendronate on fracture outcomes in postmenopausal women with low bone mass. *Bone.* 2007;40(4):843–851.

40. A 69-yr-old man is brought to the emergency department because, while eating breakfast, he started to have shaking movements of his left arm and leg without loss of consciousness. The episode lasted about a minute; afterward, the patient was sleepy and confused for 15 min. The patient smokes tobacco and has a history of COPD, diabetes, major depressive disorder, and hypertension. Medications include enalapril, paroxetine, inhaled tiotropium and inhaled fluticasone.

On examination, blood pressure is 160/100 mmHg, pulse rate is 92 per minute, and respiratory rate is 18 per minute. The rest of the examination is normal except for lethargy. MRI scan of the brain shows several lesions consistent with metastatic cancer.

Which anticonvulsant medication is the best agent for this patient?

(A) Carbamazepine
(B) Gabapentin
(C) Lamotrigine
(D) Phenobarbital
(E) Topiramate

ANSWER: C

This patient had a partial seizure secondary to metastatic disease and, therefore, treatment is indicated. When choosing an anticonvulsant medication, important considerations include effectiveness, safety and tolerability, comorbidities, other medications, ease of administration, cost, patient age, and adherence. Lamotrigine is at least as effective for partial seizure as carbamazepine, and it is better tolerated. It also has fewer drug-drug interactions than carbamazepine. Given this patient's history of other chronic medical conditions, which include hypertension and depression, and multiple medications, the preferred medication is lamotrigine (SOE=A). Gabapentin and topiramate are less effective than either lamotrigine or carbamazepine for treatment of partial seizures (SOE=A). Phenobarbital has the potential to cause significant adverse events on cognition in older adults and should be avoided.

References
1. French JA. First choice for newly diagnosed epilepsy. *Lancet.* 2007;369(9566):970–971.
2. Marson AG, Al-Kharusi AM, Alwaiah M, et al. The SANAD study of effectiveness of carbamazepine, gabapentin, lamotrigine, oxycarbazepine or topiramate for treatment of partial epilepsy: an unblinded randomised controlled trial. *Lancet.* 2007;369(9566):1000–1015.
3. Marson AG, Al-Kharusi AM, Alwaiah M, et al. The SANAD study of effectiveness of valproate, lamotrigine or topiramate for treatment of partial epilepsy: an unblinded randomised controlled trial. *Lancet.* 2007;369(9566):1016–1026.
4. Pugh MJ, Foreman PJ, Berkowitz DR. Prescribing antiepileptics for the elderly: difference between guideline recommendations and clinical practice. *Drugs Aging.* 2006;23(11):861–975.

41. A 72-yr-old man comes to the office because he wants to try a new approach for controlling his blood pressure. He has just stopped all his antihypertensive medications, because he says that he has tried many and they all have adverse events. His blood pressure (off medicine) is 140/98 mmHg. He wants to try something "natural."

Which of the following is *least* likely to lower his blood pressure?

(A) Breathing entrainment device
(B) Tai Chi
(C) White chocolate
(D) DASH (Dietary Approaches to Stop Hypertension) diet
(E) Coenzyme Q_{10}

ANSWER: C

In small studies, *RespErate*, a commercial product approved by the FDA, lowered systolic blood pressure by approximately 15 mmHg and diastolic blood pressure by 10 mmHg. The *RespErate* device uses a strap around the chest to monitor breathing and produces a series of musical notes in response to the respiratory rate. The wearer is asked to synchronize breathing with the music. Over about 2 min, the device helps the wearer slow respiratory rates from an average of 16 toward a goal of <10 breaths per minute. Slowed breathing is thought to affect the autonomic nervous system by increasing tidal volume, leading to greater cardiopulmonary stretch-receptor stimulation. This in turn reduces sympathetic efferent discharge and vasodilation (SOE=B).

In studies incorporating Tai Chi, blood pressure reductions have ranged from 3 mmHg to 32 mmHg systolic and from 2 mmHg to 18 mmHg diastolic. In one study of previously sedentary people ≥60 yr old, Tai Chi resulted in an average reduction of 7 mmHg systolic and 3 mmHg diastolic (SOE=B).

The polyphenols in dark chocolate reduce blood pressure and enhance insulin sensitivity. The presumptive mechanism is protection of the vascular endothelium by augmenting availability of nitrous oxide, thereby improving endothelium-dependent vasorelaxation (SOE=B). White chocolate contains no polyphenols; it is used as the control in these studies, and it has not been shown to reduce blood pressure.

The multicenter Dietary Approaches to Stop Hypertension (DASH) trial tested the effects of diet on blood pressure. Participants were assigned randomly to one of three groups: control (no change in diet), diet rich in fruits and vegetables, or combination diet rich in fruits and vegetables with low-fat dairy products and reduced saturated fat. In hypertensive participants, the combination diet reduced systolic blood pressure by 11.4 mmHg and diastolic by 5.5 mmHg. Blood pressure decreased in the setting of stable weight and sodium intake of approximately 3 g/day. Additional studies of DASH alone and combined with other lifestyle interventions have consistently confirmed its effectiveness (SOE=A).

Approximately 40% of people with hypertension are deficient in coenzyme Q_{10}. There is evidence that over 4–12 wk, coenzyme Q_{10} (at a dosage of 100–200 mg/d) lowers blood pressure in people with hypertension. Reductions of 6 mmHg to 19 mmHg systolic and of 2 mmHg to 16 mmHg diastolic were observed in four small, placebo-controlled trials. In four other studies comparing blood pressure before and after treatment with coenzyme Q_{10}, systolic blood pressure decreased by 12 mmHg to 21 mmHg, and diastolic pressure decreased by 9 mmHg to 15 mmHg. The presumed mechanism of action for coenzyme Q_{10}—preservation of nitric oxide in the endothelium—offers an approach to treatment of hypertension that is unique and distinct from pharmaceutic agents (SOE=B).

Additional nonpharmacologic strategies include eating a vegetarian diet; reducing alcohol and caffeine intake; increasing intake of fish oil, soy foods, and olive oil; increasing exercise; and in overweight persons, losing weight.

References

1. Anonymous. Resperate for hypertension. *Med Lett Drugs Ther*. 2007;49(1268):72.
2. Appel LJ, Moore TJ, Obarzanek E, et al. A clinical trial of the effects of dietary patterns on blood pressure. DASH Collaborative Research Group. *N Engl J Med*. 1997;336(16):1117–1124.
3. Nowson CA, Worsley A, Margerison C, et al. Blood pressure change with weight loss is affected by diet type in men. *Am J Clin Nutrition*. 2005;81(5):983–989.
4. Rosenfeldt F, Hilton D, Pepe S, et al. Systematic review of effect of coenzyme Q_{10} in physical exercise, hypertension and heart failure. *Biofactors*. 2003;18(1-4):91–100.
5. Wang C, Collet JP, Lau J. The effect of Tai Chi on health outcomes in patients with chronic conditions: a systematic review. *Arch Intern Med*. 2004;164(5):493–501.

42. Which of the following best characterizes memory loss in older adults?

(A) Older adults with self-reported memory loss are often depressed.
(B) Older adults with memory loss usually benefit from early neuropsychologic testing.
(C) Memory loss is easily detected in routine clinical practice.
(D) Older adults with self-reported memory loss can have normal cognitive function on neuropsychologic testing.

ANSWER: D

Memory loss in older adults is common but not readily recognized in the absence of screening. Older adults should routinely be screened for cognitive impairment (SOE=C).

Many older adults who self-report memory loss do well on routine memory tests and further neuropsychologic testing. However, neuropsychologic testing can identify a subgroup of these patients with measurable deficits sufficient for diagnosis of mild cognitive impairment (SOE=A). Neuropsychologic testing is not recommended for all adults with memory loss. It should be used selectively 1) for distinguishing among normal cognition in older adults, mild cognitive impairment, and early dementia; 2) for establishing a baseline in patients with mild cognitive impairment; 3) for differential diagnosis of dementia; and 4) as part of a comprehensive assessment that can contribute to management decisions and cognitive rehabilitation in mild cognitive impairment and dementia (SOE=B). Older adults with self-reported memory loss should be evaluated for depression, but most will have subjective memory loss findings only.

References

1. Chertkow H, Nasreddine Z, Joanette Y, et al. Mild cognitive impairment and cognitive impairment, no dementia: Part A, concept and diagnosis. *Alzheimer's Dementia: J Alzheimer's Assoc*. 2007;3(4):266–282.
2. Jacova C, Kertesz A, Blair M, et al. Neuropsychological testing and assessment for dementia. *Alzheimer's Dementia: J Alzheimer's Assoc*. 2007;3(4):299–317.

43. An 82-yr-old woman comes to the office because she is fatigued and worried that she is terminally ill. She is recently widowed and lives alone. History includes dyslipidemia, hypertension, and obesity; she has no psychiatric history. Medications are furosemide, simvastatin, propranolol, and aspirin. At her last visit 2 mo ago, she was concerned that she had cancer; extensive evaluation was negative. Since then, she has lost 6.8 kg (15 lb). Another set of tests are negative. She reluctantly agrees to try citalopram 40 mg, even though she insists that she is not depressed and is instead worried about her health. After 8 weeks, she is not sleeping, has lost an additional 8.2 kg (18 lb), and rarely leaves her house. She denies any desire to die—on the contrary, she fears death—yet, more and more often, she wishes for "this torture to be over."

Which of the following is the most appropriate next step?

(A) Add mirtazapine 15 mg at bedtime.
(B) Switch to another antidepressant.
(C) Increase citalopram to 60 mg.
(D) Admit to psychiatric inpatient unit for electroconvulsive therapy (ECT).
(E) Add risperidone 0.5 mg at bedtime.

ANSWER: D

This patient has major depressive disorder with psychotic features. In an 82-yr-old woman with weight loss and fatigue, a malignancy or other possible medical causes must be excluded. However, when the evaluation is negative and the patient is unable to be reassured by the evidence, the most likely diagnosis is major depressive disorder with psychosis. In older adults with major depressive disorder, the presentation of psychotic symptoms usually takes the form of somatic preoccupations. It is easy not to recognize the delusional nature of such beliefs and thereby to delay necessary treatment. Major depressive disorder is associated with high morbidity and mortality; the risks are higher when psychosis is also present, and beginning appropriate treatment without delay is of paramount importance.

ECT is the treatment of choice for major depressive disorder with psychosis in older adults, because its onset of action is faster and its effectiveness greater than that seen with pharmacologic therapy. Even though its exact mechanism of action is still unknown, ECT is safe and well tolerated in this population. The combination of antidepressant and antipsychotic medication instituted early and at an aggressive dosage can be effective for psychotic depression in older adults. ECT can be used in those patients who do not respond to medication. The main advantage of pharmacologic therapy is that it does not require hospitalization and is more acceptable to patients who might be resistant to the idea of ECT. Therefore, if started together with the citalopram (or any other second-generation antidepressant), risperidone (or any other second-generation antipsychotic) would have been an appropriate intervention for this patient. However, because her symptoms have worsened after several months, she exhibits substantial weight loss, and she is now highly dysfunctional and passively suicidal, further delay would pose an unacceptable risk for her. Even if the patient refuses ECT, hospitalization is advisable because of her severe weight loss and suicidal thoughts.

References
1. DeBattista C, Lembke A. Challenges in differentiating and diagnosing psychotic depression: phenomenology and the pursuit of optimal treatment. *Primary Psychiatry*. 2008;25(4):59–64.
2. Meyers BS, Flint AJ, Rothschild AJ, et al; STOP-PD Group. A double-blind randomized controlled trial of olanzapine plus sertraline versus olanzapine plus placebo for psychotic depression: the study of pharmacotherapy of psychotic depression (STOP-PD). *Arch Gen Psychiatry*. 2009;66(8):838–847.
3. Van der Wurff FB, Stek ML, Hoogendijk WJ, et al. The efficacy and safety of ECT in depressed older adults: a literature review. *Int J Geriatr Psychiatry*. 2003;18(10):894–904.

44. Which of the following is true regarding the role of language interpreters during clinical encounters?

(A) Interpretation by family members is optimal.
(B) Bilingual interpreter services should always be available at no cost to patients.
(C) Interpreters consistently transmit information accurately and in a culturally competent manner.
(D) Young children are effective interpreters for family members.

ANSWER: B

Effective communication between medical staff and patients depends enormously on language skills. This significantly affects access to care, adherence to treatment plans, and health outcomes. Patients with no or limited English proficiency are less likely to have a regular primary care physician; if they do have a regular physician, they are less likely to visit him or her. They are also less likely to receive appropriate preventive, dental, or ophthalmologic care, or timely physical examinations. Inability to overcome a language barrier contributes to medical error and neglect.

Federal law mandates that all healthcare organizations and providers who participate in federally funded programs such as Medicare and Medicaid provide linguistically accessible care through bilingual staff or interpreter services at all encounters, at no cost to patients. Professional interpreters can improve communication between medical staff and patients (SOE=A). They usually have knowledge of the medical terminology and the healthcare system, and because they do not know the patient personally, they are less likely to filter information or answer on behalf of the patient (SOE=A). However, interpreters are not always able to transmit crucial information accurately and in a culturally competent manner. The ability to speak a language does not imply knowledge about the culture in which that language is spoken or about the subculture of the patient. Interpreters may be able to translate information literally but may fail to recognize relevant cultural, social, or ethnic contexts.

Use of family members as interpreters seems less expensive and more convenient, and is often assumed to be preferred by patients. Family members often observe patients daily and can thereby notice significant changes in their conditions. The presence of a family member may encourage a patient to volunteer more information, or the family member may be able to expand on or clarify information. In contrast, family members may also answer questions without actually giving the patient an opportunity to answer, or they may unintentionally give inaccurate translations. They may also alter or withhold information between medical staff and the patient for personal reasons. The presence of a family member can also deter the patient from offering valuable information in order not to compromise his or her privacy. For these reasons, family members should not be used as the primary interpreters whenever possible.

It is not ethical to use children as interpreters because they are often not capable of translating technical medical terms, and because they may not be emotionally able to handle complex and sensitive medical issues. Children lack the vocabulary and the emotional maturity to serve as effective interpreters.

References

1. Barr DA, Wanat SF. Listening to patients: cultural and linguistic barriers to health care access. *Fam Med.* 2005;37(3):199–204.
2. Brach C, Fraser I, Paez K. Crossing the language chasm. *Health Aff.* 2005;24(2):424–434.
3. Flores G. Language barriers to health care in the United States. *N Engl J Med.* 2006;355(5):229–231.
4. Ngo-Metzger Q, Sorkin DH, Phillips RS, et al. Providing high-quality care for limited English proficient patients: the importance of language concordance and interpreter use. *J Gen Intern Med.* 2007;22(Suppl 2):324–330.

45. A 73-yr-old retired man is brought to the office by his daughter. Since his wife died 6 yr ago, he has lived alone in the suburban home that he has owned for 40 yr. The patient has been increasingly forgetful and has neglected his appearance and hygiene for 2 yr. There were no major changes in his physical health or social setting during this time. He shops every week and attends church when reminded. The daughter visits him most evenings, but she cannot take him into her home. Twice in the past 3 mo, he has required police assistance: the first time, for being lost while wandering on foot at night, and the second time because of a vehicular accident. He refuses to live in a nursing home. The patient's annual income from Social Security and pension is $23,000, and he has $70,000 in savings.

Medical and neurologic evaluations indicate probable Alzheimer's disease. His score is 20/30 on the Mini–Mental Status Examination.

Which of the following is the best option for his continuing care?

(A) Adult day healthcare on weekdays, with supervision by the family on nights and weekends
(B) Nursing-home placement
(C) Medicaid application to cover personal care services in the home
(D) Assisted-living in a secure dementia unit
(E) Referral to a home-health agency under Medicare Part A for dementia care

ANSWER: D

This patient has progressive dementia and is at risk of serious misadventures, injury, or death if he continues to live alone or drive. Because the daughter cannot live with the patient, assisted living in a secure unit is the best option. Many communities have a variety of facilities with locked or alarmed, staffed units designed for individuals with dementia. Although moderately expensive, assisted-living facilities are usually less costly and less restrictive than nursing homes. Between 60% and 70% of assisted-living residents have dementia.

Adult day healthcare is an excellent resource when the caregiver and patient share the same residence, because caregivers are present after hours for supervision. This arrangement would not work for this patient because he would be alone for much of each 24-hour period.

The patient opposes nursing home placement. In addition, it costs more than assisted living, and he does not require nursing home care because he is ambulatory and independent in ADLs, although he is becoming dependent in IADLs.

Medicaid application should be considered in the future. State Medicaid programs allow a small bank account and monthly income ranging from 100% to 200% of the federal poverty level, which is about $8,000 for a single individual for a year. This patient would have to spend down his assets, which would take more than a year given his savings, and he would have to make regular, substantial co-payments for personal care services to reach the Medicaid financial threshold. More importantly in this case, Medicaid personal care is intermittent, with a maximum of 8 or 10 hours per day in most cases, and safe supervision would require the presence of a family member in the home when the aides were not there.

Medicare Part A home health services can be initiated for dementia care if the patient's condition is unstable. These services are intermittent, typically at most a few hours per week, and require the regular presence of a family member or other caregiver in the home the rest of the time. This approach would not address the needs of this patient.

No matter which option is chosen, long-term care costs will become an issue for this patient. He is likely to live for at least 5 more years and will require increasing amounts of supportive care. Medicaid application should be initiated unless there is another source of funds that will pay for his long-term care.

References

1. Magsi H, Malloy T. Underrecognition of cognitive impairment in assistive living facilities. *J Am Geriatr Soc.* 2005;53(2):295–298.
2. Rosenblatt A, Samus QM, Steele CD, et al. The Maryland Assisted Living Study: prevalence, recognition, and treatment of dementia and other psychiatric disorders in the assisted living population of central Maryland. *J Am Geriatr Soc.* 2004;52(10):1618–1625.

46. A 68-yr-old resident of a nursing facility is admitted to the hospital because he has increasing pain and erythema related to a sacral pressure ulcer for which he had been receiving treatment. He has a history of stroke and right-sided hemiparesis.

On examination, vital signs are stable. There is a 3 cm × 6 cm midline sacral ulcer with a dry, black eschar covering the entire wound, surrounding warmth, and erythema. It is tender to touch, and when pressed, it exudes moderate amounts of pus.

Which of the following is the most appropriate treatment for the pressure ulcer?

(A) Hydrocolloid dressings applied every 3 to 5 days
(B) Sharp debridement of eschar
(C) Papain-urea cream applied to eschar twice daily
(D) Wet-to-dry dressings applied twice daily
(E) Hydrogel dressings applied twice daily

ANSWER: B

This patient has an unstageable pressure ulcer with a black eschar and signs of infection. He has no contraindications to local excision. The wound needs to be opened and cleansed to promote healing. The eschar requires sharp debridement with a scalpel, scissors, or forceps (SOE=C). Antibiotic therapy is required as well.

Hydrocolloid dressings are appropriate for stage II and III ulcers and provide a good environment for autolytic debridement but are contraindicated in infected ulcers (SOE=C). Papain-urea cream is a form of enzymatic debridement that dissolves devitalized tissue and is helpful with patients who cannot tolerate surgery or procedures (SOE=C), but it is also contraindicated in infected ulcers.

Wet-to-dry dressings promote mechanical debridement; they are inappropriate in the setting of an infected, unstageable ulcer. Wet-to-dry dressings can also cause damage to healing granulated tissue (SOE=B).

Hydrogel dressings are cross-linked polymer gels that are often shaped into sheets to provide and maintain a moist wound environment; they need to be combined with gauze dressings. They are appropriate for stage II, III, and IV ulcers (SOE=B). By increasing moisture content, hydrogel dressings help clean and debride necrotic tissue. They may be appropriate for treatment of this patient's ulcer, but only after the eschar has been removed, the wound cleansed, and the stage of the ulcer identified.

References

1. Bass MJ, Phillips LG. Pressure sores. *Curr Probl Surg*. 2007;44(2):101–143.
2. Bergstrom N, Bennett A, Carlson CE, et al. *Pressure Ulcer Treatment*. Clinical Practice Guideline. AHCPR Pub No 95-0653. Rockville, MD: U.S. Department of Health and Human Services, Public Health Service, Agency for Health Care Policy and Research; 1994.
3. Heyneman A, Beele H, Vanderwee K, et al. A systematic review of the use of hydrocolloids in the treatment of pressure ulcers. *J Clin Nurs*. 2008;17(9):1164–1173.
4. Langemo D, Cuddigan J, Baharestani M, et al. Pressure ulcer guidelines: "minding the gaps" when developing new guidelines. *Adv Skin Wound Care*. 2008;21(5):213–217.

47. A 79-yr-old man is brought to the office by his daughter; both are concerned about his recent deterioration and want to know his prognosis. The patient has hypertension, peripheral vascular disease, and stage IV colon cancer. Poorly differentiated adenocarcinoma of the colon, metastatic to liver and peritoneum, was diagnosed 2 yr ago. He did well after surgical resection of his tumor and treatment with bevacizumab. However, now there is increased involvement of his liver and peritoneum along with new pulmonary nodules. He has constant abdominal pain that is well controlled with a fentanyl patch and oxycodone as needed for breakthrough pain. He has become increasingly debilitated over the last 6 mo. Because of fatigue and pain, he is unable to do most IADLs, and in the last 4 wk he has become dependent in all ADLs except feeding.

Which of the following patient characteristics is most predictive of a poor prognosis?

(A) Low performance status
(B) Advanced tumor stage
(C) Multiple comorbidities
(D) Advanced age
(E) Opioid use

ANSWER: A

Performance status is the best predictor of prognosis in patients with advanced cancer (SOE=A). It is a global measure of a patient's functional capacity, or ability to maintain independence in daily life. A number of different tools are available to assess performance status, including the Karnofsky Performance Score and the Palliative Performance Scale, Version 2.

In some studies, tumor stage, comorbidity, advanced age, and opioid dependence have been shown to influence prognosis, but the findings are not consistent. These factors are usually most prognostic in less advanced disease.

References

1. Barbot A, Mussault P, Ingrand P, et al. Assessing 2-month clinical prognosis in hospitalized patients with advanced solid tumors. *J Clin Onc*. 2007;26(15):2538–2543.
2. Lamont EB, Christakis NA. Complexities in prognostication in advanced cancer. *JAMA*. 2003;290(1):98–104.
3. Maltonii M, Caraceni A, Brunelli C, et al. Prognostic factors in advanced cancer patients: evidence-based clinical recommendations—a study by the steering committee of the European Association for Palliative Care. *J Clin Onc*. 2005;23(25):6240–6248.

48. An 83-yr-old otherwise healthy woman is brought to the office by her daughter because the mother has become confused and forgetful since beginning treatment with extended-release oxybutynin 10 mg for urge urinary incontinence 6 mo ago. The incontinence has improved, yet the daughter is unwilling to continue the oxybutynin because of the increased confusion. The mother, when asked, has no new complaints about memory or cognition.

Which of the following is the most appropriate next step?

(A) Discontinue extended-release oxybutynin 10 mg; begin immediate-release oxybutynin 2.5 mg q6h.
(B) Begin memantine, titrating over 3 wk from starting dose of 5 mg/d to 20 mg/d.
(C) Begin donepezil 5 mg/d, titrating to 10 mg/d if needed.
(D) Reassure the daughter that the medication is unlikely to produce cognitive adverse events.
(E) Discontinue extended-release oxybutynin 10 mg; implement behavioral therapy for incontinence.

ANSWER: E

While most patients receiving anticholinergic bladder-relaxant therapy have no discernable cognitive decline, some will have cognitive adverse events (SOE=C). Because the symptoms may be an adverse event of medication, the agent should be discontinued (SOE=C). Adding memantine or donepezil would not be appropriate because cholinesterase inhibitors can worsen symptoms of overactive bladder in some patients.

Cognitive adverse events of oxybutynin are related to peak medication concentration (SOE=A). Immediate-release medication with the same total dosage could potentially worsen this effect.

Behavioral therapy is an effective therapy for urge incontinence (SOE=A). If this patient is not cognitively intact enough to fully participate in behavioral therapy, she might benefit from the use of toileting assistance protocols such as prompted voiding (SOE=A).

References

1. Lackner TE, Wyman JF, McCarthy TC, et al. Randomized, placebo-controlled trial of the cognitive effect, safety, and tolerability of oral extended-release oxybutynin in cognitively impaired nursing home residents with urge urinary incontinence. *J Am Geriatr Soc.* 2008;56(5):862–870.
2. Ouslander JG. Management of overactive bladder. *N Engl J Med.* 2004;350(8):786–799.
3. Scheife R, Takeda M. Central nervous system safety of anticholinergic drugs for the treatment of overactive bladder in the elderly. *Clin Ther.* 2005;27(2):144–153.

49. A 92-yr-old man who resides in an assisted-living facility has increasing shortness of breath with activity and increasing frequency of chest pain. The chest pain responds promptly to sublingual nitroglycerin. He walks daily, reads, and plays the piano. History includes severe aortic valve stenosis with preserved ejection fraction confirmed by echocardiography, paroxysmal atrial fibrillation accompanied by shortness of breath, hypertension, dyslipidemia, osteoarthritis, lumbar spine disease, gastroesophageal reflux, benign prostatic hyperplasia, and depression. Medications include furosemide, losartin, warfarin, atorvasatin, mirtazepine, tamulosin, finasteride, acetaminophen, calcium, and vitamin D.

On examination, the patient is pale and appears younger than his stated age. Weight is 84 kg (185 lb), blood pressure is 120/70 mmHg, heart rate is 76 beats per minute and regular. There is a 3/6 harsh late-peaking systolic murmur audible at the apex and left sternal edge. There are no bruits, and his lungs are clear. His score on the Mini–Mental State Exam is 29/30. The Charlson Comorbidity Index = 6.

Laboratory results:

Creatinine	1.1 mg/dL with an estimated GFR >60 mL/min
Electrolytes	normal
CBC	normal

Which of the following is the best diagnostic test to further evaluate this patient's cardiac status?

(A) Transthoracic echocardiogram
(B) Treadmill stress test
(C) Coronary angiography
(D) Persantine thallium stress test
(E) Cardiac MRI

ANSWER: C

This patient with previously diagnosed aortic stenosis presents with worsening symptoms. The only definitive therapy is valve replacement, and the information needed to guide the procedural approach is the presence or absence of concomitant coronary artery disease or mitral valve disease. The gold standard for acquiring information on coronary artery anatomy is coronary angiography (SOE=A).

Echocardiography has been performed in this patient and suggests severe aortic stenosis. Repeat transthoracic echocardiography is unlikely to contribute additional information to guide therapy because it is not highly accurate in precisely quantifying the degree of aortic stenosis, which depends on both the gradient across the valve and the flow, and because it cannot define the coronary anatomy (SOE=B). MRI can provide anatomic information on the valves and function, and limited information on very proximal coronary anatomy. However, it is expensive and does not fully delineate the coronary artery anatomy in most, if not all, cases. Both treadmill stress tests and dobutamine echocardiograms are used to determine the likelihood and area of coronary artery disease but do not define the anatomy. There tests are accompanied by increases in blood pressure and heart rate that can precipitate symptoms and heart failure. These symptoms can be catastrophic in patients with aortic stenosis, because cardiopulmonary resuscitation is unlikely to be successful in severe aortic stenosis. External cardiac compression cannot generate the very high ventricular pressures necessary to open the stenotic aortic valve. Persantine thallium testing and imaging can provide only the likelihood and area of coronary artery disease. It also carries increased risk in patients with aortic stenosis. This is due to their limited ability to further increase contractility, as well as the decrease in diastolic filling and wall tension development that accompanies reflex tachycardia precipitated by the persantine-induced drop in blood pressure. CT with calcium scoring was not offered as a choice. However, it is not very specific in older adults: vascular calcifications are common but do not correlate with the presence or absence of obstructive coronary artery disease and cannot define the coronary anatomy (SOE=D).

References

1. Rosengart, TK, Fedman T, Borger MA, et al. Percutaneous and minimally invasive valve proce- dures: a scientific statement from the American Heart Association Council on Cardiovascular Surgery and Anesthesia, Council on Clinical Cardiology, Functional Genomics and Translational Biology Interdisciplinary Working Group, and Quality of Care and Outcomes Research Interdisciplinary Working Group. *Circu- lation*. 2008;117(13):1750–1767.

2. Fisoufi F, Rahmanian PB, Castillo JG, et al. Excellent early and late outcomes of aortic valve replacement in people aged 80 and older. *J Am Geriatr Soc.* 2008;56(2):255–262.

3. The Auscultation Assistant. http://www.med.ucla.edu/ wilkes/inex.htm (accessed Nov 2009).

50. A 74-yr-old woman lives by herself in an apartment building for older adults. She has poor vision and urinary incontinence. She walks with a cane, and has fallen 3 times in the past year. She has not seen a physician in the past 6 mo, other than a visit to the emergency department after a fall. History includes hypertension, painful osteoarthritis, stroke, and frequent urinary tract infections. She takes 10 prescription medications.

Which of the following is most likely to increase this patient's life expectancy and reduce her functional impairment?

(A) Protocol-based reduction in medications
(B) Neuropsychiatric testing
(C) In-home assessment with multiple home visits
(D) Multimodality pain management
(E) Physical therapy

ANSWER: C

Comprehensive in-home geriatric assessment with multiple home visits (≥9) reduces mortality in young-old adults (ie, 65–74 yr old) who are at risk, improves functional outcome, and can reduce long-term use of nursing facilities (SOE=A). In addition, comprehensive in-home geriatric assessment for high-risk patients is associated both with improved clinical measures and with reduced emergency department and hospital use over 2 yr.

Medication reduction is a generally sound strategy in older adults, when it can be accom- plished without destabilizing serious medical conditions, but it has not been shown to affect mortality or functional outcomes. Neuropsychiatric testing is more reliable than an in-office screen for diagnosing dementia. Because this patient has no record of cognitive impairment, she should be screened using an in-office screen before referral for neuropsychiatric testing. In addition, there is no evidence that diagnosis and treatment of dementia affect mortality or ADLs.

Pain management using multiple modalities often improves symptom control in patients with chronic pain, but it has not been shown to have an impact on mortality.

As part of a multifaceted intervention, physical therapy reduces the incidence of falls and is cost-effective in high-risk patients, mostly by preventing fractures. However, physical therapy has not been shown to affect mortality.

References

1. Counsell SR, Callahan CM, Clark DO, et al. Geriatric care management for low-income seniors: a randomized controlled trial. *JAMA*. 2007;298(22):2623–2633.
2. Gitlin LN, Winter L, Dennis MP, et al. A randomized trial of a multicomponent home intervention to reduce functional difficulties in older adults. *J Am Geriatr Soc*. 2006;54(5):809–816.
3. Huss A, Stuck AE, Rubenstein LZ, et al. Multidimensional preventive home visit programs for community-dwelling older adults: a systematic review and meta-analysis of randomized controlled trials. *J Gerontol A Biol Sci Med Sci*. 2008;63(3):298–307.
4. Stuck AE, Egger M, Hammer A, et al. Home visits to prevent nursing home admission and functional decline in elderly people: systematic review and meta-regression analysis. *JAMA*. 2002;287(8):1022–1028.

51. An 82-yr-old woman is discharged to home after a 2-wk hospital stay for pneumonia. The hospitalization was complicated by atrial fibrillation with a rapid ventricular response, delirium, and development of a 4-cm, stage IV sacral pressure ulcer. The patient lives with her daughter and adult granddaughter. She has been admitted to home health care under Medicare Part A and is receiving skilled nursing and physical therapy. The hospital physician recommended twice-daily wound care; the family wants the agency to provide this care, because they are unwilling to do it themselves. According to the agency, twice-daily nursing visits are not feasible under Prospective Payment and are not needed. The agency suggests that a specialty low-air-loss mattress be ordered under Medicare Part B, that the wound care regimen be revised so that dressings can be changed every 1 or 2 days, and that the agency teach the family how to perform wound care, with regular nursing visits for dressing changes and wound assessment.

Which of the following would be the best response to the agency's request?

(A) The Medicare home health agency is required to provide twice-daily dressing changes when ordered by a physician.
(B) Medicare will not cover the specialty mattress for this patient.
(C) Prospective Payment categories are adjusted to patient need, including twice-daily care.
(D) The agency plan is reasonable and appropriate.
(E) Families should not be required to provide care.

ANSWER: D

Since 2000, Medicare Part A home health agencies have been paid prospectively for 60-day episodes of care. Care must be medically reasonable and necessary, ordered by a physician, intermittent, and safe to provide in the home. Payments are based on 80 categories (Home Health Resource Groups or HHRGs) that are defined by the patient's characteristics.

Because Prospective Payment places agencies at financial risk, agencies are permitted to manage the case using recognized care processes that are expected to obtain the specified outcomes. Typically, twice-daily visits for wound care over an extended period are neither needed in a wound of this type, nor financially sustainable: HHRGs are not adjusted to include these visits. If the agency and physician cannot agree on this issue, the agency may have to withdraw from the case.

The agency's proposed care plan is reasonable because most wounds of this type can be managed with wound care every 1 or 2 days using hydrocolloid, hydrogel, foam, or alginate dressings with or without enzymatic debriding agents.

Pressure-relieving mattresses are covered by Medicare Part B when there is a large stage III or IV wound on the trunk or torso; they can be an important part of the care plan.

Families bear a great deal of the burden in home care. Medicare payment policy clearly indicates that agencies should teach patients and families to assume responsibility for their own care, rather than rely on agency staff for providing all aspects of care.

Reference

1. Home Health Agency Center. Centers for Medicare and Medicaid Services. United States Department of Health and Human Services. http://www.cms.hhs.gov/center/hha.asp (accessed Nov 2009).

52. A 72-yr-old man comes to the office for evaluation because he has impaired fasting glucose levels. Fasting levels were between 110 and 120 mg/dL on 3 occasions. He has well-controlled hypertension. His body mass index is 29.5 kg/m².

Which of the following is most likely to prevent development of type 2 diabetes mellitus in this patient?

(A) Reduce caloric intake and increase physical activity to 150 min/week.
(B) Increase physical activity and begin metformin.
(C) Begin metformin.
(D) Reduce caloric intake.

ANSWER: A

The landmark trial from the Diabetes Prevention Program Research Group evaluated patients at risk of new-onset diabetes who were randomly assigned to 1) lifestyle intervention (goal of 7% weight loss through reducing caloric intake and increasing physical activity by 150 min/wk), 2) educational materials plus metformin 850 mg q12h, or 3) educational materials only (control). Participants were overweight and had both fasting and post-load hyperglycemia at levels not yet diagnostic of diabetes. Lifestyle intervention was the most effective approach to diabetes prevention: the incidence of diabetes in this group was reduced by >50% versus in patients who received only educational materials. The incidence of diabetes was also reduced in the group that received metformin plus educational materials versus in patients who received only educational materials, but to a lesser extent (by 25%). Intensive lifestyle intervention worked especially well for older participants. Metformin was most effective in participants with a lower body mass index and in participants with lower fasting glucose concentrations (SOE=A).

References

1. American Diabetes Association. Standards of medical care in diabetes—2008. *Diabetes Care*. 2008;31(Suppl 1):S1–11.
2. Chang AM, Halter JB. Diabetes mellitus. In: Halter JB, Hazzard WR, Ouslander JG, et al. *Hazzard's Geriatric Medicine and Gerontology*, 6th ed. NY: McGraw-Hill; 2009:1305–1324.
3. Knowler WC, Barrett-Conner E, Fowler SE, et al. Reduction in the incidence of type 2 diabetes with lifestyle intervention or metformin. *N Engl J Med*. 2002;346(6):393–403.

53. A 72-yr-old man with poorly controlled diabetes mellitus complicated by renal disease presents for transfer of care. His feet are now numb, but in the past he experienced a burning sensation.

Which examination or test is the best test to determine loss of protective sensation?

(A) 5.07 (10 gm) Semmes-Weinstein monofilament
(B) Electromyography
(C) Sharp/dull discrimination
(D) Reflex hammer
(E) Vibration sense with 128 mH

ANSWER: A

Extensive literature has been published that supports the use of the 5.07 Semmes-Weinstein monofilament for determining loss of protective sensation in diabetic patients (SOE=A). This testing is required by Medicare for reimbursement for diabetic foot care and diabetic shoes. Although sharp/dull and vibration testing are routinely performed, their reliability or predictive validity has not been confirmed. EMG testing can determine neuropathy when the neurologic lesion is proximal to the foot, but it does not perform well in patients with neuropathy in a stocking distribution. Deep tendon reflexes can assist in identifying lesions proximal to the foot and thus are not helpful in the diagnosis of diabetic peripheral neuropathy.

References

1. Screening techniques to identify people at high risk for diabetic foot ulceration: a prospective multicenter trial. *Diabetes Care*. 2000;23(5):606–611.
2. Torkington R, Van Ross ER, Whalley AM, et al. The North-West Diabetes Foot Care Study: incidence of, and risk factors for, new diabetic foot ulceration in a community-based patient cohort. *Diabet Med*. 2002;19(5):377–384.

54. A 65-yr-old woman comes to the office because over the last 5 mo she has had increasing difficulty both falling and staying asleep. Over the past year, she has also noted an uncomfortable sensation in both legs that is relieved in part with moving or rubbing her legs. The sensation usually occurs in early evening, but during the past month the sensation has become so severe that on most nights she does not fall asleep until 2 AM. Her husband has moved to another bed because her leg kicks and occasional arm movements disturb his sleep. She is so tired that she has stopped volunteering at the local library. History includes intermittent insomnia (primarily difficulty falling asleep) for about 5 yr. Treatment with sertraline was started 4 wk ago.

Which of the following is the most likely cause of this patient's sleeplessness?

(A)   Primary insomnia
(B)   Major depressive disorder
(C)   Anxiety disorder
(D)   Restless legs syndrome (RLS)
(E)   Delayed sleep phase disorder

ANSWER: D

This patient most likely has RLS exacerbated by sertraline. Diagnosis of RLS is based on the clinical history (uncomfortable sensations in the legs that are most prominent when at rest and relieved by leg movement) and on its circadian pattern (worse in the evening, and decreasing in the morning and during the day) (SOE=A). The prevalence of RLS is about 10% in most population-based surveys. It increases with age and is more common among women than men.

The patient's symptoms are more consistent with a diagnosis of RLS than of primary insomnia. Major depressive disorder is common in patients with RLS and insomnia. Although major depressive disorder and anxiety should be considered in all patients with insomnia and RLS (SOE=C), these disorders would not be the primary cause of the sensory symptoms described. SSRIs increase RLS symptoms (SOE=B); this patient's worsening symptoms were likely related to treatment with sertraline. Venlafaxine also worsens restless legs symptoms, and both fluoxetine and venlafaxine increase the number of periodic leg movements in sleep (SOE=B). Bupropion has not been shown to exacerbate symptoms of RLS or increase periodic leg movements in sleep; results from small case

studies indicate a potential benefit of bupropion for patients with RLS (SOE=B).

Delayed sleep phase disorder represents an alteration in the sleep/wake cycle in which the time of sleep onset is displaced from evening to morning time. It is associated with daytime fatigue but not difficulty staying asleep.

References

1. Allen RP, Picchietti D, Hening WA, et al. Restless Legs Syndrome Diagnosis and Epidemiology workshop at the National Institutes of Health; International Restless Legs Syndrome Study Group. Restless legs syndrome: diagnostic criteria, special considerations, and epidemiology. A report from the restless legs syndrome diagnosis and epidemiology workshop at the National Institutes of Health. *Sleep Med.* 2003;4(2):101–119.
2. Allen RP, Walters AS, Montplaisir J, et al. Restless legs syndrome prevalence and impact: REST general population study. *Arch Intern Med.* 2005;165(11):1286–1292.
3. Bassetti CL, Kretzschmar U, Werth E, et al. Restless legs and restless legs-like syndrome. *Sleep Med.* 2006;7(6):534.
4. Kim SW, Shin IS, Kim JM, et al. Bupropion may improve restless legs syndrome: a report of three cases. *Clin Neuropharmacol.* 2005;28(6):298–301.

55. Which of the following is the most likely outcome of progressive resistance strength training in geriatric rehabilitation?

(A)   Minimal gains for patients ≥85 yr old
(B)   Significant gains in health-related quality of life
(C)   Significant decline in physical disability
(D)   Significant gains in strength

ANSWER: D

Muscle weakness is common among older adults and is associated with physical disability and increased risk of falls. Progressive resistance strength training (PRT) is designed to increase strength in older adults through exercises that are performed against a specific external force that is regularly increased during training. This intervention is commonly used by physical therapists during rehabilitation for stroke and hip fracture.

In almost 70 trials with almost 4,000 subjects, PRT had a large positive effect on strength (SOE=A). Some measures of functional limitation, such as gait, showed modest improvement. However, measures of health-related quality of life and activity showed no effect of PRT on physical disability (SOE=A).

In a study of in-home PRT after hip fracture, patients in the intervention group showed more improvement in physical function and ADLs than patients performing only low-impact home exercises (SOE=B).

The patient's underlying functional status is a better determinant of outcome than age. A classic study of nursing home residents ≥90 yr old, as well as more recent studies of frail patients 70–89 yr old, showed benefits from a structured physical activity program (SOE=A). Extremely disabled patients may not benefit from these exercises, and very healthy persons may not need them. But patients in the middle, especially those with deconditioning, are likely to benefit. The risk of injury is low, such that drop outs are not significant (SOE=A).

References

1. Binder EF, Brown M, Sinacore DR, et al. Effects of extended outpatient rehabilitation after hip fracture. A randomized controlled trial. *JAMA*. 2004;292(7):837–846.
2. Fiatarone MA, Marks EC, Ryan ND, et al. High-intensity strength training in nonagenarians. Effects on skeletal muscle. *JAMA*. 1990;263(22):3029–3034.
3. Latham N, Anderson C, Bennett D et al. Progressive resistance strength training for physical disability in older people. *Cochrane Database Syst Rev*. 2003;(2):CD002759.
4. The LIFE Study Investigators. Effects of a physical activity intervention on measures of physical performance: results of the Lifestyle Interventions and Independence for Elders Pilot (LIFE-P) Study. *J Gerontol A Biol Sci Med Sci*. 2006;61A(11):1157–1165.

56. A 78-yr-old woman comes to the office because she has symptoms of mixed stress and urge urinary incontinence. She is most bothered by the urge incontinence. She is generally healthy and cognitively intact, and she does not drink caffeinated beverages or take diuretics. The patient is interested in a nonpharmacologic intervention and will not consider surgery at this point.

On physical examination, there is no evidence of uterine prolapse, cystocele, rectocele, or fecal impaction.

Which of the following is true about behavioral therapy combining urge suppression strategies with exercises to strengthen pelvic floor muscles?

(A) Improvement in symptoms correlates directly with gains in pelvic floor muscle strength.
(B) Most patients are more satisfied with drug treatment because it is easier.
(C) Drug therapy more effectively reduces the number of episodes of incontinence.
(D) Behavioral therapies are more effective in younger than in older adults.
(E) Behavioral therapy combined with antimuscarinic drug therapy is often more effective than either intervention alone.

ANSWER: E

The combination of behavioral and drug treatments results in greater improvement than either therapy alone in many patients with urge incontinence (SOE=B).

In head-to-head trials for urge-predominant urinary incontinence, behavioral treatment is associated with high rates of satisfaction, and its effectiveness is equal to or statistically better than that of treatment with bladder-relaxant agents (SOE=A).

Several studies have shown that good results with behavioral therapy are possible in older adults (SOE=A). In behavioral treatment trials that include exercises for pelvic floor muscle, gains in muscle strength have not correlated directly with improvement in symptoms (SOE=A).

References

1. Burgio KL, Kraus SR, Menefee S, et al. Behavioral therapy to enable women with urge incontinence to discontinue drug treatment. *Ann Intern Med*. 2008;149(3):161–169.
2. Burgio KL, Locher JL, Goode PS. Combined behavioral and drug therapy for urge incontinence in older women. *J Am Geriatr Soc*. 2000;48(4):370–374.
3. Goode PS, Burgio KL, Locher JL, et al. Urodynamic changes associated with behavioral and drug treatment of urge incontinence in older women. *J Am Geriatr Soc*. 2002;50(5):808–816.

57. A 75-yr-old man with hypertension that is not well controlled on hydrochlorothiazide at 25 mg/d and lisinopril at 40 mg/d comes to the office to discuss changes in his diet that would help lower his blood pressure. A 24-hour diet recall shows that he had turkey sausage and toast for breakfast, a tuna sandwich with apple wedges for lunch, and grilled fish and vegetables for dinner. He snacks on 2 or 3 bananas a day and has several glasses of nonfat milk daily in addition to 2 glasses of wine.

In addition to adjusting his medication and reducing alcohol intake, which of the following dietary changes would help lower his blood pressure?

(A) Increased intake of lowfat milk
(B) Decreased intake of bananas
(C) Decreased intake of turkey sausage
(D) Increased intake of flax seed
(E) No diet modification necessary

ANSWER: C

In advising patients with hypertension, adequate time should be spent reviewing salt intake. Reducing salt in diet can decrease systolic blood pressure by 2–8 mmHg; although the reduction is small, it has a beneficial effect on outcome (SOE=A). Patients often assume that a heart-healthy diet means avoiding fats and cholesterol (such as replacing fatty meats with chicken or turkey). Management of hypertension should emphasize limiting salt intake, through helping the patient identify hidden sources of sodium and teaching the patient how to read food labels.

There is no evidence that increasing intake of low-fat milk or flax seed, or decreasing intake of bananas will improve his blood pressure control.

Reference

1. Sacks FM, Svetkey LP, Vollmer WM, et al. DASH–Sodium Collaborative Research Group. Effects on blood pressure of reduced dietary sodium and the Dietary Approaches to Stop Hypertension (DASH) diet. DASH–Sodium Collaborative Research Group. *N Engl J Med.* 2001;344(1):3–10.

58. An 81-yr-old man comes to the office for follow-up after myocardial infarction 5 wk earlier. He has not needed nitroglycerin for angina since 4 days after the infarct. He would like to resume sexual relations with the woman he has dated since his wife died 2 yr ago. In the past year, before the infarct, he was able to maintain an erection sufficient for intercourse about half of the time. He is anxious because he is now unable to achieve erections sufficient for intercourse. History includes well-controlled hypertension with left ventricular hypertrophy, and transurethral resection of the prostate 15 yr ago for benign prostatic hyperplasia. Medications include atenolol 50 mg/d, simvastatin 40 mg/d, aspirin 81 mg/d, and nitroglycerin as needed.

On examination, peripheral pulses are diminished. His score on the Geriatric Depression Scale is 3, and he denies symptoms of depression.

Which of the following is the most appropriate next step in assessing this patient?

(A) Refer to cardiologist.
(B) Measure serum testosterone and bioavailable testosterone.
(C) Measure nocturnal penile tumescence.
(D) Refer to psychiatrist.

ANSWER: A

The probability of erectile dysfunction increases from 40% to 70% between ages 40 and 70. Dyslipidemia, hypertension, coronary artery disease, neurologic disorders (eg, stroke), use of certain medications, psychologic factors (eg, fear of failure, anxiety, unresolved grief, depression), hormonal changes, and hypogonadism can all be associated with erectile dysfunction. This patient has coronary artery disease as well as evidence of peripheral vascular disease, and thus has a significant vascular component to his erectile dysfunction. Consensus guidelines (SOE=C) have been developed for men with coronary artery disease to assess risk of sexual intercourse. Patients at low risk have asymptomatic coronary artery disease and no more than 2 of the following: controlled hypertension, mild stable angina, successful revascularization, previous uncomplicated revascularization, mild valvular disease, and heart failure with left ventricular dysfunction. This patient has more than 2 of the criteria. He is at intermediate risk and should be evaluated by a cardiologist. An exercise stress test should be ordered, because intercourse requires the ability to perform moderate metabolic equivalents of activity. Results of the test can also be used to evaluate whether the patient would benefit from treatment with phosphodiesterase inhibitors.

Generally, testosterone and bioavailable testosterone levels would not be measured immediately, unless libido is low, there is other evidence of hypogonadism, or the patient does not respond to treatment for erectile dysfunction (SOE=B). While hypogonadism increases in prevalence with age, this patient's erectile dysfunction is most likely related to vascular disease, which is the most common cause of erectile dysfunction (SOE=B).

The patient's score on the Geriatric Depression Scale does not increase his likelihood of having major depressive disorder and he denies depressive symptoms. Because he had erections before the infarct, it is unlikely that unresolved grief related to being widowed is the cause of his erectile dysfunction. Sudden death due to intercourse is rare, and results of a stress test should reassure him. Thus, psychiatric evaluation is not warranted.

References

1. Association of Clinical Endocrinologists medical guidelines for clinical practice for the evaluation and treatment of male sexual dysfunction: a couple's problem—2003 update. *Endocr Pract.* 2003;9(1):77–95.
2. Jackson G, Rosen RC, Kloner RA, et al. The second Princeton consensus on sexual dysfunction and cardiac risk: new guidelines for sexual medicine. *J Sex Med.* 2006;3(1):28–36.
3. McVary K. Clinical practice. Erectile dysfunction. *N Engl J Med.* 2007;357(24):2472–2481.
4. Seftel AD. From aspiration to achievement: assessment and noninvasive treatment for erectile dysfunction in aging men. *J Am Geriatr Soc.* 2005;53(1):119–130.

59. A 76-yr-old man is brought to the office by his older sister to establish care. His doctor recently retired, and his sister has brought his medical records, which are complete and include recent laboratory and progress notes. The patient has significant autism. He lives with his sister, who reports that over the past 3 mo he has been rocking, pacing, and yelling more often, and has hit himself twice. The behaviors have slowly increased in frequency and intensity to a degree that she has not seen for several years. His sleep is disrupted and he often paces during the night. His sister is his guardian; she reports that his care is increasingly difficult for her. She recently moved them from their family home to an apartment, and they are getting out less frequently for walks and shopping. He has no history of significant illnesses and is on no routine medications.

On examination, the patient is slightly underweight. He rocks and hums nearly constantly during the office visit. His skin is intact, and there are no bruises. The examination is essentially normal other than his repetitive behaviors.

Which of the following is the most appropriate initial step in managing the patient's behaviors?

(A) Begin quetiapine 25 mg.
(B) Begin zolpidem 5 mg at bedtime.
(C) Begin mirtazapine 15 mg.
(D) Reevaluate in 2 wk if the behavior persists.
(E) Begin methylphenidate 5 mg.

ANSWER: C

Adults with autism or autism-spectrum disorders characteristically have diminished social interaction; diminished expressive communication; repetitive and obsessive, ritualistic, or compulsive behaviors; a narrow range of interests or activities; and intolerance to change of routine or circumstances. Despite their diminished expressive ability, adults with autism can have good receptive ability and perception of the environment. Anxiety in response to change is common and can cause increased repetitive or stereotypic behaviors. Self-injurious behaviors, ranging from mild scratching to severe, potentially life-threatening injury, can begin or increase. A significant amount of clinical experience supports off-label use of second-generation antidepressants to decrease the intensity and frequency of self-injury (SOE=D).

This patient's changes in residence and familiar activities are the likely causes of his increased anxiety. The best choice among the options in this case would be to initiate a second-generation antidepressant at an appropriate dosage and carefully monitor the results.

Off-label use of the agents naltrexone and risperidone has been investigated for challenging behaviors in adults with autism, and risperidone has been approved for use in children with autism. In the choice between a relatively safe, well-studied, second-generation antidepressant, such as mirtazapine, with anxiolytic effects and a second-generation antipsychotic agent, such as quetiapine, the antidepressant offers better risk/benefit potential. If the patient's behaviors were markedly more dangerous to himself or to others, urgency may make the antipsychotic agent the wiser option.

A sedative is unlikely to produce much benefit in this case. The patient's sleep is probably disturbed by anxiety related to changes or frustrated compulsive needs. It is better to treat the anxiety that causes the behavior than to sedate an older patient.

Waiting to reevaluate the patient while someone is at risk of injury is not a good option. Although some challenging behaviors resolve with time or change in the environment, both the patient and his sister are currently at risk.

Because this patient has no evidence of attention deficit/hyperactivity disorder, methylphenidate is not an appropriate option.

Finally, the healthcare provider should ask the patient's sister about the extent of formal and informal social support available.

References

1. Aman MG. Management of hyperactivity and other acting-out problems in patients with autism spectrum disorder. *Sem Pediatr Neurol.* 2004;11(3):225–228.
2. Posey DJ, McDougle CJ. Pharmacotherapeutic management of autism. *Expert Opin Pharmacother.* 2001;2(4):587–600.
3. Rooker GW, Roscoe EM. Functional analysis of self-injurious behavior and its relation to self-restraint. *J Appl Behav Anal.* 2005;38(4):537–542.
4. Symons FJ, Thompson A, Rodriguez MC. Self-injurious behavior and the efficacy of naltrexone treatment: a quantitative synthesis. *Ment Retard Dev Disabil Res Rev.* 2004;10(3):193–200.
5. http://www.ninds.nih.gov/disorders/autism/detail_autism.htm (accessed Nov 2009).

60. A 91-yr-old resident of a nursing facility is hospitalized after he falls in his bathroom. On return to the nursing facility, he has a 4 cm × 4 cm stage III pressure ulcer on his left heel with minimal slough and exudates.

Which of the following is the best method for cleansing the wound bed of the pressure ulcer?

(A) Isotonic saline
(B) Hydrogen peroxide
(C) Povidone-iodine
(D) Acetic acid
(E) Whirlpool therapy

ANSWER: A

Ulcers are typically colonized with a mixture of bacterial flora that can lead to cellulitis, osteomyelitis, or sepsis if not adequately treated. Wounds need regular cleansing of exudates, debris, and contaminants, as well as debridement of necrotic tissue to enhance healing (SOE=C). Normal saline irrigation is standard for wound cleansing (SOE=C). Although new commercial products and cleansers show some promise in accelerating wound healing, there is no strong evidence to overturn the accepted practice of saline irrigation. Tap water is as effective as saline solutions in wound healing (SOE=B), if the water source is reliably clean.

Wound antiseptic agents (eg, hydrogen peroxide, hypochlorite solution, acetic acid, chlorhexamide, povidone-iodine, and cetrimide) have antibacterial properties but are toxic to healthy granulation tissue and should be avoided in daily care of pressure ulcers (SOE=C).

According to a recent Cochrane review, the only study that showed improved healing of pressure ulcers with whirlpool therapy had methodologic flaws, yielding no statistically significant findings when compared with usual care (SOE=B).

References

1. Bergstrom N, Bennett MA, Carlson CE, et al. *Treatment of Pressure Ulcers.* Clinical Practice Guideline, No. 15. AHCPR Pub No 95–0652. Rockville, MD: Agency for Health Care Policy and Research, U.S. Department of Health and Human Services; 1994.
2. Moore ZE, Cowman S. Wound cleansing for pressure ulcers. *Cochrane Database Syst Rev.* 2005;(4):CD004983.
3. Whitney J, Phillips L, Aslam R, et al. Guidelines for the treatment of pressure ulcers. *Wound Repair Regen.* 2006;14(6):663–679.

61. A 73-yr-old man comes to the office 3 mo after being started on tolterodine for symptoms of urinary urgency. Before starting tolterodine, he was taking a maximal dosage of terazosin, but was still getting up 4 to 6 times nightly to urinate. He has no incontinence, and no urinary complaints other than mild urgency and frequency. History includes hypertension and diabetes mellitus; there is no history of prostate surgery or urethral instrumentation. Medications include lisinopril, metformin, and tolterodine.

He is now getting up only 3 times each night to urinate but is still feeling exhausted in the morning. His wife's sleep is also being disrupted by his trips to the bathroom and by his loud snoring and kicking at night.

On physical examination, the patient is moderately obese. Blood pressure is 140/80 mmHg. He has a normal cardiovascular examination and a small prostate. Ejection fraction was normal on echocardiography performed 3 mo ago. On noninvasive testing, urinary peak flow rate is 21 mL/sec on a void of 320 mL; postvoid residual volume is 25 mL, and urinalysis is normal. Hemoglobin A_{1c} level, renal function, and prostate-specific antigen level are normal.

Which of the following is the most appropriate next step?

(A)   Switch from tolterodine to tamsulosin.
(B)   Refer for urologic evaluation.
(C)   Prescribe furosemide 20 mg in late afternoon.
(D)   Refer to a sleep disorders clinic.
(E)   Prescribe finasteride 5 mg/d.

ANSWER: D

This patient should be referred for evaluation in a sleep disorders clinic. His history suggests a sleep disorder, either periodic leg movements during sleep or sleep apnea or both (SOE=B). Patients may complain of nocturia, but the primary problem may be awakening because of a sleep disorder. He does not need a urologic evaluation, because physical examination, prostate-specific antigen level, flow rate, postvoid residual, and urinalysis are all normal.

Most nocturia is multifactorial. α-Blockers, including terazosin (nonselective) and tamsulosin (selective), treat symptoms of benign prostatic hyperplasia. This patient has not benefited from 3 mo of therapy with an α-blocker and bladder relaxant combined. A selective α-blocker may be warranted if the nonselective agent causes adverse events (hypotension, dizziness); however, selective α-blockers are not more effective than nonselective agents (SOE=A). In addition, substitution of tamsulosin for tolterodine might further increase his blood pressure. Finasteride, a 5-α reductase inhibitor, has not been shown to have efficacy in treating nocturia (SOE=A), except in certain subgroups. Its efficacy in treating symptoms of benign prostatic hyperplasia is more likely in patients who are known to have a large prostate; this patient has a small prostate and low prostate-specific antigen level (SOE=A).

Patients with nocturia due to volume overload (eg, venous insufficiency with leg edema, heart failure) sometimes benefit from administration of a rapid-acting diuretic in the late afternoon (SOE=B). This strategy reduces the amount of fluid accumulated during the day, thereby reducing mobilization of fluid while the patient is supine during sleep. Had the evidence suggestive of a sleep disorder been less strong and the patient displayed signs of fluid overload, introducing a diuretic might be appropriate.

References

1. Miller M. Nocturnal polyuria in older people: pathophysiology and clinical implication. *J Am Geriatr Soc.* 2000:48(10):1321–1329.
2. Weiss JP, Blaivas JG. Nocturia. *J Urol.* 2000;163(1):5–12.
3. Johnson TM 2nd, Jones K, Williford WO, et al. Changes in nocturia from medical treatment of benign prostatic hyperplasia: secondary analysis of the Department of Veterans Affairs Cooperative Study Trial. *J Urol.* 2003;170(1):145–148.
4. Johnson TM 2nd, Burrows PK, Kusek JW, et al. The effect of doxazosin, finasteride and combination therapy on nocturia in men with benign prostatic hyperplasia. *J Urol.* 2007;178(5):2045–2050.

62. A 75-yr-old woman calls the office to discuss a church-based screening program in which carotid arteries, abdominal aorta, and heel-bone density are evaluated using ultrasonography. She wonders whether it is worth the $85 charge.

Which of the following is the most appropriate response?

(A) The screening is a bargain, because each of these tests usually cost >$85 at the local hospital.
(B) The screening may result in expensive or potentially risky procedures.
(C) If the sensitivity is high, the screening would be valuable.
(D) The screening should be done at the local hospital.

ANSWER: B

The United States Preventive Services Task Force (USPSTF) publishes screening recommendations based on a comprehensive literature review. The USPSTF recommends screening of the abdominal aorta by ultrasonography in men 65–75 yr old who have ever smoked, because surgical repair of abdominal aortic aneurysms >5.5 cm decreases mortality (SOE=B). However, the USPSTF recommends against screening of the abdominal aorta in women, because the prevalence of abdominal aneurysm in women is low (approximately one-sixth the prevalence in men). In fact, evidence suggests that screening and early treatment in asymptomatic women results in an increased incidence of unnecessary surgery, with an increase in associated morbidity and mortality.

The USPSTF recommends screening all women ≥65 yr old for osteoporosis with dual x-ray absorptiometry (DEXA) scanning, preferably of the hip. There is substantial discordance in results between ultrasonography of the heel and central DEXA scanning, such that the former is not a useful test. The USPSTF recommends against screening for asymptomatic carotid artery stenosis in the general adult population.

While each of these tests would cost >$85 at the local hospital, it is not a good deal if the tests are unnecessary. Although undergoing unnecessary tests at the local hospital may improve the quality of the study, it does not make the tests more appropriate.

References

1. Bachman DM, Crewson PE, Lewis RS. Comparison of heel ultrasound and finger DXA to central DXA in the detection of osteoporosis. Implications for patient management. *J Clin Densitom*. 2002;5(2):131–141.
2. U.S. Preventive Services Task Force. Screening for abdominal aortic aneurysm: recommendation statement. *Ann Intern Med*. 2005;142(3):198–202.
3. U.S. Preventive Services Task Force. Screening for osteoporosis in postmenopausal women: recommendations and rationale. *Ann Intern Med*. 2002;137(6):526–528.
4. U.S. Preventive Services Task Force. Screening for carotid artery stenosis: U.S. Preventive Services Task Force recommendation statement. *Ann Intern Med*. 2007;147(12):854–859.

63. An 85-yr-old woman comes to the office for an evaluation because she recently fell. She lives independently in a rural community. She has no significant medical history and takes no medications. She has not had her vision assessed in several years.

Which of the following is true regarding visual acuity in older adults?

(A) Visual acuity should be screened every 1–2 yr.
(B) Routine eye examinations have not been shown to improve functional status.
(C) Age-related macular degeneration, glaucoma, diabetic retinopathy, and cataracts usually produce early symptoms.
(D) Visual loss has not been shown to impair postural stability or cause falls in older adults.

ANSWER: A

Over 3 million Americans have low vision, and one-third of people ≥65 yr old have some type of vision loss. Low vision is common and causes substantial functional loss in adults ≥70 yr old. Nearly all adults ≥90 yr old have a cataract, and half have had cataract surgery. Early detection of eye disease can help identify underlying medical conditions and can slow progression of vision loss. In a 5-yr observational study of Medicare beneficiaries, patients ≥65 yr old who had routine eye examinations had less decline in vision and functional status (SOE=B). The 2009 recommendation of the U.S. Preventive Services Task Force is that evidence regarding visual screening in older adults is inconclusive (SOE=C). However, this woman has fallen recently, so evaluation of vision is not screening in nature. The American Academy of Ophthalmology recommends a comprehensive eye examination every 1–2 yr for adults ≥65 yr old.

Older adults are unlikely to be aware of gradual visual loss. Glaucoma, diabetic retinopathy, age-related macular degeneration, and cataracts do not present with early symptoms, yet are common in adults ≥65 yr old. About 50% of cases of vision loss in older adults can be corrected; in 25% of cases, the loss could have been prevented. Primary care physicians should assess vision and should ask patients about reading difficulties or problems performing tasks.

In observational studies, reduced vision has been associated with increased risk of falls.

References

1. Rosenberg EA, Sperazza LC. The visually impaired patient. *Am Fam Physician*. 2008;77(10):1431–1436.
2. Sloan FA, Picone G, Brown DS, et al. Longitudinal analysis of the relationship between regular eye examinations and changes in visual and functional status. *J Am Geriatr Soc*. 2005;53(11):1867–1874.
3. U.S. Preventive Services Task Force. Screening for Impaired Visual Acuity in Older Adults. http://www.ahrq.gov/clinic/uspstf/uspsviseld.htm (accessed Nov 2009).

64. An 82-yr-old woman comes to the office because she has urine leakage when she coughs or sneezes, as well as urinary frequency and urgency. History includes COPD, hypertension, and aortic stenosis.

On pelvic examination, there is grade III pelvic prolapse. Postvoid residual volume is 200 mL.

Which of the following is most likely to be effective for this patient?

(A) Vaginal pessary
(B) Burch colposuspension
(C) Kegel exercises
(D) Oxybutynin

ANSWER: A

Support and space-filling pessaries are used to treat pelvic organ prolapse. A support pessary can be used to treat all stages of pelvic organ prolapse and stress urinary incontinence, whereas a space-filling pessary is mostly used for severe prolapse. Use of a vaginal pessary for pelvic organ prolapse is appropriate if a patient does not want surgery, if there is a

need to delay surgery, or if the patient is a poor surgical candidate (SOE=C).

Most pessaries are made of silicone, which is nonallergenic and durable, and does not retain odors. They are fit by trial and error. A ring pessary, which provides support, is the most commonly used and is likely to be successful for stage II or III prolapse. A Gellhorn pessary is more likely to be successful with stage III prolapse. After a pessary is fitted, a follow-up visit is scheduled for 1–2 wk later. The pessary is removed and cleaned, and the vagina is examined for erosions. If the patient is unable to remove and reinsert the pessary, follow-up is again scheduled in 1–2 wk, and then every 3–4 mo thereafter. Common adverse events include vaginal erosion, bleeding, and discharge. They usually occur in the setting of vaginal atrophy and can be treated or prevented by use of low-dose vaginal estrogen cream. Serious complications from vaginal pessaries are rare. For women with urinary incontinence, 1-mo efficacy is approximately 60%. In about 60% of cases, there is long-term (6–12 mo) satisfaction and continued use.

This patient's COPD and aortic stenosis make surgery, such as colposuspension, less attractive and perhaps not feasible. Kegel exercises are not indicated for the treatment of incontinence due to prolapse. Oxybutynin, which is useful in the treatment of urge incontinence, is contraindicated in the presence of a larger postvoid residual volume.

References

1. Donnelly MJ, Powell-Morgan S, Olsen AL, et al. Vaginal pessaries for the management of stress and mixed urinary incontinence. *Int Urogynecol J Pelvic Floor Dysfunct*. 2004;15(5):302–307.
2. Hanson LA, Schulz JA, Flood CG, et al. Vaginal pessaries in managing women with pelvic organ prolapse and urinary incontinence: patient characteristics and factors contributing to success. *Int Urogynecol J Pelvic Floor Dysfunct*. 2006;17(2):155–159.
3. Powers K, Lazarou G, Wang A, et al. Pessary use in advanced pelvic organ prolapse. *Int Urogynecol J Pelvic Floor Dysfunct*. 2006;17(2):160–164.
4. Shamliyan TA, Kane RL, Wyman J, et al. Systematic review: randomized, controlled trials of nonsurgical treatments for urinary incontinence in women. *Ann Intern Med*. 2008;148(6):459–473.

65. A 79-yr-old woman comes to the office because she has knee discomfort that is exacerbated by walking, and as a consequence, she undertakes little or no physical activity. She has moderate osteoarthritis of both knees and takes acetaminophen irregularly for pain.

On examination, the patient is 1.6 m (64 in) and weighs 65 kg (144 lb). She has bilateral synovial swelling and mild varus deformity of the left knee. There is no significant ligament laxity, and no joint effusions, warmth, or tenderness on palpation. She has full range of motion (extension and flexion) of both knees, but crepitus is present on the left side. Quadriceps strength is 4+/5 bilaterally. She walks slowly but with good balance.

Which of the following is the most appropriate recommendation for physical activity?

(A) Flexibility stretching exercises 1 day/wk
(B) Aquatic exercises 1 day/wk
(C) Isotonic quadriceps exercises 5 days/wk
(D) Isotonic quadriceps exercises 2 days/wk
(E) Moderate-intensity aerobic exercise, 5 days/wk

ANSWER: D

Light to moderate exercise has a preventive and perhaps restorative role in people with osteoarthritis and should be started immediately along with the pharmacologic regimen. An appropriate program includes flexibility, strengthening, and aerobic components. For this patient, stretching once per week is insufficient; she should stretch at least 3 times per week, preferably before strengthening sessions for quadriceps muscle (SOE=D). Because quadriceps muscle weakness is a risk factor in osteoarthritis, strengthening the muscle is a critical component of the physical activity program (SOE=A). Pain control with a fixed dose of acetaminophen or NSAID is likely to be necessary, as will a graded approach to exercise. Isotonic or isometric exercises should begin at a low intensity (<50% of the person's one repetition maximum) of 6 to 8 repetitions, working up to 10 to 15 repetitions daily (SOE=C). Although weight lifting can generally be conducted at 48-hour intervals, a maximum of 2 days/wk is recommended for people who have osteoarthritis (SOE=C). An aerobic exercise program will improve bone strength and contribute to weight loss, but it is highly unlikely that this patient can engage at a moderate-intensity level; she should instead start at a low-intensity level. Aquatic exercises once a week are insufficient to provide the necessary strength or endurance to meet this patient's needs (SOE=C).

Reference

1. American Geriatrics Society. Exercise prescription for older adults with osteoarthritis pain: consensus practice recommendations. AGS Panel on Exercise and Osteoarthritis. *J Am Geriatr Soc.* 2001;49(6):808–823.

66. An 82-yr-old nursing home resident is evaluated because she has increased pain in her knee. She has refused to walk for the past several days. History includes dementia, osteoporosis, atrial fibrillation, and renal insufficiency.

On physical examination, temperature is 37.4°C (99.3°F), blood pressure is 110/80 mmHg, and pulse is 78 beats per minute. The knee is warm and tender and causes pain with movement. An effusion is palpable. There is bony enlargement of the first carpal-metacarpal and distal interphalangeal joints. Radiography of the knee demonstrates joint space narrowing, chondrocalcinosis, and osteophytes of the medial compartment.

Which of the following diagnostic tests should be obtained next?

(A) Westergren sedimentation rate
(B) Arthrocentesis and synovial fluid analysis
(C) Radiography of knee while bearing weight
(D) MRI of the knee

ANSWER: B

This patient has acute monoarthritis; direct evaluation of the synovial fluid is required to ascertain its cause. The presence of chondrocalcinosis suggests crystalline arthritis (calcium pyrophosphate deposition disease). Although her low-grade fever and inability or unwillingness to walk can be manifestations of this painful arthritis, an infectious cause must be excluded by arthrocentesis. Given her history of atrial fibrillation, she may be on anticoagulant therapy. Anticoagulant therapy is not a contraindication for arthrocentesis and has not been demonstrated to increase risk. Fluid samples should be immediately viewed with a polarizing microscope for crystals, and sent for cell count, Gram stain, and culture (SOE=B).

   Arthrocentesis may yield a bloody effusion that, together with the history of osteoporosis, raises the possibility of a tibial plateau fracture. MRI is the best diagnostic test for detection of tibial plateau fracture and is useful in elucidating the integrity of ligaments and structures around and within the knee, including periarticular bone. MRI would not be helpful in distinguishing infectious from other inflammatory causes of monoarthritis. Although radiographs of the knee bearing weight are required to assess the joint space more accurately, they will not distinguish infectious from crystalline arthritis and may be difficult to obtain in a patient who is unable or unwilling to bear weight. The Westergren sedimentation rate increases with age and anemia and will not distinguish infectious from other inflammatory etiologies.

References

1. Dunn AS, Turpie AG. Perioperative management of patients receiving oral anticoagulants: a systematic review. *Arch Intern Med.* 2003;163(8):901–908.
2. Margaretten ME, Kohlwes J, Moore D, et al. Does this adult patient have septic arthritis? *JAMA.* 2007;297(13):1478–1488.
3. Prasad N, Murray JM, et al. Insufficiency fracture of the tibial plateau: an often missed diagnosis. *Acta Orthop Belg.* 2006;72(5):587–591.
4. Rosenthal AK. Update in calcium deposition diseases. *Curr Opin Rheumatol.* 2007;19(2):158–162.

67. A 78-yr-old woman is admitted to a short-term rehabilitation facility after elective replacement of her right hip. Surgery was uneventful, and she began in-hospital rehabilitation shortly thereafter.

On examination by the rehabilitation physician, there is a 6 cm × 4 cm area of nonblanching erythema on the patient's left buttock. It is boggy, purple, and painful. Skin is intact.

Which of the following describes this finding?

(A) Stage I pressure ulcer
(B) Stage IV pressure ulcer
(C) Suspected deep-tissue injury
(D) Partial-thickness ulcer
(E) Unstageable pressure ulcer

ANSWER: C

In 2007, the National Pressure Ulcer Advisory Panel added "deep-tissue injury" and "unstageable" to the classifications for staging pressure ulcers. According to the classification, this patient has a pressure ulcer that is suspicious for deep-tissue injury: it is a "purple or maroon localized area of discolored intact skin or blood-filled blister due to damage of underlying soft tissue from pressure and/or shear. The area may be preceded by tissue that is painful, firm, mushy, boggy, warmer or cooler as compared to adjacent tissue" (SOE=C).

If the damage were limited to nonblanching erythema with intact skin, it would be designated a stage I ulcer; however, the other clinical signs indicate more serious damage underneath (SOE=C). Stage IV describes full-thickness tissue loss with exposed bone, tendon, or muscle. Because this patient's skin is intact, it is not a stage II ulcer (partial-thickness ulcer or ulcer caused by other means, eg, vascular disease or maceration) (SOE=C).

Unstageable ulcers are full-thickness ulcers in which the wound bed is obscured by slough, eschar, or both. In the past, ulcers with any necrotic tissue were often described as unstageable even when the depth of the wound could be ascertained. If a wound has necrotic tissue but the depth can be visualized, then it should be staged accordingly (SOE=C).

References

1. Berlowitz DR, Brienza DM. Are all pressure ulcers the result of deep tissue injury? A review of the literature. *Ostomy Wound Manage.* 2007;53(10):34–38.
2. Black J, Baharestani M, Cuddigan J, et al. National Pressure Ulcer Advisory Panel's Updated Pressure Ulcer Staging System. *Dermatol Nurs.* 2007;19(4):343–349.
3. Doughty D, Ramundo J, Bonham P, et al. Issues and challenges in staging pressure ulcers. *Journal of the WOCN.* 2006;33(2):126–132.

68. A 65-yr-old woman comes to the office to request advice about quitting smoking. She has a 40 pack-year smoking history. She wants to know whether she is too old to benefit from quitting.

Which of the following is a benefit of smoking cessation as an older adult?

(A) Circulation improves 5 yr after cessation.
(B) Lung function improves 5 yr after cessation.
(C) She would live longer.
(D) The risk of dying from heart disease decreases to 5 times that of a nonsmoker.

ANSWER: C

Current data suggest that 9% of people >65 yr old smoke, despite increased risk of death, lung cancer, dementia, stroke, and heart attack. Of the approximately 440,000 deaths each year from smoking-related diseases, 300,000 occur in adults ≥65 yr old. Advocating for smoking cessation is an important role for physicians, and older adults are encouraged to quit when their physicians discuss the benefits with them.

Lung function and circulation begin to improve immediately after smoking cessation. Irrespective of age or length of time since quitting, former smokers have cardiovascular mortality rates similar to those of nonsmokers. Longevity studies show that among smokers who quit at age 65, men gain 1.4–12 yr of life and women gain 2.7–3.4 yr (SOE=A).

Physicians who use the 5-step approach—**ask** about smoking, **advise** to quit, **assess** a patient's willingness, **assist** the patient in developing a quitting plan, and **arrange** for follow-up—can significantly improve the health of older patients who smoke (SOE=A).

References

1. Abdullah AS, Simon JL. Health promotion in older adults: evidence-based smoking cessation programs for use in primary care settings. *Geriatrics.* 2006;61(3):30–34.
2. Taylor DH Jr, Hasselblad V, Henley SJ, et al. Benefits of smoking cessation for longevity. *Am J Public Health.* 2002;92(6):990–996.

69. Which of the following assistive devices is most appropriate for a 72-yr-old man with Parkinson's disease who has postural instability and festination?

(A) Cane
(B) Front-wheeled walker
(C) Hemi-walker
(D) Pick-up walker
(E) 4-Wheeled walker

ANSWER: B

Walking devices are extremely helpful for people with gait disorders. They increase mobility, reduce risk of falls, and facilitate independence. The walking device must be targeted to the patient's functional deficits to avoid increasing risk, and the patient must be trained, preferably by a physical therapist, to use the device safely. The patient described has the classic mobility problems of Parkinson's disease—postural instability (often associated with backward falls) and festination (gradual increasing of forward speed while walking). The device chosen should facilitate maintenance of forward center of gravity (to limit backward falls), yet not be so mobile that it could facilitate festination. A front-wheeled walker best meets these requirements.

Standard pick-up walkers and front-wheeled walkers both decrease a patient's gait speed. However, patients using the standard walker have increased freezing and slow gait speed. Front-wheeled walkers do not increase freezing and are associated with a gait speed intermediate between no walker and a standard walker (SOE=B).

A cane is not the best choice for this patient because the posturing of arms (internal rotation) could lead to tripping. A hemi-walker is used by patients with a hemiparesis. A pick-up walker promotes a very slow gait and can accentuate backward movement when lifting, thereby increasing the risk of a fall. The four-wheeled walker rolls very easily but could promote festination. For patients (with or without Parkinson's disease) who do not have festination and can use them safely, 4-wheeled walkers are preferred because they promote a more normal gait pattern (SOE=D).

References

1. Bateni H, Maki BE. Assistive devices for balance and mobility: benefits, demands, and adverse consequences. *Arch Phys Med Rehabil.* 2005;86(1):134–145.
2. Brockton J, Hefflin MD, Thomas P, et al. Estimates of medical device–associated adverse events from emergency departments. *Am J Prev Med.* 2004;27(3):246–253.
3. Constantinescu R, Leonard C, Deeley C, et al. Assistive devices for gait in Parkinson's disease. *Parkinsonism Relat Disord.* 2007;13(3):133–138.
4. Cubo E, Moore CG, Leurgans S, et al. Wheeled and standard walkers in Parkinson's disease patients with gait freezing. *Parkinsonism Relat Disord.* 2003;10(1):9–14.

70. An 86-yr-old woman comes to the office for routine evaluation. She was the primary caregiver for her husband until his death 9 mo ago. She is somewhat fatigued and has a poor appetite but does not think that she is depressed. She has had some dizziness but no falls, and she has had occasional diarrhea with incontinence but no melena or hematochezia. History includes atrial fibrillation, heart failure (left ventricular ejection fraction 40% at last measure 6 mo ago), and hypertension. Medications include atenolol, digoxin, lisinopril, and warfarin. On examination, blood pressure is 118/66 mmHg. Ventricular heart rate is 66 beats per minute. She has lost 6.4 kg (14 lb; 9% of her body weight) over the last 6 mo. The remainder of the physical examination is not substantially changed from her last visit.

Which of the following is most likely to identify the cause of her weight loss?

(A) Chest radiography
(B) Fecal occult blood testing
(C) Geriatric Depression Scale
(D) Home visit
(E) Serum digoxin level

ANSWER: E

Review of medications should be part of assessment for weight loss. Anorexia, diarrhea, and dizziness are common adverse events of digoxin toxicity. Bradycardia, ventricular arrhythmias, apathy, nausea, confusion, visual disturbances, depression, and other adverse events are also observed. These adverse events can lead to significant weight loss. There is some controversy regarding measurement of digoxin concentrations: patients may have toxicity even when concentrations are within laboratory-established norms; nonetheless, higher concentrations correlate with greater adverse events (SOE=C). If subacute digoxin toxicity is suspected, a trial of tapering the dosage may be reasonable instead of measuring the serum concentration.

Fecal occult blood testing to screen for malignancy or hemorrhage is reasonable, but adverse consequences of digoxin are more common and should be checked immediately. The Geriatric Depression Scale may be positive, but depression should not be considered endogenous until digoxin toxicity is excluded; depression will likely be refractory until toxicity resolves. A home visit may determine if the patient is caring for herself and has quality nutrition available; however, poor living conditions could be due to depression and apathy caused by digoxin toxicity. Lung cancer can cause weight loss, but there is little else in this case to suggest lung pathology.

References

1. Gheorghiade M, van Veldhuisen D, Colucci W. Contemporary use of digoxin in the management of cardiovascular disorders. *Circulation*. 2006;113(21):2556–2564.
2. Heckman GA, McKelvie RS. Necessary cautions when considering digoxin in heart failure. *CMAJ*. 2007;176(5):644–645.
3. Onder G, Penninx BW, Landi F, et al. Depression and adverse drug reactions among hospitalized older adults. *Arch Intern Med*. 2003;163(3):301–305.
4. Smellie WS, Coleman JJ. Pitfalls of testing and summary of guidance on safety monitoring with amiodarone and digoxin. *BMJ*. 2007;334(7588):312–315.

71. A 77-yr-old woman is brought to the office by her daughter because she has been seeing her dead husband and dead brother for the past 2 mo. She sometimes talks to them and they may respond to her. She has a 4-yr history of declining memory and impairment in such daily activities as shopping, paying bills, and cooking. She has a history of major depressive disorder but is neither sad nor apathetic on examination. There is no history of alcohol or substance abuse.

Examination is notable for increasing rigidity in her arms in response to progressively more rapid passive movement and a mild shuffling gait. She has no tremor or other neurologic abnormality. Her score is 18/30 on the Mini–Mental State Examination. Laboratory tests are normal. CT shows mild cortical atrophy.

Which of the following is the most likely explanation for her symptoms?

(A) Lewy body dementia
(B) Late-onset schizophrenia
(C) Major depressive disorder with psychotic features
(D) Parkinson's disease with dementia
(E) Alzheimer's disease

ANSWER: E

Psychosis of Alzheimer's disease is diagnosed if hallucinations or delusions have been present intermittently or continuously for at least 1 mo; they disrupt the patient's or another person's life; the patient meets criteria for Alzheimer's disease; and the hallucinations or delusions are not due to delirium, effects of medication, schizophrenia, or other psychiatric disorders. Psychosis is most common in the middle stages of Alzheimer's disease. Visual hallucinations are more common than auditory hallucinations. Typically, hallucinations involve people from the past (eg, deceased relatives), intruders, animals, and objects. Delusions typically involve beliefs of theft, infidelity, abandonment, and persecution. A common delusion is the belief that the person is not living in his or her home. Delusions decrease in later stages of Alzheimer's disease.

Drug therapy is generally not used for these psychoses unless the patient has considerable distress or agitation. Although risperidone and olanzapine are modestly effective, use of second-generation anti-psychotic agents is associated with increased mortality rates in patients with dementia.

Psychosis related to Alzheimer's disease is distinguished from schizophrenia by the lack of bizarre or complex delusions, more frequent visual hallucinations, and absence of prior history of psychoses. In dementia related to Parkinson's disease, a history of movement disorder precedes the dementia by a year; the psychosis can diminish after adjustment of antiparkinsonian medication. In Lewy body dementia, movement disorders and cognitive impairment arise within a year of each other. Visual hallucinations develop early in Lewy body dementia in about 40% of cases; in Alzheimer's disease, hallucinations tend to develop later, in mid stage. In major depressive disorder with psychotic features, hallucinations are not common. When they are present, they are usually mood congruent (eg, derogatory voices) and are more commonly auditory.

The increased rigidity with passive movement of the arm (paratonia) is more commonly seen in middle- and late-stage Alzheimer's disease, and also is seen in Lewy body dementia. Patients with Parkinson's disease exhibit a more uniform rigidity to passive movement and have increased muscle tone at the onset of movement. The shuffling gait is typical of the gait apraxia seen in Alzheimer's disease. It differs from the shuffling gait of Parkinson's disease and Lewy body dementia by the absence of festination, retropulsion, and en-bloc turning.

References

1. Kennedy GJ. Caution vs. closure: the use of atypical antipsychotics for the treatment of behavioral disturbances in dementia. *Primary Psychiatry*. 2005;12:16–19.
2. Manepalli JN, Gebretsadik M, Hook, J, et al. Differential diagnosis of the older patient with psychotic symptoms. *Primary Psychiatry*. 2007;14(8):55–62.
3. Prehogan A, Cohen CI. Motor dysfunction in dementias. *Geriatrics*. 2004;59(11):53–60.
4. Schneider LS, Tariot PN, Dagerman KS, et al. Effectiveness of atypical antipsychotic drugs in patients with Alzheimer's disease. *N Engl J Med*. 2006;355(15):1525–1538.

72. A 75-yr-old man needs to begin therapy with an osteoporosis agent because he fractured his hip when he fell over an area of uneven sidewalk. The consulting pharmacist recommends zoledronic acid to reduce subsequent fractures and mortality.

Which of the following considerations would preclude use of zoledronic acid in this patient?

(A) He has a low vitamin D level.
(B) He is unwilling to take an oral bisphosphonate.
(C) The fracture occurred within the past 90 days.
(D) His creatinine clearance is <30 mL/min.

ANSWER: D

In a randomized, controlled trial, once-yearly intravenous infusion of zoledronic acid, in patients with previous hip fracture, resulted in an absolute risk reduction of 5.3% in new clinical fractures (including vertebral) and an absolute risk reduction of 3.7% in death from any cause, as compared with placebo (SOE=A). The trial also showed a trend in reduction in hip fractures (2.0% with zoledronic acid vs 3.5% with placebo), although the trial was underpowered to detect a statistically significant difference.

Infusion of zoledronic acid was required within 90 days of a low-trauma fracture. Patients included in this study had a creatinine clearance >30 mL/min and were unable or unwilling to take an oral bisphosphonate. Vitamin D deficiency was corrected before the infusion. Concomitant therapy with nasal calcitonin, selective estrogen-receptor modulators, hormone replacement, tibolone, and external hip protectors was allowed at the discretion of the investigator. Patients who had previously used bisphosphonates or parathyroid hormone were able to participate after a washout period that varied according to the drug and its duration of use. These inclusions have been the subject of some controversy.

No other controlled clinical trial has previously shown efficacy of any osteoporosis medication for reducing the recurrence of fracture in patients who already had broken a hip.

References

1. Calis KA, Pucino F. Zoledronic acid and secondary prevention of fractures. *N Engl J Med.* 2007;357(18):1861–1862.
2. Lopez CA, Tasneem Z. Zoledronate, fractures, and mortality after hip fracture. *N Engl J Med.* 2008;358(9):967–968.
3. Lyles KW, Coln-Emeric CS, Magaziner JS, et al. Zoledronic acid and clinical fractures and mortality after hip fracture. *N Engl J Med.* 2007;357(18):1799–1809.

73. A 75-yr-old woman is brought to the office because she recently started having urge urinary incontinence. She has hypertension, major depressive disorder, osteoarthritis, and probable Alzheimer's disease. Three months ago she began taking donepezil 5 mg/d; the dosage was increased to 10 mg/d after 6 wk. Other medications are acetaminophen 500 mg q6h, hydrochlorothiazide 12.5 mg/d, lisinopril 10 mg/d, and citalopram 20 mg/d (increased from 10 mg 2 mo ago).

Urinalysis is negative for bacteria and leukocyte esterase, and shows 0.3 WBCs per high-power field.

Which of the following should be done next to manage this patient's incontinence?

(A) Start tolterodine.
(B) Discontinue hydrochlorothiazide.
(C) Decrease donepezil to 5 mg/d.
(D) Decrease citalopram to 10 mg/d.
(E) Discontinue lisinopril.

ANSWER: C

This patient's symptoms of urge incontinence are consistent with cholinergic stimulation of the bladder precipitated by the increased dosage of donepezil. Reducing the dosage is appropriate, because donepezil 5 mg/d is clinically effective (SOE=A) and the patient apparently tolerated it well. If the patient's function were to worsen after decreasing the dosage, the alternatives would be to discontinue donepezil or to begin medication for overactive bladder.

The patient may have new-onset incontinence related to her dementia. However, reversible drug-induced causes must be excluded. Although tolterodine is effective for urge incontinence, patients with Alzheimer's disease are more susceptible to anticholinergic effects of medications, and increased confusion or delirium could result. In addition, medications used for overactive bladder may potentially interfere with the effectiveness of cholinesterase inhibitors (eg, donepezil). Nonetheless, cholinesterase inhibitors and anticholinergics are used concomitantly in approximately 30% of adults with dementia. Although newer anticholinergic agents are reported to be more selective for bladder muscarinic receptors (eg, darifenacin) or less likely to cross the blood-brain barrier (eg, trospium), these agents should be used cautiously in patients with dementia, because the blood-brain barrier can become more penetrable with age and comorbidity.

Citalopram and lisinopril are not associated with urinary incontinence. Because the patient had previously tolerated hydrochlorothiazide, the first step should be to reduce her donepezil dosage.

References

1. Fung CH, Spencer B, Eslami M, et al. Quality indicators for the screening and care of urinary incontinence in vulnerable elders. *J Am Geriatr Soc.* 2007;55(Suppl 2):S443–449.
2. Gill SS, Mamdani M, Naglie G, et al. A prescribing cascade involving cholinesterase inhibitors and anticholinergic drugs. *Arch Intern Med.* 2005;165(7):808–813.
3. Kay GG, Abou-Donia MB, Messer WS Jr, et al. Antimuscarinic drugs for overactive bladder and their potential effects on cognitive function in older patients. *J Am Geriatr Soc.* 2005;53(12):2195-2201.
4. Sink KM, Thomas J 3rd, Xu H, et al. Dual use of bladder anticholinergics and cholinesterase inhibitors: long-term functional and cognitive outcomes. *J Am Geriatr Soc.* 2008;56(5):847–853.

74. An 88-yr-old man comes to the office because he has severe low back pain, and pain and weakness in his right leg for 2 days. Until then, he had been feeling well and was independent in all ADLs, but he now has difficulty dressing and bathing. History includes stage III prostate cancer, which was initially treated with external-beam radiation. He has been on leuprolide q3mo for the past 3 yr.

MRI of the spine shows metastatic lesions at L4-L5 with encroachment on the ventral epidural space, no spinal cord compression, and no sign of spinal instability. He is referred to a radiation oncologist for therapy for his vertebral metastases. He is started on a fentanyl patch and oxycodone as needed for breakthrough pain, along with a stool softener and senna-based laxative.

Which of the following medications should also be prescribed?

(A) Ibuprofen 800 mg po q8h
(B) One dose of pamidronate 90 mg IV over 2 h
(C) Dexamethasone 4 mg IV q6h
(D) Gabapentin 300 mg po q8h
(E) Lidocaine patch 5% topically for 12 h daily

ANSWER: C

Dexamethasone reduces both neuropathic and bone pain and is the most appropriate addition to this patient's current pain regimen. Dexamethasone inhibits production and activity of prostaglandin E_2 and vascular endothelial growth factor, thereby decreasing vasogenic edema. In animal models, reduction in vasogenic edema is associated with improved neurologic function. Although some studies have used high-dose dexamethasone, lower dosages (24 mg/d in divided doses orally or intravenously) can provide adequate improvement in ambulatory patients without spinal cord compression (SOE=D). Patients taking dexamethasone need to be monitored for potential adverse events, including hyperglycemia, insomnia, anxiety, restlessness, and delirium.

NSAIDs, such as ibuprofen, and bisphosphonates, such as pamidronate, may decrease bone pain from vertebral metastases (SOE=A). Ibuprofen needs to be used with caution in older adults because of the increased risk of GI bleeding and effects on renal function. Pamidronate can cause hypokalemia and related adverse events. The fentanyl and oxycodone should be given a trial period with titration before adding either ibuprofen or pamidronate.

Gabapentin decreases the paresthesias and burning, shooting pain that come from peripheral nerve or spinal cord injury (SOE=A). It should be used with caution in older adults because it has many potential adverse events, including somnolence and gait instability. The lidocaine patch 5% is useful for certain types of neuropathic pain and may be helpful for this patient's L4-L5 radicular pain. Neither gabapentin nor the lidocaine patch 5% significantly decreases bone pain. This patient's neuropathic pain may decrease on the opioid regimen, and dexamethasone is a better choice because it will address both his bone and neuropathic pain.

Ibuprofen and pamidronate are useful for bone pain from metastases, and gabapentin and lidocaine are effective for neuropathic pain. However, given this patient's vertebral metastases with encroachment on the ventral epidural space, potential for spinal cord compression, and current L4-L5 radicular symptoms, dexamethasone is the best adjuvant to add for pain management now and may help the patient maintain the ability to ambulate, especially if used in combination with radiation treatment (SOE=A).

References

1. Abraham JL, Banffy MB, Harris MB. Spinal cord compression in patients with advanced metastatic cancer. *JAMA*. 2008;299(8):937–946.
2. Benjamin R. Neurologic complications of prostate cancer. *Am Fam Physician*. 2002;65(9):1834–1840.
3. Moryl N, Coyle N, Foley KM. Managing an acute pain crisis in a patient with advanced cancer. *JAMA*. 2008;299(12):1457–1467.

75. A 68-yr-old woman has a chief complaint of a sore second right toe. She states the problem is worsened by wearing shoes, and she has tried no self-care. History includes hypertension, thyroid disease, and a 45 pack-year smoking history. Physical examination shows pitting edema and absent pedal pulses bilaterally. Neurologic examination is normal. Bilaterally the second digits are contracted. There is a nonulcerated hyperkeratotic lesion on the dorsal right second toe.

Which of the following treatments for this lesion are contraindicated in this patient?

(A) Sal-acid plaster patches
(B) Foam padding
(C) Stretching the shoe
(D) Vascular clearance for surgical reconstruction
(E) Pumice stone after bathing

ANSWER: A

With aging, structural problems such as hammertoes and hallux valgus deformities frequently develop. These structural changes lead to increased pressure over bony prominences. With chronic irritation, hyperkeratotic lesions, commonly called corns and calluses, develop. Treatment includes reducing the increased pressures with shoe gear modifications and foam sleeves. Surgery can effectively correct structural abnormalities if the patient is a surgical candidate. Reducing the size of the corn or callus can reduce symptoms but must be done safely, eg, through careful use of a pumice stone after bathing. The use of sal-acid or other corn/callus/wart removers are contraindicated in patients with diabetes and/or vascular disease because of the risk of ulceration (SOE=C).

Reference

1. Benvenuti F, Ferrucci L, Guralnik JM, et al. Foot pain and disability in older persons: an epidemiologic survey. *J Am Geriatr Soc.* 1995;43(5):479–484.

76. A 79-yr-old widower is seen in the office for self-reported anhedonia and depression. He has a history of affective disorder, lives alone, and has no nearby relatives. Recently his best friend died, and his social network has been getting smaller because of disabilities and deaths of associates. Three of his aquarium fish died this week, and he has not attended church for several months. He indicates that, increasingly, ADLs have become burdensome and problematic. There is no evidence of cognitive impairment on the Mini–Mental State Examination.

Which of the following is the next best step?

(A) Refer to grief counseling group.
(B) Evaluate suicide risk.
(C) Evaluate for alcohol abuse.
(D) Refer to a psychotherapist.

ANSWER: B

This patient is at high risk of suicide because of his anhedonia, past affective disorder, diminishing social network, recent losses, and increasing difficulties with ADLs. The suicide risk should be addressed immediately before other courses of treatment are considered.

In the United States, suicide rates for men increase notably into old age (SOE=A). Psychologic autopsy studies identify five factors that contribute to risk: history of affective disorder, blunted hedonic response, medical illness, stressful life events, and diminished functional status. The risk increases substantially in individuals who are without an active social network.

References

1. Conwell Y, Thompson C. Suicidal behavior in elders. *Psychiatr Clin North Am.* 2008;31(2):333–356.
2. Segal DL, Lebenson S, Coolidge FL. Global self-rated health status predicts reasons for living among older adults. *Clinical Gerontologist.* 2008;31(4):122–132.

77. A 93-yr-old woman presents with erythrocytosis, hematocrit 49, and thrombocytosis, platelet count 533. She has a history of heart failure, COPD, gastritis, and osteoarthritis. Oxygen saturation is normal at 98% on room air. On physical examination, she is noted to have a palpable spleen tip.

Which of the following is the best choice for further diagnostic evaluation at this time?

(A) Screening colonoscopy
(B) Pulmonary function tests
(C) Bone marrow biopsy
(D) Peripheral blood testing for JAK2 mutation
(E) Peripheral blood flow cytometry

ANSWER: D

The myeloproliferative disorders, including polycythemia vera, idiopathic myelofibrosis, and essential thrombocythemia, overlap considerably; the recent discovery of the Janus kinase 2 (JAK2) mutation has helped to explain the pathophysiologic mechanism of many of their clinical similarities. A single, acquired point mutation in the JAK2 gene was reported in 2005 and was found to be present in most patients with Philadelphia chromosome–negative myeloproliferative disorders. JAK2 is a cytoplasmic tyrosine kinase involved in intracellular signaling by the receptors for erythropoietin, thrombopoietin, interleukin-3, granulocyte colony stimulating factor, and granulocyte-monocyte colony stimulating factor. The acquired mutation has been demonstrated in 95% of patients with polycythemia vera, 50%–60% of patients with essential thrombocythemia or idiopathic myelofibrosis, as well as in some patients with acute leukemia, suggesting the possibility of previously undiagnosed underlying myeloproliferative disorders.

The JAK2 mutation is already widely available as an allele-specific polymerase chain reaction assay and is being used as a clinical tool in simplifying diagnostic evaluation. Proposed diagnostic criteria allow for the diagnosis of JAK2-positive disorders without requiring a bone marrow biopsy. For example, the diagnosis of JAK2-positive polycythemia requires the presence of both a mutation in JAK2 and either high hematocrit (>52% in men, 48% in women) or an increased RBC mass. The JAK2 mutation allows for a noninvasive means of establishing a diagnosis of a treatable myeloproliferative disorder and should be used in the initial diagnostic evaluation of unexplained leukocytosis, polycythemia, or thrombocytosis.

References
1. Baxter EJ, Scott LM, Campbell PJ, et al. Acquired mutation of the tyrosine kinase JAK2 in human myeloproliferative disorders. *Lancet.* 2005;365(9464):1054–1056.
2. Campbell PJ, Green AR. The myeloproliferative disorders. *N Engl J Med.* 2006;355(23):2452–2466.
3. Tefferi A. JAK2 mutations in polycythemia vera—molecular mechanisms and clinical applications. *N Engl J Med.* 2007;356(5):444–445.

78. An 80-yr-old woman comes to the office because she has lost 4.5 kg (10 lb) in the preceding year, feels that everything she does is an "effort," and has begun using her arms to lift herself from her chair. She states that she is not depressed. She is accompanied by her daughter, with whom she lives.

Physical examination is normal except that she appears tired and has a slow, steady gait. She scores one positive response on the Geriatric Depression Scale. Results of a CBC, BUN, creatinine, electrolytes, and thyroid and liver function tests are normal. Frailty is diagnosed.

Which of the following is the most appropriate next step?

(A) Begin a trial of methylphenidate.
(B) Begin protein supplements.
(C) Begin a resistance-training exercise program.
(D) Encourage increased social interaction.
(E) Initiate a palliative care approach.

ANSWER: C

The clinical syndrome of frailty presents with multiple areas of decline: weakness, low energy or exhaustion, slowed walking speed, low physical activity, and weight loss. Many studies, each using different definitions of the syndrome, have found frailty to be associated with poor clinical outcomes, such as falls, functional decline, and mortality. A few studies have addressed interventions. Resistance training increases strength and function in frail nursing-home residents (SOE=A) and in patients recovering from hip fracture (SOE=A). Methylphenidate has been studied in small trials of medically ill adults, but results have been inconsistent. Protein supplements also have not consistently improved clinical outcomes. Social isolation appears to contribute to functional decline, but interventions to

enhance social interactions have not yet been shown to improve frailty. There is emerging evidence that severe frailty may not be reversible and that palliative care may be warranted. However, palliative care is premature in this patient, because treatment has not yet been attempted.

References
1. Binder EF, Brown M, Sinacore DR, et al. Effects of extended outpatient rehabilitation after hip fracture: a randomized controlled trial. *JAMA.* 2004;292(7):837–846.
2. Chin A, Paw MJ, van Uffelen JG, et al. The functional effects of physical exercise training in frail older people: a systematic review. *Sports Med.* 2008;38(9):781–793.
3. Fiatarone MA, O'Neill EF, Ryan ND, et al. Exercise training and nutritional supplementation for physical frailty in very elderly people. *N Engl J Med.* 1994;330(25):1769–1775.
4. Fried LP, Tangen CM, Walston J, et al. Frailty in older adults: evidence for a phenotype. *J Gerontol A Biol Sci Med Sci.* 2001;56(3):M146–156.

79. A 67-yr-old man comes to the office because he has noticed increasing weakness. Over the last 4 mo, he has had difficulty getting up from a chair and has been dropping things. More recently, he has had difficulty swallowing food. On examination, atrophy and fasciculations are noted in both legs, and reflexes are hyperactive in all extremities. Babinski sign is positive bilaterally. Gag reflex is absent.

Which of the following may improve survival for this patient?

(A) Vitamin B_{12}
(B) Immunoglobulin
(C) Plasmapheresis
(D) Steroids
(E) Riluzole

ANSWER: E

Amyotrophic lateral sclerosis (ALS) is a neurodegenerative disease that involves both upper and lower motor neurons. Patients often present with difficulty walking, dysphagia, dysarthria, and foot drop. On physical examination, patients may have hyperreflexia, clonus, positive Babinski sign, weakness, and atrophy fasciculations. In most cases of ALS, cognitive function is preserved. Affected individuals develop difficulty in dealing with respiratory secretions, with a higher incidence of pneumonia, and eventually die from respiratory failure.

Although treatment for ALS is targeted at being supportive, riluzole is thought to protect against glutamate toxicity, which may be involved in the pathogenesis of ALS. Riluzole probably improves survival by 3 mo on average (SOE=B). The beneficial effects of riluzole are very modest, and it is expensive. Adverse events are quite minor and are mostly reversible after riluzole is discontinued. Vitamin B_{12} is indicated for treatment of subacute combined degeneration. Plasmapheresis and high-dose immunoglobulin are used in the treatment of Guillain-Barré syndrome. Steroids are effective in patients with myasthenia gravis. This patient's findings are most consistent with a diagnosis of ALS.

References

1. Cwik V. ALS Clinical Motor Signs and Symptoms. In: Mitsumoto H, Przedboiski S, Gordan P, eds. *ALS*. New York: Taylor and Francie; 2006:99–115.
2. Dalbello-Haas V, Florence JM, Krivickas LS. Therapeutic exercise for people with amyotrophic lateral sclerosis or motor neuron disease. *Cochrane Database Syst Rev.* 2008 Apr 16;(2):CD005229.
3. Miller RG, Mitchell JD, Lyon M, et al. Riluzole for ALS/motor neuron disease (MND). *Cochrane Database Syst Rev.* 2007 Jan 24;(1):CD001447.
4. Mitsumoto H, Rabkin JG. Palliative care for patients with amyotrophic lateral sclerosis: "prepare for the worst and hope for the best." *JAMA.* 2007;298(2):207–216.

80. A 79-yr-old man comes to the office for advice about treatment options for localized prostate cancer. The cancer was identified during transurethral resection of the prostate for presumed benign prostatic hyperplasia. His prostate-specific antigen level is 3.6 ng/mL, Gleason score is 5, clinical stage is T1. He is concerned about adverse events associated with each of the treatment options suggested by his urologist. He has a strong aversion to the possibility of incontinence, especially because he is socially active. He is open to the idea of watchful waiting. History includes mild hypertension well controlled with atenolol and hydrochlorothiazide. He had a myocardial infarction 10 yr ago with no significant functional impairment. He is on simvastatin 10 mg/d and aspirin 81 mg/d to minimize risks of coronary heart disease.

Which of the following statements is most relevant to his situation?

(A) CT of the pelvis would provide information useful in deciding on therapy.
(B) External-beam radiation therapy minimizes the risk of incontinence and impotence.
(C) Cryoablation eliminates surgical risk and is as effective as external-beam radiation therapy.
(D) Active surveillance would be as effective as radical prostatectomy.

ANSWER: D

This patient has a low-risk prostate cancer: his prostate-specific antigen level is ≤10 ng/mL, Gleason score is ≤6, and clinical stage is T1. According to current guidelines, no further imaging evaluation is needed to guide therapeutic decisions (SOE=C). There have been no studies directly comparing external-beam radiation, cryotherapy, and radical prostatectomy. Radical prostatectomy has not been demonstrated to be more effective than watchful waiting in men ≥65 yr old, and its potential negative impact on quality of life is an important consideration for many patients (SOE=B).

References

1. Thompson I, Thrasher JB, Aus G, et al. Guideline for the management of clinically localized prostate cancer: 2007 update. *J Urol.* 2007;177(6):2106–2131.
2. Wilt TJ, Macdonald R, Rutks I, et al. Systematic review: comparative effectiveness and harms of treatments for clinically localized prostate cancer. *Ann Intern Med.* 2008;148(6):435–448.

81. An 80-yr-old patient comes to the office for a routine physical examination. She has mild hearing loss and is otherwise healthy. She takes a multivitamin and calcium citrate with vitamin D, and walks 1 mile daily. She states that she wishes to live to be 100 yr old and asks for advice about following the Mediterranean diet.

Which of the following is consistent with following the Mediterranean diet?

(A) Reduce fat intake.
(B) Reduce consumption of fish.
(C) Increase consumption of poultry.
(D) Increase consumption of legumes and whole grains.
(E) Increase consumption of bread and rice.

ANSWER: D

Mediterranean diets are characterized by high intake of vegetables, legumes, fruits, and unrefined cereals; moderate to high intake of fish; low to moderate intake of dairy, mostly as cheese and yogurt; low intake of meat; and modest intake of alcohol, mostly as wine. Mediterranean diets have up to 40% fat. What makes them healthy is the balance of fats: low intake of saturated fats; high intake of monounsaturated fats, especially olive oil; and intake of polyunsaturated fats to provide sufficient omega-3 fatty acid.

The Mediterranean diet has been associated with longevity in several studies. In a recent large-scale, prospective trial conducted by the National Institutes of Health and the American Association for Retired Persons, the Mediterranean diet was associated with reduced all-cause and cause-specific mortality. In men, the multivariate hazard ratios comparing high to low conformity to diet for all-cause, cardiovascular disease, and cancer mortality were 0.79 (95% CI, 0.76–0.83), 0.78 (95% CI, 0.69–0.87), and 0.83 (95% CI, 0.76–0.91), respectively. In women with high conformity to diet, this study found decreased risks that ranged from 12% for cancer mortality to 20% for all-cause mortality (P=.04 and P <.001, respectively).

Possible mechanisms of action for the Mediterranean diet include a high antioxidant capacity and low concentrations of oxidized low-density lipoprotein; high fiber and a low omega-6 to omega-3 fatty acid ratio, which potentially prevent cancer initiation and progression; and less chronic inflammation as evidenced by lower levels of C-reactive protein, interleukin-6, homocysteine, and fibrinogen, and by lower WBC counts (SOE=B).

References

1. de Lorgeril M, Salen P. Dietary prevention of coronary heart disease: the Lyon diet heart study and after. *World Rev Nutr Diet*. 2005;95:103–114.
2. Mitrou PN, Kipnis V, Thiebaut AC, et al. Mediterranean dietary pattern and prediction of all-cause mortality in a US population: results from the NIH-AARP Diet and Health Study. *Arch Intern Med*. 2007;167(22):2461–2468.
3. Trichopoulou A, Orfanos P, Norat T, et al. Modified Mediterranean diet and survival: EPIC-elderly prospective cohort study. *BMJ*. 2005;330(7498):991.

82. A 75-yr-old woman comes to the office for follow-up evaluation after an ischemic stroke 2 mo earlier. History includes hypertension and COPD. She had a transient ischemic attack 2 yr ago, after which she has taken aspirin 81 mg/d; since the ischemic stroke 2 mo ago, she has also been taking clopidogrel 75 mg/d. Other medications are lisinopril 10 mg/d, salmeterol 1 inhalation q12h, and tiotropium 1 capsule inhaled daily.

On examination, blood pressure is 135/80 mmHg, which is similar to readings before her stroke.

Laboratory results:

Total cholesterol	250 mg/dL
Low-density lipoprotein	180 mg/dL
High-density lipoprotein	50 mg/dL
Triglycerides	80 mg/dL

Which of the following should be done next?

(A) Discontinue aspirin.
(B) Discontinue clopidogrel; increase aspirin to 325 mg/d.
(C) Discontinue aspirin and clopidogrel; start warfarin.
(D) Start lovastatin 10 mg/d.
(E) Start warfarin.

ANSWER: A

The first priority for this patient is to reduce the risk of hemorrhage by discontinuing aspirin therapy. Recent clinical trials have documented an increased risk of hemorrhage with the combination of aspirin and clopidogrel versus monotherapy, with no added clinical benefit (SOE=A). Based on the 2008 American Heart Association/American Stroke Association (AHA/ASA) update for secondary stroke prevention, combination therapy of aspirin and clopidogrel is not routinely recommended for patients with ischemic stroke or transient ischemic attack unless they have a specific indication for this therapy (eg, coronary stent or acute coronary syndrome). Although alternative antiplatelet agents are often considered for patients with noncardioembolic events that occur while taking aspirin, there are no recommendations for selection of a specific agent (eg, clopidogrel versus extended-release dipyridamole plus aspirin) for the patient in this case. Thus, clopidogrel monotherapy is a reasonable option.

For patients who have had an ischemic cerebrovascular event while taking aspirin, there is no evidence that increasing the dosage of aspirin provides additional benefit (SOE=A). Further, in patients without atrial fibrillation, anticoagulation with warfarin is not more effective than aspirin therapy for secondary stroke prevention (SOE=A).

Statins help prevent ischemic stroke in patients with coronary heart disease. Until recently, it was less clear whether statins prevent secondary stroke in patients *without* overt heart disease. Results from the Heart Protection Study suggest that, in patients with cerebrovascular disease, statin use reduced overall vascular events but had no effect on recurrent stroke. However, based on data from the Stroke Prevention by Aggressive Reduction in Cholesterol Levels (SPARCL) trial, the AHA/ASA guidelines for secondary stroke prevention now recommend aggressive statin therapy (eg, atorvastatin 80 mg in the SPARCL trial) for patients with atherosclerotic ischemic stroke or transient ischemic attack and no known coronary heart disease, to reduce the risk of stroke and cardiovascular events. A statin more potent than lovastatin (eg, atorvastatin, rosuvastatin) should be selected (SOE=A).

References

1. Adams RJ, Albers G, Alberts MJ, et al. Update to the AHA/ASA recommendations for the prevention of stroke in patients with stroke and transient ischemic attack. *Stroke.* 2008;39(5):1647–1652.
2. Bhatt DL, Fox KA, Hacke W, et al. Clopidogrel and aspirin versus aspirin alone for the prevention of atherothrombotic events. *N Engl J Med.* 2006;354(16):1706–1717.
3. Cheng EM, Fung CH. Quality indicators for the care of stroke and atrial fibrillation in vulnerable elders. *J Am Geriatr Soc.* 2007;55(Suppl 2):S431–S437.
4. Diener HC, Bogousslavsky J, Brass LM, et al. Aspirin and clopidogrel compared with clopidogrel alone after recent ischemic stroke or transient ischaemic attack in high-risk patients (MATCH): randomized, double-blind, placebo-controlled trial. *Lancet.* 2004;364(9431):331–337.

83. An 82-yr-old woman is brought to the office to establish care. She requires complete assistance with ADLs. History includes moderate vascular dementia, atrial fibrillation, and systolic heart failure; medications include warfarin, atenolol, simvastatin, and lisinopril.

On physical examination, she has a 6-cm rectangular yellow bruise on her right buttock, a 3-cm circular purple bruise on her left forearm, and a 4-cm oval red bruise on her posterior neck.

Which of the following bruise characteristics raises suspicion of physical abuse?

(A) Size
(B) Shape
(C) Number
(D) Location
(E) Color variation

ANSWER: D

Among older adults, the risk of accidental bruising is increased by gait instability, medications, thinning of the epidermis, reduced subcutaneous fat, and increased capillary fragility. Older adults are more likely to take warfarin or NSAIDs, which add to ease of bruising. However, the location of this patient's bruises on her buttocks and neck raise suspicion of mistreatment rather than accidental trauma. In one study comprising 101 people (average age, 78 yr) from the community and nursing homes who were examined daily, 108 bruises were identified during the study period. Of these, 89% were on the extremities. No bruises were seen on the ears, neck, genitalia, buttocks, or soles of the feet. On the first day of observation, 16% of bruises were predominantly yellow. Reddish coloration was observed throughout the course of the bruises.

Although the size of a bruise does not necessarily suggest mistreatment, patients are more likely to recall the circumstance surrounding a large bruise (5–20 cm) on the trunk. It is cause for concern if an older adult has a large bruise on the trunk but cannot recall how it happened or gives an explanation inconsistent with the physical examination.

The shape of the bruise can be important if it suggests a pattern or method of injury, eg, a circular cigarette burn, or circumferential abrasions around the wrists suggesting restraint. In the absence of any suspicious pattern, the shape of the bruises on this patient does not suggest mistreatment.

The number of bruises would not trigger further assessment for abuse. However, multiple bruises clustered in a pattern inconsistent with the history should raise suspicion and prompt further assessment and documentation (SOE=C).

Reference

1. Mosqueda L, Burnight K, Liao S. The life cycle of bruises in older adults. *J Am Geriatr Soc.* 2005;53(8):1339–1343.

84. A 68-yr-old woman is brought to the emergency department because she woke up from an afternoon nap with a sudden onset of rotational vertigo and clumsiness of the right arm. She feels as though the world is tilting toward the right. She is unable to walk even with assistance, and she has a headache. History includes hypertension and type II insulin-dependent diabetes. Her medications include lisinopril, metformin, and aspirin.

On examination, temperature is 37.5°C (99.5°F). Blood pressure is 180/95 mmHg, pulse is 80 beats per minute, and respiratory rate is 16 breaths per minute. She has horizontal nystagmus and a negative head thrust test. She has difficulty both with making rapid alternating movements with the right arm and with toe-tapping or heel-to-shin movements on the right leg.

Which of the following is the most likely diagnosis?

(A) Cerebellar infarct
(B) Dorsolateral medullary stroke
(C) Meniere disease
(D) Herpes zoster infection of the inner ear (Ramsay Hunt syndrome)
(E) Benign paroxysmal positional vertigo

ANSWER: A

The sudden onset of vertigo with other focal neurologic symptoms makes a stroke most likely. A diagnosis of cerebellar or posterior fossa infarction should be considered in any patient with acute onset of vertigo. The patient should undergo immediate imaging, especially given her history of headache (SOE=C). In the event of posterior fossa hemorrhage, surgical evaluation may be lifesaving (SOE=D). The nystagmus in a cerebellar infarct may look similar to a peripheral nystagmus (horizontal torsional).

A head thrust test (or head impulse test) can help distinguish vestibular neuritis from stroke (SOE=C). With rapid, passive head rotation as the patient fixes on a central target, the normal response (ie, a negative test) is an equal and opposite eye movement that keeps the eyes stationary in space. The inability to maintain fixation after head rotation that requires a corrective gaze shift is abnormal (ie, a positive test). Vertigo with a negative head thrust test suggests central stroke. A positive head thrust test suggests a peripheral cause but does not absolutely exclude a stroke.

Patients can also present with an ocular tilt reaction that can be on the same side or on the opposite side of the cerebellar infarct. Dorsolateral medullary stroke (Wallenberg's syndrome) is usually accompanied by other focal neurologic signs and symptoms, including ipsilateral Horner's pupil, ipsilateral facial pain and loss of temperature sensation, ipsilateral central facial (lower face only) weakness, and contralateral pain and loss of temperature sensation in the arms and legs. It is often associated with artery-to-artery emboli from vertebral artery atherosclerosis to the posterior inferior cerebellar artery. Meniere disease, Ramsay Hunt syndrome, and benign paroxysmal positional vertigo do not present with clumsiness of the extremities.

References

1. Baier B, Bense S, Dieterich M. Are signs of ocular tilt reaction in patients with cerebellar lesions mediated by the dentate nucleus? *Brain*. 2008;131(Pt 6):1445–1454.
2. Newman-Toker DE, Kattah JC, Alvernia JE, et al. Normal head impulse test differentiates acute cerebellar strokes from vestibular neuritis. *Neurology*. 2008;70(24 Pt 2):2378–2385.

85. A 71-yr-old woman comes to the office to establish care. She has a history of major depressive disorder and gastroesophageal reflux. On baseline dual x-ray absorptiometry (DEXA) scan taken last year, T scores were −2.3 at the lumbar spine and −2.6 at the femoral neck. Laboratory and urine tests at that time excluded secondary causes of osteoporosis. Family history includes vertebral fracture in her mother and invasive breast cancer in several relatives. Her previous physician prescribed alendronate, which the patient did not tolerate because of its GI adverse events, and calcium and vitamin D supplements.

Which of the following is the best choice for treatment of this patient's osteoporosis?

(A) Nasal calcitonin
(B) Recombinant parathyroid hormone
(C) Risedronate
(D) Raloxifene

ANSWER: D

Raloxifene reduces the risk of clinical vertebral fractures in postmenopausal women, and it also reduces the risk of invasive breast cancer (SOE=A). It is a selective estrogen-receptor modulator (SERM) that acts as an agonist in some tissues and as an antagonist in others. In the Raloxifene Use for the Heart (RUTH) Trial for postmenopausal women with cardiovascular disease or multiple risk factors, women taking raloxifene for an average of 5.6 yr had lower rates of incident vertebral fractures and breast cancer, but increased risks of fatal stroke and venous thromboembolus than women in the placebo arm. The rates for coronary heart disease were similar in both groups.

Nasal calcitonin is much less effective against osteoporosis than bisphosphonates, estrogen, or recombinant parathyroid hormone (SOE=B). Most clinicians reserve the use of recombinant parathyroid hormone for patients who have sustained new fractures while on bisphosphonate therapy or for patients with very low T scores and high risk of fracture (SOE=A). The current recommended strategy is to use recombinant parathyroid hormone for 18–24 mo, and then a bisphosphonate to maintain gains in bone mineral density.

Risedronate is less likely to be tolerated by this patient because she had intolerable GI adverse events with another oral bisphosphonate. Intravenous bisphosphonate, however, is not associated with GI adverse events. In patients who had repair of a low-trauma hip fracture, infusion of zoledronic acid once yearly was associated with significantly lower rates of new vertebral and nonvertebral fractures and death (SOE=A).

References

1. Barrett-Connor E, Mosca L, Collins P, et al. Effects of raloxifene on cardiovascular events and breast cancer in postmenopausal women. *N Engl J Med.* 2006;355(2):125–137.
2. Lyles KW, Colon-Emeric CS, Magaziner JS, et al. Zoledronic acid and clinical fractures and mortality after hip fracture. *N Engl J Med.* 2007;357:1799–1809.
3. MacLean C, Newberry S, Maglione M, et al. Systematic review: comparative effectiveness of treatments to prevent fractures in men and women with low bone density or osteoporosis. *Ann Intern Med.* 2008;148(3):197–213.

86. An 86-yr-old man is brought to the emergency department because he has altered mental status and lower abdominal pain. He has a history of dementia and is cared for at home by his daughter. Over the past few days, he has had difficulty sleeping and his daughter has given him diphenhydramine 25 mg at bedtime.

On examination, temperature is 38°C (100.4°F), blood pressure is 178/90 mmHg, and pulse is 110 beats per minute. He is confused and thrashing around in bed. There is diffuse tenderness in the abdomen and lower abdominal fullness.

Laboratory results:

BUN	120 mg/dL
Creatinine	9.8 mg/dL
Potassium	6.8 mmol/L

Which of the following is the most appropriate *immediate* next step?

(A) Electrocardiography
(B) Placement of Foley catheter
(C) Renal ultrasonography
(D) Digital rectal examination
(E) Hemodialysis

ANSWER: A

This patient has severe acute renal failure most likely due to obstructive uropathy from urinary retention caused by the anticholinergic effects of diphenhydramine. Diphenhydramine is a well-established cause of urinary retention in men (SOE=A). Emergent attention is needed for severe hyperkalemia, which is the most life-threatening feature of this patient's presentation. Hyperkalemia is common in obstructive nephropathy because of poor glomerular filtration and potassium retention. The cardiac impact of this patient's hyperkalemia will determine further treatment. In this case, electrocardiography should be obtained at once. Hyperkalemia can lead to several changes that would be evident on electrocardiography, including peaking of T waves, prolongation of the QRS complex, and development of ventricular arrhythmias, including ventricular fibrillation. If any of these findings is present, intravenous calcium should be given immediately to stabilize the cardiac membrane (SOE=B), followed by immediate measures to reduce serum potassium (eg, intravenous insulin and glucose).

Hemodialysis may be required for patients who do not produce urine and are in severe acute renal failure. However, starting hemodialysis takes several hours, and other measures must be used during the crisis.

Acute urinary retention and acute renal failure are more likely to develop when medications with anticholinergic effects are given to older men, because they are likely to have some degree of prostatic hyperplasia and possible detrusor muscle weakness. The diagnosis of urinary obstruction is suggested by the history and by the finding of a distended, tender lower abdomen (urinary bladder). Renal ultrasonography would likely show bilateral hydronephrosis and hydroureter indicative of lower urinary tract obstruction. A Foley catheter should be inserted, with a large volume of urine expected.

References

1. Athanasopoulos A, Mitropoulos D, Giannitsas K, et al. Safety of anticholinergics in patients with benign prostatic hyperplasia. *Expert Opin Drug Saf*. 2008;7(4):473–479.
2. Mahoney BA, Smith WA, Lo DS, et al. Emergency interventions for hyperkalaemia. *Cochrane Database Syst Rev*. 2005;(2):CD003235.
3. Verhamme KM, Sturkenboom MC, Stricker BH, et al. Drug-induced urinary retention: incidence, management and prevention. *Drug Saf*. 2008;31(5):373–388.

87. Which of the following statements is true of older versus younger adults with anxiety disorders?

(A) Older adults are less likely to respond to medication for anxiety disorders.
(B) Older adults are less likely to respond to psychotherapy for anxiety disorders.
(C) Older adults are less likely to cite anxiety as a primary complaint.
(D) Older adults are less likely to have an anxiety disorder.

ANSWER: C

Older adults are less likely than younger adults to cite emotional distress as a chief complaint; this may be a cohort effect specific to the current generation of patients. Thus, clinicians need to be vigilant for anxiety disorders and their associated somatic presentations.

Anxiety disorders are seen in older adults, although phobias and panic disorder are unlikely to have first onset in old age. Because they are common in young adults as well as

highly chronic and relapsing in nature, anxiety disorders are present in many older adults (SOE=C).

Age is not a determinant of responsiveness to medication or psychotherapy in anxiety disorders.

Reference

1. Lenze EJ, Wetherell JL. Anxiety Disorders. In: Blazer DG, Steffens DC, eds. *The American Psychiatric Publishing Textbook of Geriatric Psychiatry*. 4th ed. Washington, DC: American Psychiatric Publishing Inc; 2009.

88. Which of the following is the most common nonpharmacologic intervention for urinary incontinence in nursing-home residents?

(A) Briefs or pads
(B) Toileting program
(C) Indwelling catheter
(D) External catheter

ANSWER: A

In the United States, from 48% to 65% of nursing-home residents have urinary incontinence. Urinary incontinence is associated with poor health status, urinary tract infections, skin breakdown, falls and fall-related injury, decreased quality of life, poor self-rated health, and psychologic distress. The cost of care for an incontinent resident is 2.5 times that of a continent resident, including extra nursing time, cleaning supplies, and laundry. The predominant nonpharmacologic intervention for urinary incontinence in long-term settings is use of briefs or pads (84%). Less frequently used are toileting programs (39%), indwelling catheters (3.5%), and external catheters (1.2%). Despite strong evidence that toileting programs are effective, most incontinent residents do not receive the scheduled interventions documented in the care plan.

Maintaining an effective continence program in nursing homes requires system-wide involvement of nursing-home administration and staff. Physicians, nurse practitioners, nurses, and nursing assistants perceive urinary incontinence differently, depending on their involvement in its recognition, assessment, and management. More than other providers, nursing assistants perceive urinary incontinence to have a significant impact on quality of life, ranking it second only to pain. Overcoming barriers in management of urinary incontinence requires better recognition of the correlation between incontinence and poor quality of life.

References

1. Dubeau CE, Simon SE, Morris JN. The effect of UI on quality of life in older nursing home residents. *J Am Geriatr Soc.* 2006;54(9):325–333.
2. Etheridge F, Tannenbaum C, Couturier Y. A system wide formula for continence care: overcoming barriers, clarifying solutions, and defining team member's roles. *J Am Med Dir Assoc.* 2008;9(3):178–189.
3. Lawhorne L, Ouslander JG, Parmelee PA, et al. Urinary incontinence: a neglected geriatric syndrome in nursing facilities. *J Am Med Dir Assoc.* 2008;9(1):29–35.

89. An 86-yr-old man who lives alone is prepared for discharge after hospitalization for an open leg wound and cellulitis that followed a fall at home. He is a retired professor; he reports no difficulty with ambulation, ADLs, or IADLs. Notes from the emergency medical services personnel indicate that they had difficulty gaining access to the patient's apartment because of clutter, and they noted the smell of urine and visible cockroaches. The patient reports no past medical history and takes no prescription medications.

On initial examination, the patient's temperature was 38.3°C (101°F), blood pressure was 180/90 mmHg, and heart rate was 110 beats per minute; body mass index was 18 kg/m². Blood glucose level by fingerstick was 350 mg/dL. He was disheveled and wore stained and malodorous clothing. He had several bags of papers with him. On his right medial malleolus there was a 4-cm, round, clean-based open ulcer with surrounding erythema and warmth. He had erythematous patches in his intertriginous areas and long dystrophic nails. Score on the Mini–Mental State Examination was 27 (he recalled only 1 of 3 words and was unable to draw intersecting pentagons). WBC count was 13,000/μL with 90% neutrophils, BUN was 30 mg/dL, creatinine was 1.6 mg/dL, and hemoglobin A_{1c} was 9%.

He was treated with intravenous antibiotics, an antihypertensive agent, and long-acting insulin. On discharge, he refuses home care services, home-delivered meals, and all prescription medications, insisting that he can take care of himself.

Which of the following is the most likely explanation for these findings?

(A) Dementia
(B) Delirium
(C) Depression
(D) Self-neglect
(E) Delusional disorder

ANSWER: D

This patient exhibits several cardinal features of self-neglect. Although there is no uniform, validated definition, expert consensus characterizes self-neglect as the presence of at least one of the following: 1) persistent inattention to personal hygiene or environment, 2) repeated refusal of services that can reasonably be expected to improve quality of life, and 3) self-endangerment through unsafe behaviors (SOE=C). Self-neglect can also be associated with disorders of aging that lead to executive dysfunction, which in turn leads to functional impairment in the setting of absent but needed medical or social services. When the individual loses the ability to recognize potentially unsafe living conditions, self-neglect ensues. According to prevalence estimates derived from Adult Protective Services data, self-neglect constitutes the most common category of investigated reports. In 2004, over 46,000 reports of self-neglect were made to Adult Protective Services, but this likely underestimates the true prevalence.

Dementia has been associated with self-neglect in longitudinal studies of cases identified by Adult Protective Services. Memory loss, especially executive dysfunction, plus impaired judgment can inhibit self-care. Dementia can also be associated with clutter if executive dysfunction impairs the individual's ability to sort and discard unnecessary items. Although this patient has a normal score on the Mini–Mental State Examination, it may actually reflect a decrease from his baseline, given his former occupation. However, the diagnosis of dementia alone does not adequately explain his refusal of medically indicated services. Self-neglect is also seen in the absence of cognitive impairment.

The hallmarks of delirium are an acute change in mental status, symptoms that fluctuate over minutes or hours, and inattention, in addition to altered level of consciousness or disorganized thinking. Although this patient was at risk of delirium because of his age, infection, and hospitalization, he does not exhibit features of acute delirium.

Depression has also been associated with self-neglect, possibly because it can increase the risk of nonadherence to medication, or because it can result in executive dysfunction. The patient in this case, however, has no other features of depression (eg, anhedonia, difficulty concentrating, sleep or appetite disturbance, fatigue, psychomotor changes, or suicidal ideation).

Delusional disorder most often develops in mid to late life and can manifest as poor insight and judgment and disorganized thinking. If this is seen concurrently with self-neglect, it can preclude the individual from seeking help. While this patient may misperceive his own environment—leading to apathy about the state of his apartment—he does not have any evidence of paranoia or any firmly held belief in something that is not true.

References

1. Abrams RC, Lachs M, McAvay G, et al. Predictors of self-neglect in community-dwelling elders. *Am J Psychiatry*. 2002;159(10):1724–1730.
2. Dyer CB, Goodwin JS, Pickens-Pace S, et al. Self-neglect among the elderly: a model based on more than 500 patients seen by a geriatric medicine team. *Am J Public Health*. 2007;97:1671–1676.
3. Pavlou MP, Lachs MS. Self-neglect in older adults: a primer for clinicians. *J Gen Intern Med*. 2008;23(11):1891–1896.

90. Which of the following is an age-related physiologic change that predisposes older adults to syncope?

(A) Inability to excrete a dilute urine
(B) Increased baroreflex control of arterial vasoconstriction
(C) Reduced baroreflex control of heart rate
(D) Increased relaxation of the left ventricle

ANSWER: C

Syncope is a sudden, transient loss of consciousness and postural tone with relatively rapid and spontaneous recovery. Transient cerebral hypoperfusion is the underlying pathophysiologic event. Older adults are particularly vulnerable because of age-related physiologic changes in heart rate and blood pressure regulation, structure and function of the left ventricle, and ability to preserve sodium and water. Changes in physiologic function are also related to comorbidity, medical conditions such as hypertension and atherosclerosis, reduced thirst, autonomic dysfunction, and use of medications that affect blood pressure regulation. Normal aging is

characterized by 1) reduced baroreflex control of the heart rate and peripheral vascular resistance in response to an orthostatic stress; 2) reduced left ventricular compliance, which can exacerbate preload-induced changes in blood pressure; and 3) changes in renal function that impair salt and water handling and predispose to dehydration.

References

1. Arbab-Zadeh A, Dijk E, Prasad A, et al. Effect of aging and physical activity on left ventricular compliance. *Circulation*. 2004;110(13):1799–1805.
2. Jones PP, Christou DD, Jordan J, et al. Baroreflex buffering is reduced with age in healthy men. *Circulation*. 2003;107(13):1770–1774.
3. Kenney WL, Chiu P. Influence of age on thirst and fluid intake. *Med Sci Sports Exerc*. 2001;33(9):1524–1532.
4. Stugensky KM, Neuberg GW, Maurer MS. Evaluation of syncope in the elderly patient. In: Aronow WS, Fleg JL, Rich MW, et al. *Cardiovascular Disease in the Elderly*. 4th ed. New York: Informa HealthCare; 2008:673–704.

91. A 72-yr-old woman comes to the office for a routine physical examination. Skin examination reveals multiple small (<5 mm) macules and papules scattered over her body. They have smooth, well-defined borders and brown, homogeneous coloration. A lesion on her right lower leg is a 7-mm papule with more irregular borders and tan-brown heterogeneous coloration.

Which of the following is the most appropriate next step?

(A) Laser therapy
(B) Cryosurgery
(C) Observation
(D) Excision
(E) Electrodesiccation

ANSWER: D

Recognizing the clinical signs of early melanoma improves detection rates and decreases overall mortality. Melanomas that are detected early are highly curable; most are found by the patient. No single clinical feature determines or excludes a diagnosis of melanoma.

The mnemonic ABCDE is used to identify features that can indicate melanoma in pigmented lesions: **A**symmetry, **B**order irregularity, **C**olor variation, **D**iameter (>6 mm), and **E**volving or changing. A definite change in a pigmented lesion, especially a change observed over a period of months, should arouse suspicion of an evolving melanoma. Most melanomas are varying shades of brown, but black, blue, gray, white, pink, or red can be seen, and some melanomas are not pigmented.

This patient's lesion is symmetric but has irregular borders, color variation, and a diameter of 7 mm: it requires immediate biopsy with experienced pathology review (SOE=C), rather than observation.

Skin lesions that are suspicious for melanoma should not be treated with laser, cryosurgery, or electrodesiccation.

References

1. Fox GN. 10 derm mistakes you don't want to make. *J Fam Pract*. 2008;57(3):162–169.
2. Lane JE, Dalton RR, Sangueza OP. Cutaneous melanoma: detecting it earlier, weighing management options. *J Fam Pract*. 2007;56(1):18–28.
3. Markovic SN, Erickson LA, Rao RD, et al. Malignant melanoma in the 21st century, part 1: Epidemiology, risk factors, screening, prevention, and diagnosis. *Mayo Clin Proc*. 2007;82(3):364–380.

92. A 74-yr-old man undergoes initial screening colonoscopy. He is asymptomatic and has no family history of colon cancer. A fecal occult blood test is negative. A 3-cm adenomatous polyp, without atypia, is removed via polypectomy. The colonoscopy is otherwise normal.

When should colonoscopy be repeated?

(A) 6 mo
(B) 1 yr
(C) 2 yr
(D) 3 yr
(E) 5 yr

ANSWER: D

Approximately 150,000 new cases of colorectal cancer are diagnosed each year in the United States. It is the third most common cancer diagnosed among men and women and the second leading cause of death from cancer, responsible for almost 50,000 deaths annually. Cancers of the colon and rectum most commonly develop from precursor adenomatous polyps. Colonoscopy enables early detection and prevention of cancer through polypectomy. While the initial screening colonoscopy and polypectomy are the most effective for reducing the incidence of colorectal cancer in patients with adenomatous polyps, follow-up studies are recommended.

The presence of any of the following factors confers the greatest risk: ≥3 adenomas, adenoma with high-grade dysplasia or villous features, and adenoma ≥1 cm. Patients with any of these factors should have follow-up colonoscopy 3 yr after polypectomy (SOE=C). Patients with 1 or 2 tubular adenomas that are <1 cm and have no high-grade dysplasia should have follow-up colonoscopy in 5–10 yr. Patients with hyperplastic polyps that have no malignant potential should have follow-up colonoscopy at 10 yr (SOE=C).

Patients with resected colorectal cancer are at risk of both recurrent cancer and metachronous neoplasms in the colon. Repeat colonoscopy should be performed within 1 yr of resection to search for additional neoplasms (SOE=C).

References

1. Levin B, Lieberman DA, McFarland B, et al. Screening and surveillance for the early detection of colorectal cancer and adenomatous polyps, 2008: a joint guideline from the American Cancer Society, the US Multi-Society Task Force on Colorectal Cancer, and the American College of Radiology. *Gastroenterology*. 2008;134(5):1570–1595.
2. Lieberman DA, Weiss DG, Harford WV, et al. Five-year colon surveillance after screening colonoscopy. *Gastroenterology*. 2007;133(4):1077–1085.
3. Rex DK, Kahi CJ, Levin B, et al. Guidelines for colonoscopy surveillance after cancer resection: a consensus update by the American Cancer Society and the US Multi-Society Task Force on Colorectal Cancer. *Gastroenterology*. 2006;130(6):1865–1871.
4. Walter LC, Lindquist K, Nugent S, et al. Impact of age and comorbidity on colorectal cancer screening among older veterans. *Ann Intern Med*. 2009;150(7):465–473.
5. Warren JL, Klabunde CN, Mariotto AB, et al. Adverse events after outpatient colonoscopy in the Medicare population. *Ann Intern Med*. 2009;150(12):849–857.
6. Winawer SJ, Zauber AG, Fletcher RH, et al. Guidelines for colonoscopy surveillance after polypectomy: a consensus update by the US Multi-Society Task Force on Colorectal Cancer and the American Cancer Society. *CA Cancer J Clin*. 2006;56(3):143–159.

93. A 72-yr-old man is hospitalized for 7 days because he had a large, left-hemisphere stroke, and he is then admitted to a rehabilitation unit for 30 days. His neurologic improvement is minimal, and he is admitted to a nursing home for long-term care. He has health insurance coverage only through Medicare Parts A, B, and D. He has $50,000 in savings and owns a modest home.

Which of the following will be the chief source of funding for his first year in the nursing home?

(A) Medicare Part A
(B) Medicare Part B
(C) Medicare Part D
(D) Medicaid
(E) Out-of-pocket payment

ANSWER: E

Long-term care is primarily funded by out-of-pocket payment and Medicaid. After hospital discharge, Medicare Part A provides full coverage for the first 20 days, and modest coverage ($128/day in 2008) for days 21 through 100 of a nursing-home admission, provided that the patient requires nursing care. Medicare does not pay for custodial long-term care. Thus, unless a patient has long-term care insurance, he or she pays out-of-pocket for nursing-home care. As is true of many older Americans, this patient does not have long-term care insurance. Because he has some savings, he is required to first "spend down" to a minimal level of worth (which varies state to state) before he qualifies for Medicaid. After a patient has spent down and enrolled in Medicaid, Medicaid becomes the chief source of long-term care financing.

References

1. Centers for Medicare & Medicaid Services. *Medicare & You 2008*. http://www.medicare.gov/Publications/Pubs/pdf/10050.pdf, p. 111 (accessed Nov 2009).
2. Centers for Medicare & Medicaid Services. *Medicaid Eligibility*. http://www.cms.hhs.gov/MedicaidEligibility/ (accessed Nov 2009).

94. A 76-yr-old man is admitted to a nursing facility 7 days after he was hospitalized for community-acquired pneumonia. He was treated with intravenous ceftriaxone and azithromycin, and received pantoprazole for stress-ulcer prophylaxis. Intravenous ceftriaxone was continued for 3 days in the nursing facility, for a total of 10 days of therapy. During rehabilitation, his roommate becomes the third resident in the section with confirmed *Clostridium difficile* infection.

In addition to using barrier precautions, which of the following would most likely stop the spread of *C difficile* in the facility?

(A) Use of sodium hypochlorite solution to clean rooms and bathrooms of patients with *C difficile* infection
(B) Use of alcohol-containing hand products by all staff, visitors, and patients
(C) Treatment of this patient with metronidazole
(D) Treatment with metronidazole of all patients colonized with *C difficile*

ANSWER: A

Clostridium difficile is an anaerobic, gram-positive organism capable of sporulating when environmental conditions are no longer optimal to support its continued growth. This feature enables the organism to persist on dry surfaces for weeks or months. In hospitals and nursing homes, *C difficile* travels from patient to patient mainly via the hands of healthcare workers, but also via bed rails, bed pans, toilets, bathing tubs, stethoscopes, and even telephones or remote controls. Prevention and control of *C difficile*–associated diarrhea in healthcare settings require attention to hand hygiene, contact precautions for patients with suspected *C difficile* infection, judicious use of antibiotics, and environmental cleaning. Achieving high-level compliance with these measures is a major challenge for infection-control programs.

To reduce the environmental burden of *C difficile*, the CDC recommends use of sodium hypochlorite solution for disinfection of all potentially contaminated surfaces (SOE=C). In one study, this approach reduced the number of contaminated environmental areas by half. In other studies, bone marrow transplantation units and geriatric medical units had fewer healthcare-associated *C difficile* infections during a period of hypochlorite use. The recommended approach is thorough cleaning followed by disinfection using hypochlorite-based germicides (SOE=B). Direct exposure to contaminated patient-care items and to frequently touched surfaces in patients' bathrooms has been implicated as a source of infection. Transfer of pathogen to patients via hands of healthcare workers is thought to be the most likely mode of transmission. The use of barrier precautions reduces *C difficile* transmission.

Alcohol-containing hand products or routine environmental cleaning with detergents does not eradicate *C difficile* spores. Handwashing with soap and water remains the most effective means of reducing hand contamination. Evidence is insufficient to recommend routine use of probiotics for treatment or prevention of *C difficile* diarrhea. Likewise, data are insufficient to support routine treatment of asymptomatic carriers. Although colonized patients can act as a reservoir for transmission of *C difficile*, decolonization is ineffective, because most patients become recolonized within weeks. Neither metronidazole nor vancomycin is recommended for treatment of asymptomatic carriers, although vancomycin appears more effective than metronidazole in achieving transient decolonization. Vancomycin may be useful during a hospital outbreak if temporary elimination of *C difficile* is thought necessary to reduce patient-to-patient transmission. The efficacy of metronidazole or vancomycin prophylaxis to prevent *C difficile* infection in patients who are receiving other antimicrobial agents is unproved.

It is unclear whether proton-pump inhibitors increase susceptibility to infection: some studies have identified proton-pump inhibitors as a risk factor, while others have found no association between their use and subsequent *C difficile* infection.

References

1. *CDC Guidelines for Environmental Infection Control in Health-Care Facilities*; 2003. http://www.cdc.gov/ncidod/dhqp/id_Cdiff_excerpts.html (accessed Nov 2009).
2. Gerding DN, Muto CA, Owens RC Jr. Measures to control and prevent *Clostridium difficile* infection. *Clin Infect Dis*. 2008;46(Suppl 1):S43–49.
3. Makris AT, Gelone S. *Clostridium difficile* in the long-term setting. *J Am Med Dir Assoc*. 2007;8(5):290–299.

95. A 75-yr-old woman comes to the office because she has had progressive difficulty walking over the past 10 mo. The first symptom she noticed was numbness of her feet. Over the next 4 mo, the numbness became more marked, ascended her legs, and eventually involved her fingers. As these symptoms progressed, her gait became increasingly unsteady. She now needs assistance to walk and has stopped driving.

She had partial gastric resection for peptic ulcer disease at age 40. History includes hypertension and mild osteoarthritis. The hypertension is well controlled with an ACE inhibitor and a diuretic. She also takes an "energy-boosting" multivitamin supplement obtained from a local health food store.

On examination, she has leg spasticity, generalized hyperreflexia, ankle clonus, and extensor plantar responses. She has decreased perception to light touch, pinprick, and position over the toes and fingers, and reduced vibratory sense below the knees bilaterally. Her gait is ataxic, and Romberg's sign is positive. The remainder of the examination is unremarkable.

Laboratory results:

Vitamin B_{12}	220 pg/mL
Hemoglobin	11.9 g/dL
Mean corpuscular volume	88 fL
Methylmalonic acid	0.18 μmol/L
Homocysteine	13 μmol/L

Serum electrolytes, creatinine, folate, immunoelectrophoresis, a paraneoplastic panel, and serologic tests for HIV and human T-lymphotropic virus 1 are normal. MRI of the spine shows a patchy increased T2 signal in the dorsal aspect of the cord from vertebra C3 to the lower thoracic cord.

Which of the following is the most likely cause of this patient's condition?

(A) Vitamin B_{12} deficiency
(B) Zinc deficiency
(C) Copper deficiency
(D) Vitamin B_6 deficiency
(E) Vitamin A toxicity

ANSWER: C

Copper deficiency myeloneuropathy is a distinct clinical entity that is being recognized with increasing frequency. Prompt diagnosis and institution of copper replacement therapy can prevent irreversible neurologic damage (SOE=A). The presentation is that of a progressive syndrome with clinical, electrophysiologic, and radiographic evidence of a myelopathy with predilection for the posterior columns and corticospinal tracts. Findings that should raise suspicion include sensory ataxia, leg spasticity, and peripheral paresthesias. These clinical manifestations mimic vitamin B_{12} deficiency in many ways. As with vitamin B_{12} deficiency, the neurologic manifestations due to copper deficiency can be seen in the absence of hematologic manifestations. A low serum copper or ceruloplasmin level is diagnostic.

In many cases, the cause of the copper deficiency is not certain. In several case series of patients with copper deficiency–associated myelopathy, a strong association has been found between copper deficiency and a history of partial or complete gastrectomy. Copper absorption in people is believed to occur in the stomach and proximal duodenum, so that prior surgery can lead to deficiency. Copper deficiency can also be caused by chronic zinc ingestion because zinc interferes with intestinal copper absorption. For these reasons, whenever dietary zinc supplements are used, the potential of inducing copper deficiency must be considered. Although the optimal dose and frequency of administration of zinc are not known, some clinicians advocate limiting use to every other day or even less frequently.

This patient's signs, symptoms, and clinical disease course are consistent with vitamin B_{12} deficiency. However, the low-normal vitamin B_{12} level and the normal serum methylmalonic acid and homocysteine levels make this diagnosis less likely. Measurement of serum methylmalonic acid and homocysteine is a sensitive method of screening for vitamin B_{12} deficiency, because their serum concentrations are increased early in vitamin B_{12} deficiency (SOE=A).

It is unlikely that either zinc or vitamin B_6 deficiency is the cause of the problems manifested by the patient in this case. Zinc deficiency can produce a wide array of signs and symptoms, including alterations in taste and smell, alopecia, immune dysfunction, hypogonadism, and delayed wound healing.

However, it is not known to cause the subacute combined systems degeneration seen in this case. The same is true for vitamin B_6. Although many frail or chronically ill older adults have low blood levels of vitamin B_6, overt clinical signs and symptoms of deficiency are rarely apparent. When they are seen, they are often vague and difficult to differentiate from signs and symptoms of other concurrent disease processes. The most common signs and symptoms include dermatitis, glossitis, major depressive disorder, confusion, convulsions, nervousness, irritability, insomnia, and muscle weakness. Vitamin B_6 deficiency can also cause anemia. In states of severe deficiency, difficulty can develop with walking. However, the spectrum of neurologic abnormalities seen in this case is not characteristic of vitamin B_6 deficiency.

Vitamin A toxicity can also produce a wide spectrum of signs and symptoms, including headache, photophobia, nausea, vomiting, abdominal pain, drowsiness, irritability, seizures, and desquamation after 24 hours. Chronic toxicity affects skin, mucous membranes, and musculoskeletal and neurologic systems. The musculoskeletal and neurologic manifestations include pain and tenderness (particularly in the long bones), migratory arthritis, idiopathic intracranial hypertension, blurred vision, and frontal headache, which is often the first indication of toxicity. Although patients with vitamin A toxicity may have difficulty ambulating, they would not have signs of subacute combined systems degeneration as seen in this case.

References
1. Kumar N. Copper deficiency myelopathy (human swayback). *Mayo Clin Proc*. 2006;81(10):1371–1384.
2. Kumar N, Ahlskog JE, Klein CJ, et al. Imaging features of copper deficiency myelopathy: a study of 25 cases. *Neuroradiology*. 2006;48(2):78–83.
3. Madsen E, Gitlin JD. Copper deficiency. *Curr Opin Gastroenterol*. 2007;23(2):187–192.
4. Prodan CI, Bottomley SS, Vincent AS, et al. Hypocupremia associated with prior vitamin B_{12} deficiency. *Am J Hematol*. 2007;82(4):288–290.

96. A 70-yr-old woman is referred for evaluation of fatigue and muscle aches. Symptoms include muscle pain in her neck and shoulders, difficulty falling asleep, and forgetfulness. She calls herself a "worrier" and says that her worrying has been more pronounced since she retired from an office job 5 yr ago. She describes brief periods of low mood, none longer than an hour in a given day. History includes major depressive disorder. She currently takes no medication.

Physical examination is normal. Her score on the Mini–Mental State Examination is 30/30.

Which of the following is the most likely diagnosis?

(A) Panic disorder
(B) Major depressive disorder
(C) Early Alzheimer's dementia
(D) Obsessive-compulsive disorder
(E) Generalized anxiety disorder

ANSWER: E

Generalized anxiety disorder is the most common anxiety disorder in older adults. It often escapes detection and treatment, in part because older adults often lack insight about the excessive quality of their anxiety. Its core feature is chronic worry (lasting at least 6 mo) that is distressing or impairing and that is perceived as difficult to control. Associated features can include muscle tension, insomnia, difficulty concentrating (often perceived by older adults as a memory complaint), fatigue, restlessness, and irritability. Older adults with generalized anxiety disorder usually avoid mental health treatment and instead visit their primary care provider or a medical specialist, focusing on the associated features of anxiety as the chief complaint.

As they do with other emotional issues, older patients with generalized anxiety disorder may downplay or deny the disorder when asked directly. A more productive discussion may result from asking how the patient feels when under stress; what sorts of issues trigger this kind of stress; and how often they feel anxious, worried, or concerned.

Generalized anxiety disorder carries a considerable human and economic burden in older adults. The impairment in quality of life is similar to that seen in major depressive disorder or other medical disorders, and use of healthcare resources is greater (SOE=B). Treatment options include third-generation antidepressants (such as citalopram,

escitalopram, or sertraline) and psychotherapy. Among psychotherapeutic options, cognitive-behavioral therapy is likely the most effective for generalized anxiety disorder, but relaxation training (usually a component of cognitive-behavioral therapy) alone is also effective and widely available (SOE=B).

The absence of persistent ("most of the day") mood disorder and high score on the Mini–Mental State Examination make major depressive disorder and early Alzheimer's dementia unlikely. The absence of intrusive anxiety-provoking thoughts relieved by ritualized behaviors and the absence of panic attacks make obsessive-compulsive and panic disorder unlikely.

References

1. Ayers CR, Sorrell JT, Thorp SR, et al. Evidence-based psychological treatments for late-life anxiety. *Psychol Aging*. 2007;22(1):8–17.
2. Beekman AT, Bremmer MA, Deeg DJ, et al. Anxiety disorders in later life: a report from the Longitudinal Aging Study Amsterdam. *Int J Geriatr Psychiatry*. 1998;13(10):717–726.

97. An 86-yr-old woman comes to the office because over the past 2 mo she has had increasing aches and pains and difficulty climbing the stairs to her home. She is still independent in all IADLs, but she has limited her activities and stays home most of the time. History includes dyslipidemia, systolic hypertension, and mild osteoarthritis; medications are chlorthalidone 12.5 mg/d, atenolol 25 mg/d, and atorvastatin 40 mg/d.

On examination, sitting blood pressure is 150/80 mmHg with heart rate 60 beats per minute and regular; standing blood pressure is 144/78 mmHg with heart rate 62 beats per minute. There is a 2/6 diamond-shaped murmur at the aortic area. The quadriceps muscles are tender, and there is mild pedal edema. She has difficulty getting up from a chair. Electrolytes, creatinine, and creatine kinase concentrations are within normal limits. Low-density lipoprotein cholesterol is 120 mg/dL.

What is the most appropriate next step?

(A) Increase chlorthalidone to 25 mg/d.
(B) Add acetaminophen 1 gram q8h.
(C) Add sertraline 25 mg/d.
(D) Discontinue atenolol.
(E) Discontinue atorvastatin.

ANSWER: E

The patient's muscle pain, tenderness, difficulty climbing stairs, and difficulty getting up from a chair strongly suggest statin-induced myopathy. Women are more likely than men to have statin-induced myopathy; other risk factors are older age, smaller body frame, frailty, multisystem disease (including chronic renal insufficiency, especially if due to diabetes), coadministration of certain medications (eg, fibrates, macrolide antibiotics), hypothyroidism, and alcohol abuse (SOE=B). Risk also increases perioperatively and with higher statin doses. In an observational study of patients (30% of whom were ≥65 yr old) receiving statin therapy, 10% had muscle symptoms.

Symptoms of myopathy are often nonspecific and can be difficult to differentiate from viral illnesses or other types of musculoskeletal disorders in older adults. Assessment of muscle strength can be helpful, such as the ability to get up from a chair or climb stairs.

Discontinuation of the statin, with follow-up assessment, is warranted and will help establish the diagnosis of statin-induced myopathy (SOE=A). Although an increase in creatine kinase concentration is often seen with statin-induced myopathy, a normal concentration does not exclude the diagnosis (SOE=B). In patients with statin-induced myopathy in whom statin therapy is clearly indicated, substitution of a different statin at a low dosage would be the recommended next step (SOE=C). Diagnoses such as depression, polymyalgia rheumatica, arthritis, and other musculoskeletal diseases should be considered if discontinuing the statin or substituting a different statin at a low dosage does not lead to clinical improvement.

Treating this patient symptomatically with acetaminophen, increasing chlorthalidone, adding sertraline, or stopping atenolol would not address the underlying cause of her problem. The longer she has myopathy, the more likely she is to have a reduced quality of life and/or functional reserve.

Statin treatment in older adults is effective in patients with established coronary artery disease or prior stroke for secondary prevention (SOE=A). Use of statins in patients ≥80 yr old who do not have cardiovascular disease is currently debated. The aggressiveness of lipid lowering should be based on remaining life expectancy, because primary prevention benefits of statin therapy have been estimated to require at least 4 yr of treatment and should be accompanied by monitoring for adverse events (SOE=C).

References

1. Bruckert E, Hayem G, Dejager S, et al. Mild to moderate muscular symptoms with high-dosage statin therapy in hyperlipidemic patients—the PRIMO Study. *Cardiovasc Drugs Ther*. 2005;19(6):403–414.
2. Grundy S. Promise of low-density lipoprotein-lowering therapy for primary and secondary prevention. *Circulation*. 2008;117(4):569–573.
3. Pasternak RC, Smith SC Jr, Bairey-Merz CN, et al. ACC/AHA/NHLBI clinical advisory on the use and safety of statins. *J Am Coll Cardiol*. 2002;40(3):567–572.
4. Sever PS, Dahlof B, Poulter NR, et al; ASCOT investigators. Prevention of coronary and stroke events with atorvastatin in hypertensive patients who have average or lower-than-average cholesterol concentrations, in the Anglo-Scandinavian Cardiac Outcomes Trial—Lipid Lowering Arm (ASCOT-LLA): a multicentre randomised controlled trial. *Lancet*. 2003;361(9364):1149–1158.

98. An 83-yr-old woman requests advice about activities to reduce the likelihood of developing dementia. She lives in a continuing-care community and is independent in ADLs and IADLs. She has had no falls.

On examination, she is alert and has a normal Mini–Mental State Examination score.

Which of the following is most likely to benefit cognition?

(A) Flexibility and stretching classes
(B) Moderate-intensity aerobic exercises
(C) Strength training
(D) Balance exercises

ANSWER: B

Physical activity is one of the most important means of health promotion in relation to cognition. In observational studies, people who are physically active are less likely than sedentary people to experience cognitive decline and dementia (SOE=A). Moderate-intensity aerobic exercises (150 min/wk) have been shown to produce at least as much cognitive benefit as cholinesterase inhibitor agents in patients with Alzheimer's dementia, over comparable follow-up periods (SOE=A). Other forms of physical activity are important to overall health but are not associated with improved cognitive performance (SOE=C). Moreover, multimodal exercise programs can be more difficult to adhere to over prolonged periods.

References
1. Baker M, Kennedy D, Bohle P, et al. Efficacy and feasibility of a novel tri-modal robust exercise prescription in a retirement community: a randomized controlled trial. *J Am Geriatr Soc.* 2007;55(1):1–10.
2. Larson E, Wagner L, Bowen J, et al. Exercise is associated with reduced risk for dementia among persons 65 years of age and older. *Ann Intern Med.* 2006;144(2):73–81.
3. Lautenschlager N, Cox K, Flicker L, et al. Effect of physical activity on cognitive function in older adults at risk for Alzheimer disease. *JAMA.* 2008;300(9):1027–1037.

References
1. Centers for Medicare & Medicaid Services. *Medicare & You 2008.* http://www.medicare.gov/Publications/Pubs/pdf/10050.pdf, pp. 17–18 (accessed Nov 2009).
2. Kaiser Family Foundation. *Medicare at a Glance.* In: *Talking About Medicare: Your Guide to Understanding the Program, 2009.* http://www.kff.org/medicare/7067/ataglance.cfm (accessed Nov 2009).

99. A 79-yr-old woman comes to the office because she has a fever and a cough. History includes hypertension, dyslipidemia, stable coronary disease, and osteoarthritis. She is enrolled in traditional Medicare Parts A and B; physicians in the office are participating Medicare providers. On physical examination, it is evident that a CBC is needed to exclude bacterial infection. The patient explains that she is financially strapped and needs to know what her out-of-pocket costs will be for the office visit and blood work. Today's visit is her fifth this year; the office visits have been her only medical encounters for the year.

How much is the patient's out-of-pocket cost for this visit?

(A)   Nothing
(B)   20% of the office visit fee and 0% of the laboratory fee
(C)   20% of the office visit fee and 20% of the laboratory fee
(D)   20% of the office visit fee and 100% of the laboratory fee
(E)   100% of the office visit fee and 100% of the laboratory fee

ANSWER: B

Outpatient services for this patient are covered through Medicare Part B. Because this is her fifth office visit this year, by this time she likely has paid all of her Part B deductible. After the deductible is paid, Medicare Part B covers 80% of office visits and 100% of diagnostic laboratory fees. The patient would be responsible for the other 20% of the office visit. In this case, CMS would reimburse the participating Medicare provider directly for 80% of the office visit and 100% of the laboratory fees, and the patient would then be billed for the remaining 20% of the office fee.

100. An 85-yr-old woman is brought to the emergency department by her family because of increasingly erratic behavior. Normally, she functions independently, but over the past few days she has been forgetful, confused, and disoriented. History includes pneumonia 6 mo ago, hypertension, and gastroesophageal reflux. Medications include hydrochlorothiazide, omeprazole, lisinopril, and a multivitamin.

On examination, her vital signs are within normal limits. She is inattentive and scores 16/30 on the Mini–Mental State Examination.

Laboratory results:

Sodium	128 mmol/L
Potassium	3.2 mmol/L
BUN	10 mg/dL
Creatinine	0.8 mg/dL
Urine sodium	80 mmol/L
Urine osmolality	450 mOsm/kg

Which of the following is the most likely cause of this patient's hyponatremia?

(A)   Syndrome of inappropriate arginine vasopressin secretion
(B)   Water intoxication
(C)   Hydrochlorothiazide
(D)   Omeprazole
(E)   Volume depletion and poor oral intake

ANSWER: C

Hyponatremia—an excess of total body water relative to sodium—is the most common electrolyte problem in older adults, with a prevalence as high as 14%. Symptoms of hyponatremia are generally manifested in the CNS and can include somnolence, cognitive impairment, seizures, and possibly coma. The symptoms are due to swelling of neurons caused by the change in osmotic gradient between the cells and the extracellular fluid. Most patients, however, exhibit no or few symptoms.

Thiazide diuretics are among the most common antihypertensive medications prescribed, and their use has increased since studies have found them highly effective in preventing serious cardiovascular outcomes in hypertensive patients. They are clearly implicated in causing many electrolyte abnormalities, including hyponatremia (SOE=B). Older adults seem particularly vulnerable: in one study, 26% of cases of hyponatremia in patients ≥65 yr old were attributable to thiazide diuretics. Older women are especially susceptible; the reason is unclear but may be related to the low-calorie, low-protein diet ("tea and toast") common in this population. The "tea and toast" diet leads to a lower urinary osmolar clearance and impaired free-water clearance. The exact pathogenesis of the condition is unknown. It may be caused by a combination of impaired urinary diluting ability, sodium loss, intracellular potassium depletion, and increases in arginine vasopressin (AVP) from mild volume depletion. The effects are often compounded by the concomitant sodium restriction that is prescribed for treatment of hypertension. More severe hyponatremia can be seen in patients who are ingesting large quantities of water. Thiazide diuretics must be discontinued in any patient presenting with hyponatremia.

The syndrome of inappropriate arginine vasopressin secretion (SIADH) is the causative factor in up to 26% of cases of hyponatremia. In the absence of thiazide diuretic use, SIADH is the likely diagnosis if renal function, adrenal function (ie, cortisol levels), pituitary and thyroid function, cardiac function, and hepatic function are all normal. Patients with SIADH have urine osmolality >100 mOsm/kg and urine sodium >20 mmol/L in the setting of euvolemia. In addition, the serum sodium concentration improves with restriction of water alone. SIADH is not diagnosed in patients on long-term diuretic therapy, because the volume depletion induced by the diuretic leads to secondary AVP secretion.

Water intoxication can lead to hyponatremia by overwhelming the capacity of the kidney to excrete water. Generally, renal excretory capacity is >8–12 L/d, so the water intake has to be excessive. Water intoxication is generally seen in patients with severe psychiatric disorders (psychogenic polydipsia).

Numerous medications are associated with development of hyponatremia through SIADH. The most common of these are third-generation antidepressants, anticonvulsants, and some antidiabetes agents. Case reports have associated many other medications with SIADH, but the instances are too anecdotal to attribute causation. For example, while omeprazole has been associated in case reports with SIADH, the incidence is likely extremely low, given the large number of patients who take omeprazole long-term. In the current case, thiazide use is a far more likely cause of the hyponatremia.

Hyponatremia can develop in patients with poor oral intake and volume depletion through activation of AVP. Generally, these patients appear clinically volume depleted and have very low levels of urine sodium.

References

1. Bissram M, Scott FD, Liu L, et al. Risk factors for symptomatic hyponatremia: the role of pre-existing asymptomatic hyponatremia. *Intern Med J*. 2007;37(3):149–155.
2. Friedman E, Shadel M, Halkin H, et al. Thiazide-induced hyponatremia. Reproducibility by single-dose challenge and an analysis of pathogenesis. *Ann Intern Med*. 1989;110(1):24–30.
3. The ALLHAT Officers and Coordinators for the ALLHAT Collaborative Research Group. Major outcomes in high-risk hypertensive patients randomized to angiotensin-converting enzyme inhibitors or calcium-channel blockers vs. diuretic. The antihypertensive and lipid-lowering treatment to prevent heart attack trial (ALLHAT). *JAMA*. 2002;288(23):2981–2997.

101. Which of the following is true regarding Medicare Advantage plans?

(A) Additional reimbursement is available to providers through a fee-for-service mechanism.

(B) Enrollees tend to be sicker and have higher medical costs than other Medicare beneficiaries.

(C) Patients can access any physician in the community, as with standard Medicare programs.

(D) Medicare Advantage plans receive payments that are higher than traditional fee-for-service Medicare plans.

ANSWER: D

Medicare Advantage plans are managed-care programs that served 22% of the Medicare population in 2009. These programs receive a capitated payment from Medicare. The capitation places them at financial risk, thereby giving them an incentive both to identify and help avert illness (and costs) in high-risk patients and to promote good health in participants with no chronic illness. Neither physicians nor other providers receive additional fee-for-service payments from Medicare. A 2007 study found that payments to Medicare Advantage plans are about 12% higher than average fee-for-service costs in the same area. Because patients may go only to physicians and other providers who contract with the Medicare Advantage plan in an area, access to providers may be more limited than with traditional fee-for-service Medicare. Older adults who choose Medicare Advantage plans are generally healthier and have lower medical costs than adults who opt for fee-for-service Medicare.

References

1. Berenson RA, Horvath J. Confronting the barriers to chronic care management in Medicare. *Health Affairs* Web Exclusive 2003. W3:37–53. http://www.dmaa.org/members/downloads/ConfrontingtheBarrierstoChronicCareManagement.pdf (accessed Nov 2009).
2. The Kaiser Family Foundation. *Medicare Advantage*. Washington DC: The Kaiser Family Foundation; 2009.
3. MedPAC (Medicare Payment Advisory Commission). *Medicare advantage benchmarks and payments compared with average Medicare fee-for-service spending*. MedPAC, Washington DC; 2007.

102. A 66-yr-old man who lives in a residential care facility is brought to the office to establish care, because his current internist is no longer comfortable managing his needs. He has severe mental retardation; its cause is unknown. His guardian is not significantly involved in his care. The patient is nonverbal except he yells when excited or agitated. His caregivers report that his agitation and need for one-on-one attention contribute to high staff turnover. Most nights he has discontinuous sleep, causing his behavior to deteriorate further the next day. He slaps his head, always in the same spot, apparently to communicate needs, seek attention, or provide self-stimulation. The caregivers note no medical concerns other than hard feces and constipation.

History includes cerebral palsy. The patient takes amitriptyline 25 mg at night for sleep and quetiapine 25 mg q12h. He is on no other medications, and this regimen has not changed for >2 yr. He ambulates only with assistance and can eat, drink, and take medication by mouth with caution. He is restless and seems uncomfortable in his wheelchair. Recent laboratory evaluation and ECG were normal.

Which of the following should be started?

(A) Increase amitriptyline to 50 mg before bed.
(B) Stop amitriptyline and begin zolpidem 5 mg.
(C) Increase quetiapine schedule to 25 mg q8h.
(D) Decrease quetiapine schedule to 25 mg before bed.
(E) Educate caregivers regarding effect of sleep disorders on behavior.

ANSWER: B

Disruptive behaviors are difficult to address in people with developmental disabilities who cannot verbalize their needs. Lack of sleep seems to worsen this patient's disruptive behaviors. The use of amitriptyline as a sleep aid is ineffective for him and may contribute to his constipation. A reasonable first step would be to stop amitriptyline and initiate a sleep medication that will not contribute to his constipation. This intervention alone may improve his sleep, increase his comfort, and decrease disruptive behavior, allowing his caregivers to respond with appropriate behavioral interventions (SOE=D).

Increasing the dose of amitriptyline at night may improve sleep but would also increase adverse events. The increased dose is likely to worsen constipation and other anticholinergic effects, and has potential for serious adverse cardiac problems. Lingering next-day lethargy might also worsen health or problem behaviors.

Decreasing the dosage of quetiapine may improve the patient's constipation but is unlikely to improve his sleep.

In this case, education of caregivers on medication and behavioral management issues would be a reasonable option if that alone would solve the patient's problems. Inconsistent or inappropriate responses by caregivers to difficult behaviors can create or perpetuate problems. However, the disrupted sleep and constipation are prominent problems for this patient that can be addressed promptly.

Further changes in management should await results of this intervention.

References
1. Harding J, Wacker DP, Berg WK, et al. Evaluation of relations between specific antecedent stimuli and self-injury during functional analysis conditions. *Am J Ment Retard.* 2005;110(3)205–215.
2. Lieberman JA. Managing anticholinergic side effects. *Prim Care Companion J Clin Psychiatry.* 2004;6(Suppl 2):20–23.
3. Rooker GW, Roscoe EM. Functional analysis of self-injurious behavior and its relation to self-restraint. *J Appl Behav Anal.* 2005;38(4):537–542.
4. http://www.effectivehealthcare.ahrq.gov (accessed Nov 2009).

103. An 82-yr-old woman comes to the office for a routine visit. She recently moved in with her daughter, who manages her medications. Last week, she tripped on the step at the entry to the kitchen, fell, and fractured her wrist. She has mild dementia, hypertension, dyslipidemia, osteoarthritis, and a history of duodenal ulcer. She has early cataracts in both eyes and wears glasses with multifocal lenses. Medications include donepezil, metoprolol, hydrochlorothiazide, simvastatin, omeprazole, a multivitamin, and acetaminophen.

On examination, blood pressure is 140/70 mmHg when the patient lies down, and 130/74 mmHg when standing. The remainder of the examination is unchanged from previous visits. She completes the Timed Up and Go test in 12 seconds.

Which of the following would decrease the likelihood of another fall?

(A) Treatment of postural hypotension
(B) Wearing single-distance glasses while walking
(C) Use of a cane or walker for better balance
(D) Review of medications

ANSWER: B

This patient has recently moved and is likely not yet familiar with her daughter's house and the step up to the kitchen. The multifocal lenses in her eyeglasses put her at risk of tripping (SOE=A). Multifocal lenses impair contrast sensitivity and depth perception because the wearer looks down through the near-vision, lower segment of the lens. Studies have shown that people wearing multifocal lenses are more likely to trip on a step because of inaccurate judgment of the step height; changing to single-distance eyeglasses improves judgment of foot placement.

The decrease in the patient's systolic blood pressure when she moves from lying down to standing position is <20 mmHg and does not meet the criterion for postural hypotension. Although her strength and balance have not been tested in detail, her 12-second Timed Up and Go test time indicates good walking and transfer ability, making the need for an assistive device unlikely.

A regimen of more than four medications increases a person's risk of falling. Medication review, with the goal of possibly reducing the number or dosage of medications, is a good strategy for managing fall risk. However, the information presented does not suggest that medications were a primary contributing factor to this patient's fall.

References
1. Johnson L, Buckley JG, Harley C, et al. Use of single-vision eyeglasses improves stepping precision and safety when elderly habitual multifocal wearers negotiate a raised surface. *J Am Geriatr Soc.* 2008;56(1):178–180.
2. Lord SR. Visual risk factors for falls in older people. *Age Ageing.* 2006;35(Suppl 2):ii42–ii45.
3. Tinetti ME. Clinical practice. Preventing falls in elderly persons. *N Engl J Med.* 2003;348(1):42–49.

104. A 70-yr-old woman comes to the office because she has had a malodorous vaginal discharge for 1 wk. She has vulvovaginal burning, itching, and soreness that have intensified over the past few months. At menopause 15 yr ago, she had similar symptoms, minus the discharge, and hot flashes. She was treated with cyclic oral estrogen and progesterone, but she stopped hormone replacement therapy after several years because she was concerned about adverse events. After the hot flashes abated, she had increasing vaginal soreness, pain, and burning after intercourse. In the past 10 yr, she has had 2 urinary tract infections, the most recent >1 yr ago. She recently tried application of aloe vera gel in an effort to relieve the itching, without effect. She does not wish to go back on hormone therapy.

On examination, there is redness and erythema in the vulvovaginal area, sparse pubic hair, and decreased vaginal moisture. Insertion of an adult speculum is moderately difficult and results in slight bleeding. Mucosa appears inflamed. Occasional vaginal petechiae are evident, and there are some fissures on the vaginal walls. There are no vaginal folds. No growths, plaques, or suspicious structures are seen or palpated. Serosanguineous discharge is present, with a pH of 6.8. A vaginal smear taken from the upper lateral third of the vagina reveals increased parabasal cells, an inflammatory exudate, and classic "blue blobs" (basophilic structures).

Which of the following is the most likely explanation for these findings?

(A) Candidiasis
(B) Atrophic vaginitis
(C) Psoriasis
(D) Vaginal cancer

ANSWER: B

With menopause, loss of estrogen results in atrophy of vulvar and vaginal epithelium. In vaginal atrophy, the number of superficial mature cells of the vagina are reduced, with a shift in cell structure to parabasal cells with a high nuclear to cytoplasmic ratio. These cells do not produce much glycogen, on which lactobacilli depend. Vaginal pH becomes higher than 4.5 because of decreased lactic acid production, and lactobacilli become fewer or disappear. There may be a shift toward coliform organisms. Vaginal rugae smooth out, the mucosa thins, and fissures may develop. Vaginal smears show WBCs and decreased or no lactobacilli (SOE=A).

Candidiasis usually causes a cheesy discharge with hyphae, not a serosanguineous discharge. It is usually seen at a younger age, or in the setting of diabetes or recent antibiotic use (SOE=B). This patient has no history of psoriasis. When psoriasis is present, its spread is symmetric, it does not involve the vagina, and it causes scaly red lesions. Cervical or vaginal cancer, although uncommon in this age group, can also be associated with a serosanguineous discharge. Usually, there is evidence of suspicious lesions, new growths, or areas of induration, any of which should be biopsied. Because no suspicious lesions were seen or palpated, vaginal cancer is unlikely. The 2003 guidelines from the U.S. Preventive Services Task Force recommend discontinuing screening for cervical cancer after age 65 if previous results were consistently normal (SOE=B). However, a Pap smear would be prudent in the presence of a serosanguineous discharge (SOE=B).

References
1. Bachmann G, Lobo RA, Nachtigall L, et al. Efficacy of low-dose estradiol vaginal tablets in the treatment of atrophic vaginitis: a randomized controlled trial. *Obstet Gynecol.* 2008;111(1):67–76.
2. Nwokolo NC, Boag FC. Chronic vaginal candidiasis. Management in the postmenopausal patient. *Drugs Aging.* 2000;16(5):335–339.
3. Sirovich BE, Welch HG. The frequency of pap smear screening in the United States. *J Gen Intern Med.* 2004;19(3):243–250.
4. U.S. Preventive Services Task Force. *Cervical Cancer Screening.* January 2003. Rockville, MD: Agency for Healthcare Research and Quality. Available at: http://www.ahrq.gov/clinic/uspstf/uspscerv.htm (accessed Nov 2009).

105. Which one of the following statements about smoking and older adults is true?

(A) Older smokers who quit gain substantial health benefits.
(B) Most smokers will attempt to quit only if they are supported by counseling or pharmacologic treatments.
(C) Older hospitalized patients are as likely as younger inpatients to receive smoking cessation interventions.
(D) Medicare does not cover tobacco cessation counseling for beneficiaries who have smoking-related illnesses.
(E) Brief interventions delivered by healthcare professionals do not affect rates of smoking cessation.

ANSWER: A

Approximately 1 in 10 older adults currently smokes. Quitting at an older age can yield substantial health benefits: compared with adults who continue smoking, men ≥65 yr old who quit gain 1.4–2 yr in longevity, and women ≥65 yr old who quit gain 2.7–3.7 yr. Improvements are observed in comorbid conditions as well (SOE=B).

The vast majority of smokers who attempt to quit each year do so without benefit of either behavioral or pharmacologic treatments. Among adults hospitalized for acute myocardial infarction, older adults who smoke are significantly less likely to receive interventions for smoking cessation than younger patients who smoke. Physicians are less aggressive when counseling older adults about smoking cessation.

In 2005, CMS estimated that 10% of its total annual budget is spent on smoking-related illnesses. As a result of the analysis, CMS now covers cessation counseling for Medicare beneficiaries who have smoking-related illnesses or who are taking medications that are affected by tobacco use. Medicare's prescription drug benefit now covers physician-prescribed smoking cessation treatments.

There is substantial evidence that brief interventions by healthcare providers can affect smoking cessation rates. The 5-step intervention is one such evidence-based approach: 1) **ask** about smoking at every visit; 2) **advise** every smoker to stop; 3) **assess** the patient's readiness to quit; 4) **assist** patients, whether they are ready to quit or not; and 5) **arrange** for a follow-up visit to readdress smoking cessation.

References

1. Brown DW, Croft JB, Schenck AP, et al. Inpatient smoking-cessation counseling and all-cause mortality among the elderly. *Am J Prev Med*. 2004;26(2):112–118.
2. Rice VH, Stead LF. Nursing interventions for smoking cessation. *Cochrane Database Syst Rev*. 2008;(1):CD001188.
3. Shiffman S, Brockwell SE, Pillitteri JL, et al. Individual differences in adoption of treatment for smoking cessation: demographic and smoking history characteristics. *Drug Alcohol Depend*. 2008;93(1-2):121–131.
4. Taylor DH, Hasselblad V, Henley J, et al. Benefits of smoking cessation for longevity. *Am J Public Health*. 2002;92(6):990–996.
5. http://www.cms.hhs.gov/SmokingCessation/ (accessed Nov 2009).

106. An 80-yr-old man with diabetes and osteoporosis comes to the office for consultation regarding his pain regimen. He has severe pain related to diabetic neuropathy and back pain related to multiple compression fractures. He takes hydrocodone/acetaminophen 2 tablets q6h, which helps the back pain but does little for the neuropathic pain.

Which of the following medications is an appropriate alternative to hydrocodone/acetaminophen for control of this patient's pain?

(A) Meperidine
(B) Propoxyphene
(C) Butorphanol
(D) Nalbuphine
(E) Methadone

ANSWER: E

Using a single agent for this patient's two different types of pain—nociceptive and neuropathic—would be ideal. Opioids have some efficacy in treating neuropathic pain, although tricyclic antidepressants and anticonvulsants are more effective (SOE=A).

Of the medications listed, methadone is the most appropriate. In addition to having mu-opioid receptor activity, methadone has antagonist activity at the NMDA receptor, making it useful in cases of opioid tolerance and neurotoxicity. Methadone inhibits reuptake of both norepinephrine and serotonin, making it potentially more effective than other opioids in the treatment of neuropathic pain, although this claim is debated (SOE=C). Methadone should be used cautiously because it has complicated pharmacokinetics and can cause prolongation of the QT_c interval (SOE=C).

Neither propoxyphene nor meperidine is recommended for use in older adults (SOE=B). Propoxyphene can accumulate in older adults and cause ataxia, dizziness, tremulousness, and seizures; it has never been shown to offer more analgesia than placebo. Meperidine is metabolized to normeperidine, which has no analgesic properties but can accumulate in patients with decreased kidney function, causing tremulousness, myoclonus, and seizures. Mixed agonist-antagonist agents such as nalbuphine and butorphanol can cause restlessness and tremulousness, and therefore should be avoided in older adults (SOE=C).

References

1. Barry PJ, O'Keefe N, O'Connor KA, et al. Inappropriate prescribing in the elderly: a comparison of the Beers criteria and the improved prescribing in the elderly tool (IPET) in acutely ill elderly hospitalized patients. *J Clin Pharm Ther*. 2006;31(6):617–626.
2. Eisenberg E, McNicol ED, Carr DB, et al. Efficacy and safety of opioid agonists in the treatment of neuropathic pain of nonmalignant origin: systematic review and meta-analysis of randomized controlled trials. *JAMA*. 2005;293(24):3043–3052.

3. Wong MC, Chung JW, Wong TK, et al. Effects of treatments for symptoms of painful diabetic neuropathy: systematic review. *BMJ.* 2007;335(7610):87–93.
4. Nicholson AB. Methadone for cancer pain. *Cochrane Database Syst Rev.* 2007;(4):CD003971.

107. A 75-yr-old man who has recently entered a hospice program is evaluated for chest pain. He has an esophageal stent and has had chemotherapy for esophageal cancer. He is having difficulty swallowing solids and has mild nausea and shortness of breath. He receives morphine 30 mg po q3h. Over the past 24 hours, he has also received 4 doses of morphine 10 mg IV for breakthrough pain. He is alert but has difficulty swallowing pills.

On examination, he has sufficient subcutaneous fat to allow use of a fentanyl patch.

Which of the following would be an appropriate starting dose of fentanyl for replacement of the oral pain regimen?

(A) 25 mcg/h topical, q72h
(B) 50 mcg/h topical, q72h
(C) 75 mcg/h topical, q72h
(D) 125 mcg/h topical, q72h

ANSWER: D

Transdermal fentanyl can be extremely effective for patients with persistent pain who have difficulty taking oral medications. Because this patient has chronic pain, can tolerate opioids, and is having difficulty swallowing, transdermal fentanyl would be an appropriate analgesic for him. The patch requires 12–24 h to achieve full analgesic effect, or to wear off after removal, so this patient should continue to receive hydromorphone IV for 12–24 h until the fentanyl starts to take effect. Fentanyl is not appropriate when patients have intermittent fevers or diaphoresis, because these may cause variable absorption. Also, patients who have little or no subcutaneous fat may not absorb fentanyl adequately. Fentanyl should not be used in opioid-naive patients.

Opioid conversion can be facilitated by equianalgesic calculators (many are available on line). Although many equianalgesic calculators are available, many conversion tables represent an oversimplification of pharmacologic principles that cannot substitute for clinical experience and caution. Conversion from intravenous morphine to a different agent requires several steps:

1) Calculate the total dose of morphine that the patient has received over the past 24 hours. This patient has received 240 mg oral morphine over the past 24 hours (30 mg q3h = 240 mg in 24 hours) plus 10 mg IV morphine × 4 doses × 3 (conversion of IV to oral) = 120 mg.

So, the total dose of morphine in this case is 240 mg + 120 mg = 360 mg oral morphine (equivalents) over 24 hours.

2) Convert the total oral dose equivalent of morphine to fentanyl equivalent (transdermal fentanyl is generally one-half the total 24-hour oral morphine dose). In this case, 360 mg oral morphine equals 180 mcg fentanyl.

3) Reduce the fentanyl dose by 25% because patients cannot tolerate a new opioid as well as the old opioid. In this case, 25% of 180 mcg fentanyl = 45 mcg; 180 − 45 = 135 mcg fentanyl. 125 mcg is the closest answer.

4) Breakthrough pain treatment should continue at 10% of the total daily dose: morphine 10 mg IV q2h prn, or morphine 30 mg po q2h prn.

References
1. Arcuri E. Pharmacological management of cancer pain in the elderly. *Drugs Aging.* 2007;24(9):761–776.
2. Quigley C. Opioid switching to improve pain relief and drug tolerability. *Cochrane Rev.* 2004;(3):1–34.

108. A 75-yr-old man was admitted to the hospital for an elective left total-knee replacement for intractable pain. He was scheduled to undergo surgery 2 mo earlier, but surgery was delayed because of deep venous thrombosis in his right leg treated with warfarin. The warfarin was discontinued 5 days before admission, and he received bridging low-molecular-weight heparin. Total knee replacement was performed without complication, and oral warfarin was restarted at 10 mg/d along with the bridging low-molecular-weight heparin. Three days after surgery, his INR is 9.5. There is no evidence of bleeding, and his hematocrit is stable. Orders are written for close observation for evidence of hemorrhage and for repeat INR in 24 hours.

Which of the following is the most appropriate next step?

(A) Discontinue warfarin.
(B) Discontinue warfarin; administer vitamin K, 10 mg SC q6h for 4 doses.
(C) Discontinue warfarin; immediately transfuse 4 units of fresh frozen plasma.
(D) Discontinue warfarin; administer 1 dose of vitamin K, 5 mg po.
(E) Omit next warfarin dose, then restart warfarin at 25% of earlier dose.

ANSWER: D

In older adults, initial oral dosing of warfarin at 5 mg/d will achieve an INR >2 in 4–5 days and will help avoid over-anticoagulation—and the associated risk of hemorrhage—seen with higher dosing regimens (SOE=A).

Warfarin dosing should be immediately held if the INR exceeds 9, and if there is no evidence of active bleeding, the patient should receive a dose of vitamin K 5–10 mg po. The INR should be repeated in 24 h. If bleeding is evident, the patient should receive a slow intravenous infusion of vitamin K along with fresh frozen plasma to correct the iatrogenic coagulopathy and promote hemostasis. Because this patient demonstrates no evidence of active bleeding, intravenous vitamin K and fresh frozen plasma are not indicated (SOE=C).

Warfarin can be restarted at a lower dose only after the INR is in a therapeutic range. Repeated dosing of subcutaneous vitamin K is not warranted and can make subsequent anticoagulation difficult when restarting warfarin (SOE=C).

A history of previous response to warfarin dosing would have been helpful in this case, as would a history of the patient's dietary patterns and intake of herbal compounds.

References

1. Ansell J, Hirsh J, Hylek E, et al; American College of Chest Physicians. Pharmacology and management of the vitamin K antagonists: American College of Chest Physicians Evidence-Based Clinical Practice Guidelines (8th Edition). *Chest*. 2008;133(6 Suppl):160S–198S.
2. O'Donnell M, Kearon C. Perioperative management of oral anticoagulation. *Clin Geriatr Med*. 2006;22(1):199–213.
3. Van Walraven C, Oake N, Wells PS, et al. Burden of potentially avoidable anticoagulant induced hemorrhage and thromboembolic events in the elderly. *Chest*. 2007;131(5):1508–1515.

109. Which of the following has been shown to be of benefit in reducing pressure ulcers in acute-care settings?

(A) Standard nutritional supplements for older patients
(B) Specialized foam mattress hospital bed
(C) Patient rotation q4h on regular hospital mattress
(D) Specialized foam-mattress overlay on operating table
(E) Standard sheepskin overlay on hospital bed

ANSWER: D

The prevalence of pressure ulcers in acute-care settings ranges from 0.4% to 38% based on observational studies. Patients with pressure ulcers have a mortality risk 2–6 times greater than patients with intact skin. In 2000 and 2001, pressure ulcers were cited as 1 of the top 3 in-hospital errors that lead to patient deaths; in an effort to improve care, as of October 2008 CMS no longer reimburses hospitals for costs due to pressure ulcers that develop during hospitalization.

In 2006, in a systematic review of trials of different interventions, evidence was sufficient to support use of specialized foam-mattress overlays on operating tables to reduce pressure ulcers (SOE=B). There was no difference in prevention of pressure ulcers between specialized foam mattresses and regular hospital beds (SOE=B). Special support surfaces may allow patients to be turned less frequently than q2h, but turning q4h has not been shown to reduce pressure ulcers. Specialized sheepskin overlays, which are thicker and denser than standard sheepskin overlays, help prevent pressure ulcers; standard sheepskin overlays do not (SOE=B).

The relationship between nutritional intake and prevention of pressure ulcers is based on limited evidence. Which specific nutrients offer the best protection is unclear. Evidence is mounting that nutritional supplementation for malnourished patients prevents wounds and helps healing (SOE=C), but there is no strong evidence that it benefits healthy older adults.

References

1. Ayello EA, Lyder CH. Protecting patients from harm: preventing pressure ulcers in hospital patients. *Nursing.* 2007;37(10):36–40.
2. Langemo D, Anderson J, Hanson D, et al. Nutritional considerations in wound care. *Adv Skin Wound Care.* 2006;19(6):297–303.
3. Reddy M, Gill S, Rochon P. Preventing pressure ulcers: a systematic review. *JAMA.* 2006;296(8):974–984.

110. An 86-yr-old woman is hospitalized for symptoms of abdominal pain, poor appetite, and weight loss that have progressed over the last 3 mo. History includes coronary artery disease and type 2 diabetes mellitus. Her physical functioning has declined: she can walk only a few steps and is dependent in all ADLs except feeding.

CT of the abdomen and chest strongly suggest metastatic pancreatic cancer.

The patient has undergone multiple procedures and hospitalizations in the past, and she states that she does not want further diagnostic studies or interventions. The patient and her daughter are interested in hospice.

Which of the following services is covered under the Medicare Hospice Benefit?

(A) Room and board in a long-term care facility
(B) Nursing care in a postacute-care nursing facility
(C) Hospital bed and bedside commode for home
(D) Private-duty caregiver at home
(E) Medications for diabetes mellitus and coronary artery disease

ANSWER: C

Patients with Medicare Part A are eligible for the Medicare Hospice Benefit if they have a chronic or terminal illness with a life expectancy of ≤6 mo. Once a patient chooses hospice care, he or she signs off Medicare Part A and signs on for the Medicare Hospice Benefit. This benefit covers a variety of services related to the terminal diagnosis, including the provision of durable medical equipment, such as a hospital bed and a bedside commode.

The benefit does not cover room and board in a long-term care facility. Patients may live in a house, an adult congregate-living facility (such as an assisted-living facility) for board

and care, or a long-term care facility. Room and board is typically paid for by personal funds or through Medicaid.

The hospice benefit does not cover nursing care in a postacute-care nursing facility. There are 4 levels of hospice care: routine home care, continuous home care, inpatient respite care, and general inpatient care. Most patients using the hospice benefit receive routine home care. Patients with pain or other symptoms that cannot be managed at home may require general inpatient care in a freestanding hospice unit or in a dedicated bed at a hospital or long-term care facility until the patient's symptoms are under control.

While the hospice benefit includes services from a variety of health professionals, it does not cover private-duty caregivers. It covers home-health aides, homemaker services, nursing visits, physician visits, social services, counseling, physical therapy, occupational therapy, and speech therapy if indicated. The hospice benefit covers medications for comfort and palliation needed because of the terminal illness, not for cure of the terminal illness. The hospice benefit does not cover medications for nonterminal conditions.

References

1. American Academy of Hospice and Palliative Medicine. *The Medicare Hospice Benefit.* http://www.aahpm.org/pdf/mhb.pdf (accessed Nov 2009).
2. Centers for Medicare and Medicaid Services. *Medicare Hospice Benefits.* www.medicare.gov/publications/Pubs/pdf/02154.pdf (accessed Nov 2009).

111. A 92-yr-old man with Alzheimer's disease is brought to the office by his daughter because over the past several months he has become increasingly aggressive toward his wife and home health aide. His daughter is worried about their safety and asks that he be given medication to control his aggression. Discussion ensues regarding different psychotropic options.

Which of the following is associated with increased mortality?

(A) Antipsychotic agents
(B) Antidepressant agents
(C) Mood stabilizers
(D) Anticholinesterase agents

ANSWER: A

The FDA mandates that second-generation antipsychotic agents carry a black-box warning of increased risk of mortality when taken by patients with dementia. Most placebo-controlled studies of dementia patients treated with second-generation antipsychotic agents (eg, olanzapine, aripiprazole, quetiapine, risperidone) report greater mortality (SOE=A), primarily from cardiac effect or infection. It is not clear what mechanism underlies this risk. In one meta-analysis, the absolute risk of death for dementia patients exposed to antipsychotic agents was 3.5%, while the absolute risk in patients given a placebo was 2.3%, yielding an NNH (number needed to harm) of 83 for that outcome.

Several studies suggest that the risk of death in patients with dementia is higher with first-generation than with second-generation antipsychotics. A recent meta-analysis comparing second-generation agents with haloperidol identified a relatively higher mortality risk with haloperidol. In a 12-mo study comparing first- or second-generation antipsychotics with nonantipsychotic psychotropic medications in outpatients with dementia, antipsychotic agents were associated with significantly higher mortality rates (23%–29%) than nonantipsychotic psychotropics (15%) (SOE=B). The study did not differentiate among cerebrovascular, cardio-vascular, or infection-related deaths in patients taking antipsychotics versus other psychotropic drugs. However, not all studies have replicated this finding, and no pathophysiologic mechanism has been clearly identified. It is not known whether the association between higher mortality and antipsychotic use reflects a direct medication effect or the pathophysi-ologic process associated with the symptoms that necessitated their use.

References

1. Kales HC, Valenstein M, Kim HM. Mortality risk in patients with dementia treated with antipsychotics versus other psychiatric medications. *Am J Psychiatry*. 2007;164(10):1568–1576.
2. Schneider LS, Dagerman KS, Insel P. Risk of death with atypical antipsychotic drug treatment for dementia: meta-analysis of randomized placebo-controlled trials. *JAMA*. 2005;294(15):1934–1943.
3. Schneeweiss S, Setoguchi S, Brookhart A, et al. Risk of death associated with the use of conventional versus atypical antipsychotic drugs among elderly patients. *CMAJ*. 2007;176(5):627–632.
4. Wang PS, Schneeweiss S, Avorn J, et al. Risk of death in elderly users of conventional vs. atypical antipsychotic medications. *N Engl J Med*. 2005;353(22):2335–2341.

112. A 55-yr-old man with Down syndrome is brought to the office by his caregivers because over the past year he has become confused and forgetful and has needed increasingly more frequent prompts for his assigned tasks. Although they do not have specific written records, the caregivers think that his speech and movement have slowed, that he is more socially withdrawn, and that he is having more outbursts with peers and staff. In the last 4 mo, he has twice lost his balance and fallen. He has been physically healthy overall and is on no medications. His last routine physical examination was 8 mo ago, at which time there were no indications of any problem.

During the visit, the patient seems shy and anxious and has a congruent affect. He has no complaints. His expressive abilities are limited and consistent with his low-moderate level of mental retardation.

Which of the following options is the most appropriate next step?

(A) Order head CT.
(B) Perform office-based, appropriate cognitive testing.
(C) Begin fluoxetine.
(D) Begin donepezil and, if well-tolerated, add memantine.
(E) Refer patient to a psychiatrist who specializes in neurodevelopmental disabilities.

ANSWER: B

Patients with developmental disabilities are now surviving to middle age and presenting with geriatric conditions, such as dementia and osteoporosis. This patient has symptoms consistent with dementia in Down syndrome. Early symptoms in patients both with and without Down syndrome include more short-term than distant memory loss, forget-fulness, and confusion. Patients with Down syndrome also have earlier frontal lobe symptoms, such as slowing of speech, language, and motor activities; social withdrawal; and problems with sleep, balance, and emotional regulation (SOE=B). This patient displays many of the symptoms of dementia, but diagnostic tests and additional history are needed before determining an appropriate treatment strategy. The cognitive testing necessary in this situation is available through psychology and psychiatry services and does not require consultation with a specialist in neurodevelopmental disabilities.

Despite the caregivers' report of falls, brain imaging is not likely to yield additional clinically useful information. Although some of the patient's symptoms suggest depression, more information would be needed before making a diagnosis of depression.

The degree of severity and patient values should guide treatment for dementia. The patient's presentation suggests mild rather than moderate or severe dementia. A medication regimen that combines two agents is not an appropriate first choice. In addition, cognitive assessment must be performed first.

References

1. Deb S, Braganza J. Comparison of rating scales for the diagnosis of dementia in adults with Down's syndrome. *J Intellect Disabil Res.* 1999;43(Pt 5):400–407.
2. Deb S, Hare M, Prior L. Symptoms of dementia among adults with Down's syndrome: a qualitative study. *J Intellect Disabil Res.* 2007;51(Pt 9):726–739.
3. Deb S, Hare M, Prior L, et al. Dementia screening questionnaire for individuals with intellectual disabilities. *Br J Psychiatry.* 2007;190:440–444.
4. Margallo-Lana ML, Moore PB, Kay DWK, et al. Fifteen-year follow-up of 92 hospitalized adults with Down's syndrome: incidence of cognitive decline, its relationship to age and neuropathology. *J Intellect Disabil Res.* 2007;51(6):463–477.

113. An 86-yr-old female resident of an assisted-living facility has urinary frequency, urgency, urge incontinence, leakage of urine when bending over and walking up or down stairs, and a sensation of incomplete bladder emptying. History includes hypertension, mild Alzheimer's disease, and lumbosacral degenerative joint disease, for which she uses a walker. Medications include a cholinesterase inhibitor, a thiazide diuretic, and an angiotensin-receptor blocker.

On physical examination, there is mild atrophic vaginitis, a moderate cystocele, normal rectal sphincter tone, and no fecal impaction. While the patient is standing, a cough test for stress incontinence is positive. She voids 100 mL; postvoid residual volume is 225 mL. Urinalysis is positive for trace of protein.

Which of the following is the most likely diagnosis?

(A) Stress incontinence
(B) Diuretic-induced incontinence
(C) Cholinesterase inhibitor–induced incontinence
(D) Detrusor hyperactivity with impaired bladder contractility
(E) Urinary retention and incontinence due to cystocele

ANSWER: D

This patient's symptoms and findings on examination are typical of detrusor hyperactivity with impaired bladder contractility. Affected patients have two simultaneous abnormalities of bladder function: involuntary bladder contractions, and weakness of the detrusor muscle resulting in incomplete bladder emptying with involuntary (and voluntary) bladder contractions (SOE=A). Detrusor hyperactivity with impaired bladder contractility can cause several different symptoms, as in this patient, and can mimic stress incontinence.

Diuretics can exacerbate symptoms of detrusor hyperactivity, but a thiazide diuretic is unlikely to be the primary cause of symptoms in this patient. Cholinesterase inhibitors can increase bladder contractility and possibly contribute to symptoms of overactive bladder (SOE=B). In older women with severe pelvic prolapse, urethral obstruction can develop, causing difficulty with bladder emptying (SOE=C). This patient, however, does not have severe pelvic prolapse. Even some obstruction of her urethra due to the cystocele would not account for all of her symptoms.

References

1. Holroyd-Leduc JM, Tannenbaum C, Thorpe KE, et al. What type of urinary incontinence does this woman have? *JAMA.* 2008; 299(12):1446–1456.
2. Resnick NM, Yalla SV. Detrusor hyperactivity with impaired contractile function. An unrecognized but common cause of incontinence in elderly patients. *JAMA.* 1987;257(22):3076–3081.
3. Taylor JA 3rd, Kuchel GA. Detrusor underactivity: clinical features and pathogenesis of an underdiagnosed geriatric condition. *J Am Geriatr Soc.* 2006;54(12):1920–1923.

114. A 65-yr-old woman is brought to the office by her niece because she believes that a neighbor has been coming into her apartment to steal items such as paper towels and sponges. She has called the police several times to report these thefts, and she complains regularly to her niece. This behavior began about 6 mo ago. The niece reports that her aunt has always been a little suspicious of other people. There is no history of alcohol or substance abuse. She has no hallucinations or depressive symptoms, and she has no other medical disorders. She is able to conduct her normal daily activities. Physical examination is normal except that she displays some mild memory loss. MRI is unremarkable.

Which of the following is the most likely explanation for her symptoms?

(A) Late-onset schizophrenia
(B) Delusional disorder
(C) Alzheimer's disease
(D) Bipolar disease
(E) Paranoid personality disorder

ANSWER: B

Delusional disorder is characterized by nonbizarre delusions involving situations that can occur in real life, such as theft, suffering from a disease, spousal infidelity, or being followed. According to the *Diagnostic and Statistical Manual of Mental Disorders, 4th Edition, Text Revision* it is rare; its precise prevalence is unknown, but it is estimated to be 0.03% in the general population, typically beginning in middle to late adulthood. Findings are mixed regarding the association of delusional disorder with hearing loss. Antipsychotic agents often are effective, especially in agitated delusional patients (SOE=C), but patients with delusions typically deny their illness. Consequently, they commonly do not adhere to medication regimens. Cognitive-behavioral therapy may also be effective. Modified electroconvulsive therapy has been reported as successful for refractory cases.

Delusional disorder is differentiated from schizophrenia by a lack of prominent auditory or visual hallucinations and by the absence of deterioration in areas of functioning outside the delusional scope. It can be distinguished from dementia by absence of cognitive and functional impairment, and from mood disorders by delusions preceding any mood disturbances. Although a history of schizotypal or paranoid personality disorders is more common in delusional disorder, the latter can be distinguished from personality disorders by the presence of delusions.

Delusional disorders can be difficult to differentiate from paranoid schizophrenia, but the latter has more bizarre delusions and auditory hallucinations. Poor psychosocial functioning in delusional disorder is directly related to the delusional beliefs.

References

1. Desai AK, Grossberg GT. Differential diagnosis of psychotic disorders in the elderly. In Cohen CI, ed. *Schizophrenia into Later Life*. Washington, DC: American Psychiatric Publishing; 2003.
2. Jeste DV, Dunn LB, Lindamer LA. Psychoses. In: Sadovoy J, Jarvik LF, Grossberg GT, et al, eds. *Comprehensive Textbook of Geriatric Psychiatry*. New York: WW Norton; 2004.
3. Manepalli JN, Gebretsadik M, Hook J, et al. Differential diagnosis of the older patient with psychotic symptoms. *Primary Psychiatry*. 2007;14(8):55–62.

115. An 86-yr-old man comes to the office to establish care. His wife died 10 yr ago; he recently moved to the area to be closer to his children and grandchildren. History includes visual impairment secondary to macular degeneration, osteoarthritis of the hip and knee, insomnia, benign prostatic hyperplasia, and mild nocturia. Medications include aspirin and tamsulosin daily, and meloxicam and temazepam, each 3 or 4 times weekly. His alcohol history comprises 1 highball each night before dinner and 1 glass of wine with dinner. At least once a week, the patient has a second glass of wine during dinner. The patient reports that his current pattern of drinking has remained the same for the past 40 yr. His CAGE (**C**ut down, **A**nnoyed, **G**uilty, **E**ye opener) score is 0 of 4.

On examination, he has decreased visual acuity, an enlarged prostate, and an antalgic gait.

Which one of the following is the most appropriate intervention?

(A) Recommend continuing alcohol intake at this level.

(B) Recommend restricting alcohol intake to no more than 1 drink per day.

(C) Measure liver enzyme levels to assess for alcohol-related liver impairment.

(D) Defer discussion of alcohol consumption until relationship with patient is more established.

(E) Defer renewing prescriptions for meloxicam and temazepam until he agrees to abstain from alcohol.

ANSWER: B

Although light to moderate alcohol consumption has been associated with cardioprotective benefits in both middle-aged and older adults, it also poses substantial risk (SOE=A). Alcohol-related risk increases with age, due in part to age-related physiologic changes (decreased volume of distribution and gastric alcohol dehydrogenase levels) that result in higher blood alcohol levels in older adults than in younger adults. Thus, current guidelines recommend no more than 1 drink per day for people ≥65 yr old. This patient meets criteria for at-risk drinking: he has an average of 15 drinks per week, and regularly uses medications (a benzodiazepine and an NSAID) that may interact negatively with alcohol and increase his risk of alcohol-related morbidity.

Liver function tests have limited sensitivity as markers of alcohol-related liver injury in older adults and would not help to establish a diagnosis in this particular case. Failing to address the patient's alcohol consumption at the initial visit would be inappropriate, particularly given his comorbidity and medication list. Furthermore, his insomnia may be exacerbated by his alcohol intake. Substantial research has demonstrated that brief interventions can lead to substantial and sustained reductions in alcohol consumption, and should be instituted at the time of screening if at all possible (SOE=A).

Although elimination of either alcohol or benzodiazepines would be optimal, a stepwise approach to reducing both is more realistic than immediate abstinence.

References

1. Merrick EL, Horgan CM, Hodgkin D, et al. Unhealthy drinking patterns of older adults: prevalence and associated characteristics. *J Am Geriatr Soc.* 2008;56(2):214–223.

2. Moore AA, Whiteman EJ, Ward KT. Risks of combined alcohol/medication use in older adults. *Am J Geriatr Pharm.* 2007;5(1):64–74.

3. Reid MC, Guo Z, Van Ness PH, et al. Are commonly ordered lab tests useful screens for alcohol disorders in older male veterans? *Subst Abuse.* 2005;26(2):25–32.

4. http://www.americangeriatrics.org/products/positionpapers/alcoholPF.shtml (accessed Nov 2009).

116. A 78-yr-old widowed woman is in a nursing facility after hemicolectomy for metastatic cancer. She is dependent in ADLs, and her medical prognosis is poor. She presents herself as a woman who had unparalleled success in her career and numerous offers of marriage. Her brother reports that her lifelong tendency to become enraged after perceived slights has alienated her from her children and other relatives. Although at times she is tearful, she enjoys making herself the focus of unit activities. She has not had changes in sleep or appetite. As her medical problems worsen, she is increasingly demanding and verbally abusive of nursing staff.

Mental status examination reveals normal rate of speech and psychomotor activity, and cognitive examination is normal.

Which of the following is the most likely diagnosis?

(A) Bipolar disorder, manic type
(B) Histrionic personality disorder
(C) Major depressive disorder
(D) Narcissistic personality disorder

ANSWER: D

This patient has personality disorder, which is characterized by a long-standing, pervasive pattern of disturbances in emotionality, cognition, interpersonal functioning, and impulse control that cause significant distress or impaired functioning. Patients with narcissistic personality disorder tend to exaggerate achievements, seek admiration, and exhibit arrogant behavior and limited empathy toward others. In late life, such behaviors and traits become particularly troublesome when interpersonal environmental demands change. Unavoidable dependency, transition to institutional living, and the need to rely on others to meet one's daily needs always require time to achieve a new equilibrium. But when the need to adjust is compounded by chronic interpersonal vulnerabilities, persistent dysequilibrium can be the result. When a "situational adjustment reaction" seems extreme or overlong, a personality disorder should be considered.

Patients with histrionic personality disorder display excessive emotionality and seek attention but do not have the inflated sense of self-importance or entitlement seen with narcissistic personality disorder.

Patients with bipolar disorder, manic type, can demonstrate persistently elevated or irritable mood during an episode, which can manifest as inflated self-esteem, as well as excessive engagement in pleasurable activities, decreased need for sleep, and increased rate of speech.

Because the patient is not pervasively dysphoric, enjoys daily activities, and does not report changes in sleep or appetite, major depressive disorder is unlikely.

References

1. Agronin ME, Maletta GJ, eds. *Principles and Practice of Geriatric Psychiatry*. Philadelphia, PA: Lippincott Williams & Wilkins; 2006.
2. Oxman TE. Personality disorders. In: Blazer DG, Steffens DC, eds. *The American Psychiatric Publishing Textbook of Geriatric Psychiatry*. 4th edition. Washington, DC: American Psychiatric Publishing Inc; 2009.
3. Zweig RA. Personality disorders in older adults: managing the difficult patient. *Clinical Geriatrics*. 2003;11:22–25.

117. How many of the 78 million "baby boomers" are predicted to develop Alzheimer's disease in their lifetime?

(A) 5 million (6%)
(B) 10 million (13%)
(C) 15 million (19%)
(D) 20 million (26%)
(E) 25 million (32%)

ANSWER: B

The predicted prevalence of Alzheimer's disease after age 55 is 13% for the "baby boomer" cohort, higher for women (17%) than for men (9%) because of women's longer life expectancies. This translates into 10 million cases of Alzheimer's disease among adults born between 1946 and 1964. The rates increase when all types of dementia are considered. Dementia of some type is predicted to develop in about 14 million baby boomers

(18%). Furthermore, the lifetime risk of dementia will increase if the number of deaths due to other causes (eg, heart disease, cancer, stroke) continues to decline. By 2050, between 11 and 16 million people ≥65 yr old will have Alzheimer's disease. Over 60% of that group will be ≥84 yr old.

The causes of dementia and their prevalence vary with age. Based on cross-sectional population surveys, in adults ≥70 yr old who have dementia, 70% appear to have Alzheimer's disease, 17% have vascular dementia, and 13% have dementia related to other causes. In people ≥90 yr old, 80% of cases will be Alzheimer's disease, up from 47% of cases in adults 71–79 yr old who have dementia.

References

1. Alzheimer's Association. *2008 Alzheimer's Disease Facts and Figures*. Chicago, IL and Washington, DC: Alzheimer's Association; 2008.
2. Cummings JL. Alzheimer's disease. *N Engl J Med*. 2004;351(1):56–67.
3. National Institute on Aging. *Alzheimer's Disease Fact Sheet*. Washington, DC: National Institute of Health; 2006.

118. A 69-yr-old woman comes to the office because she has had anorexia, nausea, and vague lower abdominal pain associated with the onset of constipation 1 wk earlier. She also believes she has had a low-grade fever.

On examination, she appears uncomfortable. Temperature is 37.2°C (99.0°F), blood pressure is 130/80 mmHg, pulse is 90 beats per minute, and respiratory rate is 14 breaths per minute. She has suprapubic fullness and abdominal tenderness with localized guarding but no rebound. Bowel sounds are decreased. Laboratory results are normal except for mild anemia and a WBC count of 12,000/μL with a left shift. Radiography demonstrates a nonspecific ileus pattern.

Which of the following studies should be performed next?

(A) Barium enema
(B) Ultrasonography of pelvis
(C) CT of abdomen and pelvis
(D) Small-bowel series
(E) Colonoscopy

ANSWER: C

The prevalence of diverticulosis increases with age and is estimated to be 70% among adults ≥80 yr older. Diverticulitis (inflammation of a diverticulum) is the most common clinical complication of diverticular disease, affecting 10%–25% of patients with diverticula. Most diverticula (80%) are located in the sigmoid and descending colon regions of the large intestine. Diverticulitis is commonly accompanied by gross or microscopic perforation and usually involves the sigmoid or descending colon.

Contained perforation can result in abscess formation, fistulization, small-bowel obstruction from adhesions, and after repeated episodes, large-bowel obstruction from fibrotic narrowing of the colon lumen. Free perforation will likely lead to frank peritonitis.

Diverticulitis typically causes left lower-quadrant abdominal pain, although the location of the pain can be variable because of the redundancy of the sigmoid colon. Leukocytosis is generally present, and low-grade fever and obstipation are common. Urinary symptoms may occur with adjacent bladder irritation.

CT is recommended as the initial radiologic examination (SOE=C). It has high sensitivity (approximately 93%–97%) and specificity approaching 100% for the diagnosis. It also allows the extent of disease to be delineated. CT can also reveal other disease processes that cause lower abdominal pain, such as appendicitis or carcinoma, and may be of value in predicting the need for surgery. In patients with evidence of abscess on CT, conservative therapy often fails; CT findings can be used to stratify cases that should be referred for early surgical intervention.

Because of the risk of perforation or other exacerbation, colonoscopy and sigmoidoscopy are contraindicated. While limited-contrast studies of the descending colon and rectum with water-soluble contrast media can help distinguish between diverticulitis and carcinoma, barium enema should be avoided during the acute attack because of possible leakage of barium into the peritoneal cavity. Ultrasonography can be used to diagnose acute colonic diverticulitis, but its use is limited by what has been described as "the unhappy triad" of too much pain, too much gas, and too much fat.

References
1. Comparato G, Pilotto A, Franze A, et al. Diverticular disease in the elderly. *Dig Dis.* 2007:25(2):151–159.
2. Jacobs DO. Diverticulitis. *N Engl J Med.* 2007;357(20):2057–2066.
3. Parro-Blanco A. Colonic diverticular disease: Pathophysiology and clinical picture. *Dig.* 2006;73(Suppl 1):47–57.
4. Sheth AA, Longo W, Floch MH. Diverticular disease and diverticulitis. *Am J Gastroenterol.* 2008;103(6):1–7.

119. An active, 70-yr-old moderately obese woman presents with a chief complaint of a painful left heel over the last few months. She has pain on first getting out of bed and after periods of rest. She denies any previous treatments. Past medical history is unremarkable. Physical examination of the left heel reveals pain at the medial tuberosity of the calcaneus. Dorsiflexion at the ankle joint is decreased but pain free, and foot structure is normal. A radiograph of her left heel is unremarkable.

What is the most likely diagnosis?

(A) Heel spur
(B) Calcaneal stress fracture
(C) Partial tear of Achilles tendon
(D) Posterior tibial tendonitis
(E) Plantar fasciitis

ANSWER: E

Plantar fasciitis is a common condition seen after age 40 and is usually diagnosed through symptoms and physical examination findings. Patients typically have pain on rising in the morning and after periods of rest. During periods of nonactivity, the plantar ligament shortens; subsequently, the first few steps cause a sudden stretch, resulting in significant pain that usually decreases as the ligament is lengthened. An associated factor is ankle equinus or reduction in dorsiflexion of the ankle joint demonstrated on physical examination. This leads to increased stress on the plantar fascia during walking. Pain is usually maximal at the insertion of the plantar fascia on the medial tuberosity of the calcaneus. A pain-free range of motion in the ankle excludes a partial Achilles tear, because this tear is associated with end-range pain. Normal radiographs exclude heel spur and most calcaneal stress fractures; although stress fractures can be missed on plain radiographs, pain due to a stress fracture would not improve with ambulation. A normal foot structure and symptoms not worsening during ambulation (as the medial arch is stressed) exclude tendonitis.

References
1. Young CC, Rutherford DS, Niedfeldt MW. Treatment of plantar fasciitis. *Am Fam Physician*. 2001;63(3):467–474, 477–478.
2. Cole C, Seto C, Gazewood JD. Plantar fasciitis: evidence-based review of diagnosis and therapy. *Am Fam Physician*. 2005;72(11):2237–2242.

120. A 75-yr-old man is evaluated because he has sudden onset of shortness of breath; sharp, pleuritic left-sided chest pain; and cough productive of blood-tinged sputum. He had elective hip replacement surgery 6 days ago. He has been (and is) wearing pneumatic compression devices on both legs. He has a 20-yr history of COPD. He is taking a proton-pump inhibitor for a duodenal ulcer diagnosed 2 wk ago and albuterol as needed.

On examination, temperature is 38.0°C (100.4°F), blood pressure is 165/90 mmHg, heart rate is 110 breaths per minute, and respiratory rate is 26 breaths per minute. There is no accessory muscle use. He has slight expiratory wheezing. There is no jugular venous distension. A left-sided S4 gallop is audible. The abdomen is soft without masses or hepatosplenomegaly. There is no cyanosis, clubbing, edema, or thigh or calf pain.

WBC count is 13,800/µL, with 85% polymorphonuclear cells and 6% bands. Enzyme-linked immunosorbent assay reports D-dimer <500 ng/mL.

Arterial blood gas on room air:

pH	7.48
PaO_2	70 mmHg
$PaCO_2$	30 mmHg

An ECG reveals sinus tachycardia. Chest radiography reveals left lower-lobe atelectasis or infiltrate. Ventilation-perfusion (V/Q) scan indicates a low probability for pulmonary embolism. Bilateral lower-extremity Doppler ultrasonography demonstrates no evidence of deep vein thrombosis (DVT).

Which of the following is the most appropriate next step?

(A) Treat with heparin.
(B) Place an inferior vena cava filter.
(C) Treat with antibiotics and steroids.
(D) Obtain CT of chest.
(E) Obtain CT angiography of chest.

ANSWER: E

The individual symptoms, signs, laboratory data, and predisposing factors for pulmonary thromboembolism (PTE) are neither sensitive nor specific (SOE=A). When the clinical presentation suggests the possibility of PTE, pretest probability must be determined. In a validated clinical decision rule (Wells score), points are assigned based on history and clinical signs and symptoms. Pretest probability is based on total points (SOE=A). This patient's total Wells score is 6.5 (heart rate >100 beats per minute = 1, immobilization = 1.5, hemoptysis = 1, PTE more likely than alternative diagnosis = 3), indicating a high probability for PTE.

The results of all investigations must be interpreted in light of this high pretest probability. D-dimer is highly sensitive for DVT and PTE. Because several conditions (eg, sepsis, recent surgery, liver disease, malignancy) can increase D-dimer, the test is not specific for DVT or PTE. Consequently, a negative D-dimer (<500 ng/mL) by enzyme-linked immunosorbent assay, in the setting of low or intermediate probability of DVT or PTE, makes DVT and PTE unlikely (SOE=A). In this case, however, with the high pretest probability of PTE, the normal D-dimer does not result in a post-test probability low enough to preclude further evaluation, so the test result is not useful (SOE=A).

The only clinically useful results of a V/Q scan are normal and high probability. Because a V/Q scan is highly sensitive, a normal scan provides compelling evidence against PTE (SOE=A). In patients with a high pretest probability for PTE, a high probability V/Q scan confirms the diagnosis (SOE=A). V/Q scans other than normal or high probability require additional diagnostic evaluation (SOE=A). In this patient, the low-probability V/Q scan does not exclude PTE. In the Prospective Investigation of Pulmonary Embolism Diagnosis (PIOPED), 40% of patients with a low-probability V/Q scan in whom the clinical suspicion of PTE was high had angiographically confirmed PTE.

The sensitivity and specificity for diagnosing *symptomatic* proximal DVT by Doppler ultrasonography is ≥95% (SOE=A). However, its sensitivity and specificity in the setting of *asymptomatic* proximal DVT ranges from 47% to 62%. Again, a negative result cannot exclude PTE in this patient.

In almost all circumstances, prolonged treatment of PTE (eg, with inferior vena cava filter or heparin) requires objective documentation. Although treatment with heparin is recommended during evaluation for suspected PTE, in this case heparin is contraindicated because of the patient's recent history of a duodenal ulcer. CT of the chest could be useful for diagnosing pulmonary causes of this patient's presentation other than PTE, ie, pulmonary infiltrate consistent with pneumonia. However, given the high pretest probability of PTE, CT angiography is required to exclude PTE.

References

1. Qaseem A, Snow V, Barry P, et al, for the Joint American Academy of Family Physicians/American College of Physicians Panel on DVT/PE and Current Diagnosis of VTE in Primary Care: a Clinical Practice Guideline from the AAFP and the ACP. *Ann Fam Med.* 2007;5(1):57–62.
2. Rathbun SE, Whitsett TL, Veseley SK, et al. Clinical utility of D-dimer in patients with suspected pulmonary embolism and nondiagnostic lung scans or negative CT findings. *Chest.* 2004;125(3):851–855.
3. Stein PD, Fowler SE, Goodman LR, et al. Multidetector computed tomography for acute pulmonary embolism. *N Engl J Med.* 2006;354(22):2317–2327.

121. A 72-yr-old man with mild dementia returns to the office because he has had difficulty both falling and staying asleep for the past 4 mo. In addition, he has had vivid dreams a few times per month. His sleep disturbance emerged shortly after another physician prescribed a new medication.

Which of the following is most likely to cause these symptoms?

(A) Buspirone
(B) Trazodone
(C) Donepezil
(D) Melatonin
(E) Ramelteon

ANSWER: C

In older adults, medications are a common cause of insomnia or they can exacerbate preexisting insomnia. Donepezil, an acetylcholinesterase inhibitor commonly used for treatment of cognitive function in patients with Alzheimer's disease, has been shown to disturb sleep, as well as increase rapid eye movement (REM) sleep. REM sleep is the stage most commonly associated with

dreaming; vivid dreams have been reported by patients when they have taken donepezil in the evening.

Activation of cholinergic systems increases wakefulness and alertness, as well as REM sleep, and can contribute to sleep disturbances. In clinical trials, insomnia and vivid dreams have been identified as potential adverse events of donepezil (SOE=A). In a study examining the use of donepezil and hypnotic agents in older adults with Alzheimer's disease living in the community, use of hypnotic agents was higher among patients prescribed donepezil.

Buspirone, an anxiolytic medication, and trazodone, a sedating antidepressant, are unlikely to cause insomnia (SOE=B); indeed, trazodone is often used off-label for treatment of insomnia (SOE=B). Melatonin is a nutritional supplement with sleep-promoting properties (SOE=B), and ramelteon is a melatonin-receptor agonist hypnotic medication that does not promote insomnia (SOE=A).

References

1. Dunn NR, Pearce GL, Shakir SA. Adverse effects associated with the use of donepezil in general practice in England. *J Psychopharmacol.* 2000;14(4):406–408.
2. Kavirajan H, Schneider LS. Efficacy and adverse effects of cholinesterase inhibitors and memantine in vascular dementia: a meta-analysis of randomised controlled trials. *Lancet Neurol.* 2007;6(9):782–792.
3. Roman GC, Rogers SJ. Donepezil: a clinical review of current and emerging indications. *Expert Opin Pharmacother.* 2004;5(1):161–180.
4. Roth T, Seiden D, Sainati S, et al. Effects of ramelteon on patient-reported sleep latency in older adults with chronic insomnia. *Sleep Med.* 2006;7(4):312–318.
5. Stahl SM, Markowitz JS, Gutterman EM, et al. Co-use of donepezil and hypnotics among Alzheimer's disease patients living in the community. *J Clin Psychiatry.* 2003;64(4):466–472.

122. A 79-yr-old man comes to the office because he has increasing difficulty understanding conversations with his grandchildren.

Which of the following is the most likely diagnosis?

(A) Presbycusis
(B) Sociocusis
(C) Ototoxicity
(D) Acoustic neuroma

ANSWER: A

Approximately 40%–50% of adults ≥75 yr old have age-related hearing loss (presbycusis); it is the third most common chronic condition and contributes to cognitive and physical decline. Characteristic pathologic changes in the temporal bone correlate with six types of presbycusis, each having a distinctive pattern of hearing loss. The hearing loss is sensorineural, bilateral, symmetric, and gradual in onset. Manifestations include difficulty understanding speech, especially in noisy situations. Older adults with presbycusis report that they can hear people speaking but cannot make out the words.

Sociocusis refers to non–workplace-related hearing loss due to exposure to noise. Ototoxicity refers to the toxic effects of medications on the sensory and balance structures of the inner ear. Aminoglycosides, salicylates, and cisplatin are toxic to the hearing mechanism and can cause hearing or balance problems. Older adults are often susceptible to ototoxicity, especially when kidney function is compromised. Hearing testing and laboratory tests can be used to monitor the early onset of ototoxic effects. Presbycusis is more common than ototoxicity.

Acoustic neuroma usually causes unilateral hearing loss.

It is often difficult for audiologists to determine from the audiogram whether hearing loss is due solely to the effects of aging, because environmental factors and ototoxicity are also associated with loss that is sensorineural and affects primarily high-frequency hearing.

References

1. Agrawal Y, Platz E, Niparko J. Prevalence of hearing loss and differences by demographic characteristics among U.S. adults. *Arch Intern Med.* 2008;168(14):1522–1530.
2. Lam B, Lee D, Gomez-Marin O, et al. Concurrent visual and hearing impairment and risk of mortality. The National Health Interview Survey. *Arch Ophthalmol.* 2006;124(1):95–101.
3. Lee F, Matthews L, Dubno J, et al. Longitudinal study of pure-tone thresholds in older persons. *Ear Hear.* 2005;26(1):1–11.
4. Yueh B, Collins M, Souza P, et al. Screening for Auditory Impairment–Which Hearing Assessment Test (SAI-WHAT): RCT design and baseline characteristics. *Contemp Clin Trials.* 2007;28(3):303–315.

123. A 90-yr-old woman comes to the office because, over the past year, she has had increasing difficulty walking. Her gait is slower, and she feels as if she might fall backward at times. She has hypertension, hypothyroidism, and osteoarthritis, and she had coronary artery bypass surgery 10 yr ago, with no recurrence of angina.

On examination, she has moderate dorsal kyphosis and arthritic changes in her fingers and knees. Strength and reflexes are symmetric. She has some increased muscle tone. She uses her arms to push up from the chair; once standing, she has difficulty starting to walk. Her gait is symmetric, with a normal base, but her foot clearance and stride length are both decreased. She turns slowly and carefully, with an increased number of steps.

Which of the following is the most likely cause of her gait abnormality?

(A) Osteoarthritis
(B) Proprioceptive deficits
(C) Cerebrovascular disease
(D) Parkinson's disease
(E) Cautious gait

ANSWER: C

This older patient has known vascular disease. The difficulty starting to walk, the slow gait with decreased foot clearance, and the tendency to fall backward suggest subclinical cerebrovascular disease (SOE=A). Her advanced age and history of hypertension place her at risk of microvascular disease affecting cerebral white matter and of lacunar infarcts. More advanced cerebrovascular disease can result in vascular parkinsonism, with poor standing balance, rigidity, masked face, parkinsonian gait, and cognitive impairment.

The patient has osteoarthritis, yet she does not have evidence of pain on walking and does not complain of her legs "giving way." Her gait is symmetric; with painful osteoarthritis, there is usually some gait asymmetry. Proprioceptive deficits, with loss of position sense, lead to a wide-based, steppage gait, which she does not have. The typical gait of Parkinson's disease involves initial hesitation, then small, shuffling steps with no arm swing and difficulty with balance. Associated findings would include tremor, masked face, and cogwheel rigidity. Fear of falling can lead to a slow, cautious gait, with decreased step length. Although this patient is probably being cautious because she fears falling, she has objective abnormalities, including difficulty rising from a chair, difficulty with starting to walk, and decreased foot clearance.

References

1. Alexander NB. Gait disorders in older adults. *J Am Geriatr Soc.* 1996;44(4):434–451.
2. Gilman S. Parkinsonian syndromes. *Clin Geriatr Med.* 2006;22(4):827–842.

124. An 89-yr-old man presents to you complaining of generalized weakness. General physical examination and neurologic examination are normal. He lives with his wife in a rural community, is independent in ADLs and IADLs, and rarely drives. He has avoided medical care for most of his life. He is on no medications other than calcium, vitamin D, and aspirin 81 mg/d.

Laboratory tests:

Hemoglobin	11.9 g/dL
Hematocrit	35%
Mean corpuscular volume	102 mm^3
Serum B$_{12}$	200 pg/mL (low normal)
Methylmalonic acid	300 nmol/L (increased)
Homocysteine	18 μmol/L (increased)
RBC folate	normal
Ferritin	250 ng/mL

What is the best next step?

(A) Prescribe oral vitamin B$_{12}$ 1000 mcg/d.
(B) Administer vitamin B$_{12}$ 1000 mcg IM weekly for 8 wk, followed by 1000 mcg IM monthly.
(C) Administer a 3-part Schilling test.
(D) Recommend upper and lower endoscopy to exclude pernicious anemia and bacterial overgrowth syndrome.

ANSWER: A

Many patients with B$_{12}$ deficiency have no or mild hematologic or neurologic symptoms. In one study, less than one-third of patients with documented B$_{12}$ deficiency had anemia or macrocytosis (SOE=B). The diagnosis of vitamin B$_{12}$ deficiency can be made with relative certainty (specificity of ≥95%) when the serum concentration is <200 pg/mL (<148 pmol/L) (SOE=B). For indeterminate result (200–300 pg/mL (148–241 pmol/L), increased methylmalonic acid and homocysteine concentrations can help establish the diagnosis with a sensitivity of 94% and specificity of 99% (SOE=A).

Causes of B$_{12}$ deficiency include pernicious anemia, history of gastrectomy, malabsorption syndromes, ileal resection or bypass, pancreatic insufficiency, diet, and a number of medications (eg, proton-pump inhibitors). While many authors argue that a cause for B$_{12}$ deficiency must be found, it has never been demonstrated that identifying a cause for B$_{12}$ deficiency improves clinical outcomes (SOE=B). The clinician needs to think carefully about whether finding the cause of B$_{12}$ deficiency will be helpful in managing a particular patient. Anti-intrinsic factor antibodies are highly specific for pernicious anemia and can help establish the diagnosis. Schilling tests are rarely necessary (SOE=C).

Recommended options for vitamin B$_{12}$ replacement include oral or sublingual delivery of 500–2000 mcg/d, intranasal administration of 500 mcg/wk in one nostril, and intramuscular or deep subcutaneous delivery of 30 mcg/day for 5 to 10 days, followed by a maintenance dose of 100–200 mcg/mo; parenteral and oral options have equivalent efficacy in most patients, even in the absence of intrinsic factor (SOE=B). A response to therapy should be documented, and in the rare patient in whom oral therapy is not effective, the dosage should be increased or parenteral therapy should be substituted (SOE=C).

In this patient, who lives in a rural area, does not drive, and is not an enthusiastic consumer of medical care, a trial of oral B$_{12}$ therapy should be initiated. Parenteral therapy would be a reasonable alternative if the patient were able to get into the clinic or receive injections at home, or if he did not respond to oral therapy. A Schilling test would be unlikely to influence therapy in this patient who is otherwise asymptomatic. Endoscopy and colonoscopy are not indicated in an 89-yr-old man with no evidence of iron deficiency anemia (SOE=B).

References

1. Eussen SJ, de Groot LC, Clarke R, et al. Oral cyanocobalamin supplementation in older people with vitamin B$_{12}$ deficiency: a dose-finding trial. *Arch Intern Med.* 2005;165(10):1167–1172.
2. Lane LA, Rojas-Fernandez C. Treatment of vitamin B$_{12}$-deficiency anemia: oral versus parenteral therapy. *Ann Pharmacother.* 2002;36(7-8):1268–1272.
3. Sehl ME, Naeim A, Charette SL. Macrocytosis in the elderly. *Clin Geriatrics.* 2008;16:36–43.

4. Sharabi A, Cohen E, Sulkes J, et al. Replacement therapy for vitamin B$_{12}$ deficiency: comparison between the sublingual and oral route. *Br J Clin Pharmacol.* 2003;56(6):635–638.
5. Vidal-Alaball J, Butler CC, Cannings-John R, et al. Oral vitamin B$_{12}$ versus intramuscular vitamin B$_{12}$ for vitamin B$_{12}$ deficiency. *Cochrane Database Syst Rev.* 2005;(3):CD004655.

125. Which of the following is most likely to reduce the incidence of in-hospital falls?

(A) Use of bed alarms to alert staff
(B) Use of specially colored, nonslip slipper-socks
(C) Use of four siderails
(D) Team discussion of patient's risk factors
(E) Individualized exercise programs to improve balance

ANSWER: D

In-hospital falls can result in several complications, including fear of future falls, injury, and increased length of stay. There is little evidence to support a particular intervention to reduce falls in the acute-care setting. The best evidence available supports care planning by nursing staff to reduce risk factors for individual patients (SOE=B).

Bed alarms that ring either in the patient's room or at the central nurses' station can be effective alerts. However, hospital staff may not remember to activate the alarms or respond in time to prevent a fall. Colored, nonslip slipper-socks, along with wrist bands and room markers, are used to identify patients at risk of falling, but there has been no study demonstrating that this single intervention is effective. The use of restraints, including four siderails, has not been shown to reduce the incidence of falls and may increase the risk of fall injuries. In-hospital exercise programs have not been shown to prevent falls.

References

1. Coussement J, De Paepe L, Schwendimann R, et al. Interventions for preventing falls in acute- and chronic-care hospitals: a systematic review and meta-analysis. *J Am Geriatr Soc.* 2008;56(1):29–36.
2. Cumming RG, Sherrington C, Lord SR, et al. Cluster randomised trial of a targeted multifactorial intervention to prevent falls among older people in hospital. *BMJ.* 2008;336(7647):758–760.
3. Healey F, Monro A, Cockram A, et al. Using targeted risk factor reduction to prevent falls in older in-patients: a randomized controlled trial. *Age Ageing.* 2004;33(4):390–395.

4. Oliver D, Connelly JB, Victor CR, et al. Strategies to prevent falls and fractures in hospitals and care homes and effect of cognitive impairment: systematic review and meta-analyses. *BMJ.* 2007;334(7584):82–87.

126. A 92-yr-old woman is brought to the office by her daughter because she is moving more slowly and unsteadily. She has not had any falls. She lives with her family and she is independent in ADLs. Until 2 yr ago, she took walks 3 times a week. Now her aerobic activity is limited to climbing 7 household steps about twice daily. She has a distant history of breast cancer and mild osteoarthritis. Medications include acetaminophen, vitamin D, and calcium.

On examination, vital signs are normal. There is no tremor or rigidity, and motor strength is symmetric and only slightly reduced. She stands unassisted but sways on standing and reaches out for contact assistance. She walks across the examination room without assistance but reaches out to touch the examination table. Her Mini–Mental State Examination score is normal.

Which of the following is the most appropriate next step?

(A) Establish a graduated balance-training program.
(B) Establish a high-intensity quadriceps strengthening program with 10 to 15 repetitions per session.
(C) Establish a moderate-intensity walking program of ≥1,000 steps per day.
(D) Establish a high-intensity walking program of ≥5,000 steps per day.
(E) Prescribe pain medication to be taken immediately before exercise.

ANSWER: A

This patient is at risk of falls and loss of function. She has not engaged in exercise over the past 2 yr, and her balance has deteriorated significantly. She requires a comprehensive physical activity program. However, the program should be initiated slowly to reduce the risk of injury and to improve the likelihood of adherence. Graduated balance-training exercises should begin immediately, with static exercises such as single-leg stands and side-to-side weight shifts, and dynamic exercises such as tandem walk and heel walk (SOE=C). Strengthening exercises of the quadriceps and hip flexors would be beneficial but should not be high intensity (ie, maximum that can be lifted). The aerobic component of the program should start at low intensity. Setting a goal based on number of steps per day is not useful, even with a pedometer, because it is difficult to translate number of steps into minutes of continuous exercise (SOE=C). Pain medication can be used if needed, but there is no indication that pain is limiting her activity.

References

1. Ackermann RT, Williams B, Nguyen HQ, et al. Healthcare cost differences with participation in a community-based group physical activity benefit for Medicare managed care health plan members. *J Am Geriatr Soc.* 2008;56(8):1459–1465.
2. American Geriatrics Society. Exercise prescription for older adults with osteoarthritis pain: consensus practice recommendations. AGS Panel on Exercise and Osteoarthritis. *J Am Geriatr Soc.* 2001;49(6):808–823.
3. Nelson ME, Rejeski WJ, Blair SN, et al. Physical activity and public health in older adults: recommendations from the American College of Sports Medicine and the American Heart Association. *Med Sci Sports Exerc.* 2007;39(8):1435–1445.

127. A 68-yr-old man comes to the office because he has had pain in his feet, knees, hands, wrists, and shoulders for the past 4 mo. The foot pain has limited his ability to walk, causing him to retire from postal work. He has joint stiffness that is most problematic on awakening and persists for 2 h. He has been taking OTC acetaminophen.

On examination, both forefeet appear enlarged, with tenderness and fullness along the undersurface of the metatarsal phalangeal joints. There is swelling, erythema, and tenderness of the metacarpophalangeal joints, wrists, elbows, and knees. Erythrocyte sedimentation rate is 64 mm/h, and serum creatinine is 2.3 mg/dL; the anticyclic citrullinated peptide (anti-CCP) antibody level is moderate.

In addition to physical therapy, what would be the best initial therapy for late-onset rheumatoid arthritis?

(A) Methotrexate
(B) Prednisone
(C) Antitumor necrosis factor
(D) NSAID

ANSWER: A

Late-onset, seropositive, inflammatory rheumatoid arthritis can result in aggressive joint destruction, osteoporosis, and profound functional limitations. Physical therapy should be initiated early to restore and maintain function and to prevent falls in older adults with all forms of arthritis, particularly in light of the accelerated bone loss seen with rheumatoid arthritis.

Data on disease-modifying antirheumatic drugs (DMARDs) suggest that older adults can benefit from methotrexate, hydroxychloroquine, and sulfasalazine if liver function and blood counts are monitored and if rechecked regularly. Of these medications, methotrexate is the preferred first-line DMARD (SOE=A). Data for biologic agents (antitumor necrosis factor therapies) are limited but suggest that their use is not associated with greater infectious complications in older adult patients. However, antitumor necrosis factor therapies are not first-line agents and should be reserved for patients at risk of destructive arthritis who do not respond to other DMARDs. Greater risk of infectious complications has been observed with prednisone when prescribed at high dosages or for long durations. Prednisone can be used for short-term symptom control when starting DMARD therapy.

NSAIDs are not recommended for older patients and would not be first-line therapy in any case. In addition, this patient's creatinine is 2.3 mg/dL, which precludes NSAID use.

Use of DMARD or biologic therapies for seronegative forms of polymyalgia rheumatica and remitting symmetric seronegative synovitis with peripheral edema (ie, the "RS3PE" syndrome) is not supported by evidence. Also, older adults with a history of disease that is no longer clinically active do not require aggressive medical management.

References

1. Combe B, Landewe R, Lukas C, et al. EULAR recommendations for the management of early arthritis: report of a task force of the European Standing Committee for International Clinical Studies Including Therapeutics (ESCISIT). *Ann Rheum Dis.* 2007;66(1):34–45.
2. Fleischmann R, Iqbal I. Risk:benefit profile of etanercept in elderly patients with rheumatoid arthritis, ankylosing spondylitis or psoriatic arthritis. *Drugs Aging.* 2007;24(3):239–254.
3. Geusens P. Osteoporosis: clinical features. *Minerva Med.* 2008;99(2):167–175.

4. Turkcapar N, Demir O, Atli T, et al. Late onset rheumatoid arthritis: clinical and laboratory comparisons with younger onset patients. *Arch Gerontol Geriatr.* 2006;42(2):225–231.

128. A 79-yr-old Asian-American woman is brought to the office because she has increasing forgetfulness; apathy; and behavioral changes of irritability, agitation, and aggression. Her primary caregiver reports that she is disruptive, occasionally screaming at imaginary people, and is frequently becoming combative. The patient has Alzheimer's disease but no history of psychosis or major depressive disorder. Physical examination, CBC, and serum chemistries are normal.

Which of the following is the next best step?

(A) Treat with a first-generation antipsychotic agent.
(B) Treat with a second-generation antipsychotic agent.
(C) Admit to a psychiatric unit for further evaluation.
(D) Review behavioral interventions with the caregiver.

ANSWER: D

The behavior reported by the caregiver could lead to nursing-home admission and requires rapid intervention. However, treatment with either a first- (SOE=B) or second-generation antipsychotic (SOE=A) is more often associated with adverse events necessitating discontinuation than with meaningful benefit. As a result, antipsychotics are not considered first-line treatment for agitation among individuals with dementia and should not be started until behavioral interventions have proved inadequate. Admission to a psychiatric unit before exhausting behavioral and pharmacologic interventions is premature. It may be necessary ultimately but will initially exacerbate disorientation and combativeness. Consensus suggests that a cholinesterase inhibitor is the first-line pharmacologic treatment combined with behavioral interventions when objectionable behaviors either are not the expressions of the patient's unmet needs or exceed the caregiver's tolerance.

References
1. Schneider LS, Tariot PN, Dagerman KS, et al. Effectiveness of atypical antipsychotic drugs in patients with Alzheimer's disease. *N Engl J Med.* 2006;355(15):1525–1538.
2. Sink KM, Holden KF, Yaffe K. Pharmacologic treatment of neuropsychiatric symptoms of dementia: a review of the evidence. *JAMA.* 2005;293(5):596–608.
3. Teri L, Logsdon RG, Peskind E, et al. Treatment of agitation in AD: a randomized, placebo-controlled clinical trial. *Neurology.* 2000;55(9):1271–1278.
4. Trinh NH, Hoblyn J, Mohanty S, et al. Efficacy of cholinesterase inhibitors in the treatment of neuropsychiatric symptoms and functional impairment in Alzheimer's disease: a meta-analysis. *JAMA.* 2003;289(2):210–216.

129. A 68-yr-old man is brought to the office by his son for follow-up evaluation. The patient is a widower who lives in his own apartment. He has type 2 diabetes mellitus, peripheral vascular disease, ischemic cardiomyopathy, and macular degeneration. A visiting nurse comes weekly, and his son and daughter-in-law help him with shopping and chores at home. He has been hospitalized three times over the past 2 mo, most recently for cellulitis of his right foot. The patient drove until 2 mo ago, when his first hospitalization occurred. He also gave his checkbook to his son, "just for a little while, until I get better."

The son voices concern about the father's ability to live independently. The patient becomes visibly upset and states that he will never leave his home. He suggests that his son is after his Social Security money.

Which of the following is the most appropriate next step?

(A) Evaluate for cognitive impairment.
(B) Evaluate for possible financial exploitation and for mistreatment or abuse.
(C) Initiate discussion regarding advance directives.
(D) Perform comprehensive geriatric assessment.
(E) Arrange for a daily home health aide.

ANSWER: D

This patient has had functional decline and is at high risk of rehospitalization. Because his physical, mental, and social status have changed, comprehensive geriatric assessment is appropriate. Comprehensive assessment includes functional, psychosocial, cognitive, economic, and environmental domains, as well as a thorough medical evaluation and discussion of advance directives. Comprehensive assessment also includes investigation of existing financial supports and the ability of the patient and family to manage finances.

The assessment can be done at home or in the office, hospital, or nursing facility. Most comprehensive geriatric assessments are performed in an outpatient setting and may require more than one visit. A multidisciplinary team (eg, geriatrician, nurse, social worker, physical and occupational therapists, and others) works closely with the patient and family or other care provider. Goals of care are determined and reevaluated during follow-up visits. While comprehensive assessment may reveal functional deficits, it is premature to arrange for a home health aide.

When geriatric evaluation and management are targeted to high-risk older adults, studies show less functional decline and improved mental health at no additional cost (SOE=A). Many studies show a trend of improved survival, but a comprehensive meta-analysis of randomized, controlled trials did not demonstrate a survival benefit for outpatient comprehensive assessment (SOE=A).

References

1. Caprio TV, Williams TF. Comprehensive geriatric assessment. In: Duthie EH, Katz PR, Malone ML, eds. *Practice of Geriatrics*. 4th ed. Philadelphia: Saunders; 2007:41–53.
2. Kuo HK, Glasser-Scandrett K, Dave J, et al. The influence of outpatient comprehensive geriatric assessment on survival: meta-analysis. *Arch Geront Geri*. 2004;39(3):245–254.

130. Which of the following statements is true?

(A) Aged skeletal muscle cells are more likely than younger skeletal muscle cells to undergo apoptosis (cell death) as a result of physical inactivity.

(B) The reductions in skeletal muscle tone and contractility that occur with aging are due primarily to changes in muscle mass.

(C) Muscles do not lose any tone with aging if they are exercised regularly.

(D) The rate and extent of muscle changes is determined almost entirely by exercise and does not have a genetic component.

ANSWER: A

Loss of muscle mass and declines in muscle function with aging are the major clinical features of sarcopenia. The pathophysiology of this highly prevalent condition remains unknown.

Older animals are more likely to develop apoptosis of skeletal muscle cells in response to physical inactivity. Declines in muscle quality with aging include decreased regen-erative potential and increased tissue fibrosis. Muscle stem cells (satellite cells) from aged mice have a greater tendency to convert from a myogenic to a fibrogenic lineage as they begin to proliferate. Moreover, this conversion appears to be mediated by circulating factors present in serum from aged mice that induce Wnt signaling. Age-related reductions in muscle tone and contractility result from both aging changes in the nervous system as well as changes involving the quality of the muscle tissue. The rate and extent of muscle changes seems to be, at least in part, genetically determined and is also influenced by physical activity.

References

1. Brack AS, Conboy MJ, Roy S, et al. Increased Wnt signaling during aging alters muscle stem cell fate and increases fibrosis. *Science*. 2007;317(5839):807–810.
2. Loeser RF, Delbono O. Aging of the muscles and joints. In: Halter JB, Hazzard WR, Ouslander JG, et al, eds. *Hazzard's Principles of Geriatric Medicine and Gerontology, 6th ed*. New York: McGraw Hill; 2009:1355–1368.
3. Marzetti E, Leeuwenburgh C. Skeletal muscle apoptosis, sarcopenia and frailty at old age. *Exp Gerontol*. 2006;41(12):1234–1238.

131. A 72-yr-old woman is brought to the office by her daughter. The patient has COPD that is well controlled on tiotropium. It is winter, and many people in the community have been ill with respiratory viruses. The health department has identified sporadic influenza, respiratory syncytial virus, human metapneumovirus, rhinovirus, and coronaviruses, but no clear "outbreak" has been identified. Her illness started about a week ago with temperature to 37.8°C (100.0°F) and upper respiratory symptoms of a mild sore throat and hoarseness, but no rhinorrhea, myalgias, or cough. On examination, she has mild wheezes bilaterally. A chest radiograph demonstrates the COPD changes noted previously and a new interstitial infiltrate.

Which organism is the most likely cause of her pneumonia?

(A) Influenza
(B) Respiratory syncytial virus
(C) Parainfluenza virus
(D) Coronavirus
(E) Rhinovirus

ANSWER: C

Respiratory viral infections are common in older adults in the community. Winter respiratory season carries risk of each of the viruses listed and all can cause viral pneumonia, but clinical clues can help differentiate them. In the midst of the peak influenza season and an identified outbreak in the community, the pretest probability for any respiratory illness being due to influenza is very high. However, outside an outbreak, there is no clearly most prevalent organism. This patient's illness is of subacute onset and lacks myalgias, cough, or rhinorrhea, but hoarseness is prominent and there are mild wheezes. She has underlying COPD, so any of these viruses can cause bronchospasm. Wheezing is often seen with respiratory syncytial virus, but rhinorrhea is common as well. Influenza usually starts abruptly with high fever and myalgias. Coronaviruses and rhinoviruses also nearly universally have shorter incubation periods and result in nasal symptoms. In contrast, parainfluenza virus is often subacute and results in hoarseness; laryngitis is common. Only influenza has clearly effective therapy (oseltamivir or zanamivir) if administered early in the course of illness.

References

1. Falsey AR. Community-acquired viral pneumonia. *Clin Geriatr Med*. 2007;23(3):535–552.
2. Johnstone J, Majumdar SR, Fox JD, et al. Viral infection in adults hospitalized with community-acquired pneumonia: prevalence, pathogens, and presentation. *Chest*. 2008;134(6):1141–1148.

132. A 75-yr-old woman comes to the office because she perceives hearing loss. On examination, both of her ears are impacted with cerumen.

Which of the following types of hearing loss results from impacted cerumen?

(A) Conductive
(B) Sensorineural
(C) Mixed
(D) Functional

ANSWER: A

Conductive hearing loss can be caused by occlusion of the outer ear (external auditory canal) by impacted cerumen, which is common in older adults. Other causes of conductive hearing loss include middle ear effusion, otosclerosis, Eustachian tube obstruction, and tumor of the middle ear or nasopharyngeal region. The prevalence of middle ear abnormalities and hearing loss is higher in older adults with osteoarthritis who have no family history of hearing loss, no noise exposure, and no chronic middle ear effusion than in older adults without arthritis.

The audiogram, a graph of hearing level (loudness) as a function of frequency (pitch), describes the nature, severity, and configuration of an individual's hearing loss. The audiologist plots hearing level by frequency for right and left ears. The ability to hear tones transmitted by air and bone conduction is tested. Assessment of hearing by air conduction yields information about the status of the outer, middle, and inner ear; the eighth cranial nerve; and the central auditory pathways, including the brain. Assessment of hearing by bone conduction tells the audiologist about the status of the cochlear (sensorineural) mechanism. If there is a difference between thresholds for air and bone conduction, with bone conduction normal or better than air conduction, the individual has a conductive hearing loss.

In sensorineural hearing loss, both air and bone conduction are depressed to the same degree and are at the same point on the audiogram. Sensorineural hearing loss is associated with presbycusis, tumors of the eighth cranial nerve, Meniere disease, ototoxicity, and noise exposure. High-frequency sensorineural hearing loss due to aging, noise exposure, or ototoxic agents is usually treated with nonmedical interventions. These interventions are designed to enhance audibility of high-frequency, low-intensity consonants, which is key to understanding speech. Tinnitus and vertigo can accompany sensorineural hearing loss, or they can be symptoms of medical conditions.

Mixed hearing loss develops when hearing for air- and bone-conducted signals is depressed below normal, with air conduction significantly worse than bone conduction. In older adults with presbycusis, new onset of a middle ear infection or impacted cerumen may temporarily cause mixed hearing loss. Mixed and conductive types of hearing loss can require referral to an otolaryngologist and are often reversible.

Functional hearing loss is diagnosed when audiometric test results appear unreliable or inconsistent with behavior, and when findings appear to lack validity. Individuals who attempt to feign hearing loss often perform inconsistently on audiometric tests, resulting in a diagnosis of functional hearing loss.

References

1. Bagai A, Thavendiranathan P, Detsky A. Does this patient have a hearing impairment? *JAMA.* 2006;295(4):416–428.
2. Rawook V, Harrington B. Middle ear admittance and hearing abnormalities in individuals with osteoarthritis. *Audiol Neurotol.* 2007;12(2):127–136.

133. A 72-yr-old man is seen for preoperative assessment in anticipation of a prostate biopsy. He has asymptomatic aortic stenosis with a stable III/VI holosystolic murmur and type II diabetes mellitus controlled by diet. He is allergic to penicillin but has taken cephalexin or clindamycin for dental procedures in the past without difficulty.

Which of the following is the most appropriate recommendation regarding endocarditis prophylaxis for the biopsy?

(A) No prophylaxis
(B) Oral cephalexin
(C) Intravenous cefazolin
(D) Oral cephalexin plus oral clindamycin
(E) Intravenous cefazolin plus intravenous clindamycin

ANSWER: A

In 2007 the American Heart Association revised its endocarditis prophylaxis recommendations to recognize the rarity of seeding of heart valves associated with various procedures. Antibiotic prophylaxis is no longer recommended for GI or genitourinary procedures. It is still recommended for a limited number of respiratory and skin/soft tissue procedures, for dental procedures that include manipulation of gingival tissue or the periapical tooth region, and for procedures that involve perforation of the oral mucosa. Prophylaxis under any circumstance is now recommended *only* for patients with prosthetic heart valves or in whom prosthetic material was used for repair, and for patients with a history of endocarditis (SOE=B). Patients with unrepaired congenital heart disease or with repaired congenital heart disease who still have a residual defect should also receive prophylaxis under any circumstance. Patients with congenital heart disease repaired with prosthetic material or a device should receive prophylaxis under any circumstance *only* in the first 6 mo after repair.

Reference

1. Wilson W, Taubert KA, Gewitz M, et al. Prevention of infective endocarditis: guidelines from the American Heart Association. *Circulation.* 2007;116(15):1736–1754.

134. A 67-yr-old woman comes to the office for advice regarding diet. She recently had a modified radical mastectomy for stage I breast cancer. She chose this approach because she wanted to avoid radiation and chemotherapy. She has always had a healthy lifestyle. She asks whether there are any dietary changes she could make to avoid recurrence of breast cancer.

Which of the following is most likely to reduce breast cancer recurrence?

(A) Increase soy foods.
(B) Drink 4 cups of green tea daily.
(C) Restrict fats to <10% of diet.
(D) Follow a strict vegetarian diet.

ANSWER: B

Green tea has been shown to reduce the recurrence of stages I and II breast cancer. A meta-analysis of 13 studies indicated a lower risk of breast cancer with green (but not black) tea consumption. There are multiple mechanisms for the role of tea in cancer prevention: tea has antioxidant and antiangiogenic properties, and it suppresses proliferation of neoplastic cells, inhibits formation of N-nitroso compounds, inhibits cell division by telomerase inhibition, upregulates intracellular gap junction communication, interferes with estrogen metabolism, and increases apoptosis in cancer cells. The recommended amount for cancer prevention is 4 to 5 cups daily (SOE=B).

The recommendation to eat soy foods is controversial for women who have had breast cancer. Epidemiologic data support soy food as preventive of breast cancer only if it is consumed during adolescence. In vitro data show both tumor growth and suppression with exposure to soy (SOE=C).

The Women's Health Initiative did not show a statistically significant reduction in recurrence of breast cancer with a low-fat diet. In this 8-yr study, women were asked to reduce fat to 20% of total calories. Only 31% of the women were able to meet the goal at year 1, and only 14% at year 6; the result was an underpowered study (SOE=A).

A strict vegetarian diet has not been assessed for prevention of breast cancer. There is epidemiologic evidence of increased risk with beef and with any burnt animal flesh (SOE=D).

References

1. Michels KB, Mohllajee AP, Roset-Bahmanyar E, et al. Diet and breast cancer: a review of the prospective observational studies. *Cancer.* 2007;109(12 Suppl):2712–2749.
2. Prentice RL, Caan B, Chlebowski RT, et al. Low-fat dietary pattern and risk of invasive breast cancer: The Women's Health Initiative Randomized Controlled Dietary Modification Trial. *JAMA.* 2006;295(6):629–642.
3. Sun CL, Yuan JM, Koh WP, et al. Green tea, black tea and breast cancer risk: a meta-analysis of epidemiological studies. *Carcinogenesis.* 2006;27(7):1310–1315.

135. An 83-yr-old woman comes to the office because she has shortness of breath when she exercises and general fatigue and weakness. She reports no abdominal pain, change in bowel function, rectal bleeding, passage of black feces, or chest pain.

Examination is normal except for stool, which is positive for occult blood.

Laboratory results:
Hemoglobin	8.9 g/dL
Mean corpuscular volume	75 fL
Ferritin	10 ng/mL

Upper intestinal endoscopy and colonoscopy are normal, and no potential bleeding source is identified.

Which of the following studies should be done next?

(A) Angiography
(B) CT enteroclysis
(C) Small-bowel barium radiography
(D) Double-balloon enteroscopy
(E) Capsule endoscopy

ANSWER: E

In approximately 5% of patients with GI bleeding, no source is found on conventional upper and lower endoscopy. The most common cause of obscure blood loss in patients ≥40 yr old is arteriovenous malformation of the small intestine. Occult small-bowel bleeding can be detected by capsule endoscopy in up to 88% of cases (SOE=B). Capsule endoscopy and double-balloon enteroscopy have the same level of effectiveness in diagnosis of

small-bowel disease, including obscure GI bleeding. Each technique detects lesions not always seen by the other. The procedures can be complementary, but capsule endoscopy should be the initial diagnostic test because it is noninvasive, easily tolerated, and provides a view of the entire small bowel; it also is useful in determining the initial route of double-balloon enteroscopy (SOE=C).

Initial capsule endoscopy appears to be superior to angiography for the immediate investigation in patients with obscure intestinal bleeding, and is superior to CT enteroclysis in detection of potential bleeding lesions. Capsule endoscopy is more effective in finding the bleeding site than push enteroscopy. Barium radiography of the small bowel can reveal masses and structural abnormalities but would be unlikely to reveal arteriovenous malformations, the most likely cause of bleeding in an 83-yr-old woman.

References

1. Kamalaporn P, Cho S, Basset N, et al. Double-balloon enteroscopy following capsule endoscopy in the management of obscure gastrointestinal bleeding: outcome of a combined approach. *Can J Gastroenterol.* 2008;22(5):491–495.
2. Li XB, GE ZZ, Dai J, et al. The role of capsule endoscopy combined with double-balloon enteroscopy in diagnosis of small bowel diseases. *Chin Med J.* 2007;120(1):30–35.
3. Pasha SF, Leighton JA, Das A, et al. Double-balloon enteroscopy and capsule endoscopy have comparable diagnostic yield in small-bowel disease: a meta-analysis. *Clin Gastroenterol Hepatol.* 2008;6(6):671–676.
4. Saperas E, Dot J, Videla S, et al. Capsule endoscopy versus computed tomographic or standard angiography for the diagnosis of obscure gastrointestinal bleeding. *Am J Gastroenterol.* 2007;102(4):731–737.

136. A three-member geriatrics practice serves patients in two nursing homes and a private office. A researcher meets with the senior physician to recruit the practice for enrolling patients with heart failure into a nonblind, uncontrolled trial of a newly approved β-blocker. The trial is meant to test patient dosing preferences. The pharmaceutical company will provide the medications, keep the records, and do all follow-up for the research. The company will interact directly with the patients after obtaining their names and contact information from the practice, and the researcher does not need access to the patients' medical records. The contact physician will be listed as a coauthor of an article if the group refers at least 20 patients over the coming year. The group will get a payment of $1,000 per patient enrolled.

Which of the following statements is true?

(A) The research design will likely answer the question of patient dosing preference.
(B) Including the referring physician as a coauthor is appropriate in publications of multicenter trials.
(C) Entering patients into the trial requires documented informed consent by the patient or by a legal surrogate.
(D) Approval of the research by an Institutional Review Board authorized under the Office for Human Research Protections is sufficient legal oversight for the patient.
(E) No disclosure is needed for the financial agreement.

ANSWER: C

The lack of a control group, the offer of authorship, the substantial financial inducement, the lack of engagement of the patient or physician in evaluating the data, the vagueness of the data collected, and the inattention to the patient's baseline condition indicate that this project is marketing disguised as research. Such projects are an effective strategy for manufacturers to familiarize physicians with a new product and encourage switching patients to it. Converting the physician and patient to the product more than balances the initial cost to the manufacturer. Results from most of these trials are never published, or are published in journal supplements controlled by the manufacturers.

Physicians are often flattered to be asked to join in research and believe that the financial inducements are appropriate. If the physician is inclined to participate, he or she could investigate the endeavor by asking to see the protocol and analytic plan and the researcher's record of publication, by requesting that the protocol be reviewed by a reputable academic group or by the state or national professional organization, and by reviewing the submission to and the consent of the ethics review board for protection of the research participants. If there is any concern about the validity of the research, then any risk to patients is unjustified. One approach to ensuring the appropriateness of involvement is to establish a standard procedure to notify patients of any situation (including payments) that might appear to compromise the physician's ability to advocate for the patient's best interests. If making that information available to patients would be uncomfortable or unacceptable, participating in the research is unwise.

A physician who chooses to go forward with this plan would have to recognize an obligation to a high standard of informed consent. Believing that the new medication actually offers an advantage is worth telling the patient, of course, but the patient has to know that the physician may have a conflict of interest.

The design of the study is not likely to address any merits of the new drug. Sequential, nonblind, nonrandomized designs are unlikely to be sensitive to small effects, and at least two elements are being tested simultaneously: the different medication and the daily dosing.

Citing the physician as a coauthor on any ensuing publication is contrary to the obligations of authorship.

The approval of the Institutional Review Board for the project does not settle the legal issues for the physician and patient. The physician maintains an obligation to serve the patient well; such responsibility would not be voided solely with the Board's approval of the research and its consent process.

If the party proposing such an arrangement is unwilling to have it made public, the physician should not participate. Almost all contracts involving patient well-being are readily discoverable, and a clause that penalized physicians for sharing information with their patients would be scandalous.

References

1. International Committee of Medical Journal Editors.
   Uniform Requirements for Manuscripts Submitted to
   Biomedical Journals: Writing and Editing for
   Biomedical Publication. Updated October 2007.
   http://www.icmje.org/index.html (accessed Nov 2009).
2. Rao JN, Cassia LJ. Ethics of undisclosed payments to
   doctors recruiting patients in clinical trials. *BMJ.*
   2002;325(7354):36–37.
3. Ross JS, Lackner JE, Lurie P, et al. Pharmaceutical
   company payments to physicians: early experiences
   with disclosure laws in Vermont and Minnesota.
   JAMA. 2007;297(11):1216–1223.

137. An 88-yr-old black woman with peripheral
arterial disease is admitted to the hospital
because she has gangrene in 2 toes and
soft-tissue infection of her distal foot. She is a
widow and lives alone; her daughter visits at
least weekly.

On admission, her blood pressure is 140/80
mmHg, respiratory rate is 16 breaths per
minute, pulse is 90, and temperature is 38°C
(100.4°F). She is acutely confused and
inattentive. Her speech is rambling.

Which of the following factors is most likely to
increase her risk of in-hospital functional
decline and nursing home placement?

(A) Marital status
(B) Race
(C) Gender
(D) Delirium

ANSWER: D

Factors that predict both in-hospital functional
decline (as measured by ability to perform
ADLs) and nursing-home placement include
older age, dependence in IADLs, delirium, and
other cognitive impairment, such as dementia
(SOE=B). Factors more predictive of
nursing-home admission than of functional
decline include living alone and patient and
family preference for institutional care. Gender,
race, and marital status have less influence as
predictors of either outcome.

The effect of race on in-hospital functional
decline has been examined. There was no
difference between older black and older white
patients in improvement in ADLs by the time
of hospital discharge or by 90 days after
discharge. At the same time points, however,
improvement in IADLs was significantly less
likely among black patients than among white
patients.

References

1. Boyd CM, Xue QL, Guralnik JM, et al. Hospitalization
   and development of dependence in activities of daily
   living in a cohort of disabled older women: the
   Women's Health and Aging Study I. *J Gerontol A Biol
   Sci Med Sci.* 2005;60(7):888–893.
2. Hoogerduijn JG, Schuurmans MJ, Duijnstee MS, et al.
   A systematic review of predictors and screening
   instruments to identify older hospitalized patients at
   risk for functional decline. *J Clin Nurs.*
   2007;16(1):46–57.
3. Sands LP, Landefeld CS, Ayers SM, et al. Disparities
   between black and white patients in functional
   improvement after hospitalization for an acute illness.
   J Am Geriatr Soc. 2005;53(10):1811–1816.

138. Which of the following is true of the
relationship between gambling and age?

(A) Rates of participation increase with age.
(B) Older adults who are recreational
    gamblers report poorer physical health
    than older adults who do not gamble.
(C) Older adults gamble more to win money
    than to relieve boredom.
(D) Gambling in later life is strongly
    associated with alcohol and other
    substance disorders.
(E) Naltrexone decreases the urge to gamble
    among older adults.

ANSWER: D

A recent analysis of the National
Epidemiologic Survey on Alcohol and Related
Conditions found strong associations between
gambling (both recreational and problem) and
alcohol and nicotine disorders among all adults
(SOE=B). This finding supports screening for
substance use disorders among older gamblers
(SOE=C).

Participation in gambling has increased
among older adults over the past decade,
probably because of the greater number of
casinos. Nonetheless, age remains inversely
associated with rates of participation in
gambling.

Despite similar levels of chronic illness,
older adults who are recreational gamblers (ie,
people who gamble but do not meet criteria for
problem or pathologic gambling) report better
mental and physical functioning than older
adults who do not gamble. One plausible
mechanism for this finding is that gambling
keeps older adults socially active, which could
translate into better perceived mental and
physical functioning. Older gamblers are more
likely to cite relief from boredom as a reason
to gamble than winning money.

Naltrexone has not been shown to decrease the urge to gamble.

References

1. Clarke D. Older adults' gambling motivation and problem gambling: a comparative study. *J Gambl Stud.* 2008;24(2):175–192.
2. Desai RA, Desai MM, Potenza MN. Gambling, health and age: data from the National Epidemiologic Survey on Alcohol and Related Conditions. *Psychol Add Behav.* 2007;21(4):431–440.
3. Desai RA, Maciejewski PK, Dausey DJ, et al. Health correlates of recreational gambling in older adults. *Am J Psychiatry.* 2004;161(9):1672–1679.
4. Pietrzak RH, Morasco BJ, Blanco C, et al. Gambling level and psychiatric and medical disorders in older adults: results from the National Epidemiologic Survey on Alcohol and Related Conditions. *Am J Geriatr Psych.* 2007;15(4):301–313.
5. http://www.gamblersanonymous.org/ (accessed Nov 2009).
6. http://www.ncpgambling.org/ (accessed Nov 2009).

139. A 74-yr-old man comes to the office for a routine examination. He feels well except for occasional discomfort in his left knee. He exercises 3 days per week, with strength training (lifting weights) for 60 min and running on a treadmill for 10–15 min. He engages in no other aerobic physical activity. History includes diabetes and hypertension; he has no history of angina or coronary artery disease. Medications include pioglitazone, glipizide, lisinopril, hydrochlorothiazide, and atorvastatin. On this regimen, systolic blood pressure has consistently ranged from 140 mmHg to 150 mmHg, and diastolic blood pressure has ranged from 70 mmHg to 80 mmHg.

On examination, he is 1.7 m (68 in) tall and weighs 83.9 kg (185 lb). Blood pressure is 142/74 mmHg.

Which of the following would you recommend?

(A) Reduce duration of weight lifting to 30 min, 3 days/wk.
(B) Begin balance exercises for at least 30 min, 3 days/wk.
(C) Begin moderate-intensity aerobic exercises for at least 30 min, 5 days/wk.
(D) Begin flexibility exercises for at least 30 min, 5 days/wk.
(E) Begin high-intensity aerobic exercises for at least 60 min, 3 days/wk.

ANSWER: C

This patient has diabetes and hypertension, which are significant risk factors for decreased functional status, morbidity, and mortality. His blood pressure and weight are high. Physical activity reduces the risk of cardiovascular disease, reduces blood pressure, improves glycemic control, and assists with weight loss and weight maintenance (SOE=A). The patient's current exercise regimen is inadequate: he needs to increase his aerobic exercise to at least 10 min of continuous activity per session, at least 30 min/day, at least 5 days/wk (SOE=B). The choice of aerobic exercises depends on his preference.

Overweight people who undertake an appropriate aerobic exercise program are at risk of sarcopenia due to weight loss. To counter this risk, the patient should continue strength training. However, he should focus on number of sets and repetitions, rather than on duration of the training period (SOE=C). Balance exercises are unnecessary in a person with steady gait and no history of falls (SOE=D). Flexibility exercises can be coordinated with his aerobic and strength-training program (SOE=D), but increased aerobic exercise is most important for this patient.

While high-intensity aerobic exercise of 60 min/day, 3 days/wk is an alternative regimen to control this patient's medical problems and reduce his risk of future decline, he should not increase suddenly from his current 10–15 min/day aerobic exercise to 60 min. In addition, his left knee may not tolerate high-intensity aerobic exercise (eg, running), although swimming may be an option.

References

1. American Geriatrics Society. Exercise prescription for older adults with osteoarthritis pain: consensus practice recommendations. AGS Panel on Exercise and Osteoarthritis. *J Am Geriatr Soc.* 2001;49(6):808–823.
2. Galvao DA, Taafe D. Resistance exercise dosage in older adults: single- versus multiset effects on physical performance and body composition. *J Am Geriatr Soc.* 2005;53(12):2090–2097.
3. Nelson ME, Rejeski WJ, Blair SN, et al. Physical activity and public health in older adults: recommendations from the American College of Sports Medicine and the American Heart Association. *Med Sci Sports Exerc.* 2007;39(8):1435–1445.

140. A 94-yr-old nursing home resident with Alzheimer's disease is evaluated because she has been disturbing other patients by screaming for help and banging on her recliner throughout the day for the past 4 wk.

Which of the following is most likely to reduce the patient's agitation?

(A) Nonpharmacologic intervention
(B) Second-generation antidepressant
(C) Second-generation antipsychotic agent
(D) Cholinergic agent

ANSWER: A

Nonpharmacologic interventions are first-line treatment in management of agitated behavior in patients with dementia (SOE=B). Analysis of the behavioral pattern can help identify stimuli or unmet needs that can trigger agitation. For example, specific environmental triggers, such as bathing, dressing, and under- or over-stimulation can cause increased agitation, as can reversible precipitants, such as pain and medical illness. Treating the pain or reconfiguring the environment may reverse or reduce agitation.

Once offending stimuli and unmet needs have been addressed, use of a second-generation antipsychotic agent is a second-line strategy for managing agitation. Use of second-generation antidepressants is another approach to managing agitation. Citalopram is somewhat effective in reducing irritability and disruptive vocalizations over 4–6 wk. In placebo-controlled studies in patients treated with fluvoxamine, no significant improvement was seen in irritability, anxiety, panic, restlessness, and mood. Reports have been mixed for other antidepressants, such as trazodone (SOE=C).

First-generation antipsychotic agents are somewhat effective for agitation but poorly tolerated (SOE=B). Their use is associated with high risk of extrapyramidal symptoms, tardive dyskinesia, hypotension, sedation, anticholinergic adverse events, and cognitive and functional impairment. Second-generation antipsychotics, such as risperidone, aripiprazole, and olanzapine, can also help reduce agitation and are associated with a lower incidence of extrapyramidal symptoms but high incidence of other adverse events (SOE=B). Safety concerns for these agents include metabolic syndrome, stroke risk, and increased mortality.

A review of the effect of cholinesterase inhibitors and memantine on cognition in patients with dementia incidentally found that several studies noted positive outcomes on a variety of behavioral measures (SOE=B). Mood symptoms appeared most responsive to cholinesterase inhibitors; improvements in aggression and agitation were observed most with memantine. There was great variability between studies. In general, trials with negative behavioral outcomes primarily involved institutionalized patients. As a whole, cholinesterase inhibitors and memantine appear to have a greater role in prevention, rather than treatment, of behavioral disturbance.

References

1. Cummings JL, Mackell J, Kaufer D. Behavioral effects of current Alzheimer's disease treatments: a descriptive review. *Alzheimers Dement.* 2008;4(1):49–60.
2. Hogan DB, Bailey P, Black S, et al. Diagnosis and treatment of dementia: 5. nonpharmacologic and pharmacologic therapy for mild to moderate dementia. *CMAJ.* 2008;179(10):1019–1026.
3. Schneider LS, Tariot PN, Dagerman KS, et al. Effectiveness of atypical antipsychotic drugs in patients with Alzheimer's disease. *N Engl J Med.* 2006;355(15):1525–1538.
4. Sink KM, Holden KF, Yaffe K. Pharmacological treatment of neuropsychiatric symptoms of dementia: a review of the evidence. *JAMA.* 2005;293(5):596–608.
5. Zarit S, Femia E. Behavioral and psychosocial interventions for family caregivers. *Am J Nursing.* 2008;108(9 Suppl):47–53.

141. A 72-yr-old man with chronic emphysema is being discharged home after spending 3 wk on a ventilator after a probable viral infection. The patient receives oxygen at home. Several months ago, he was on a ventilator for a few days. During preparations for discharge, the patient emphatically states that he does not want ventilator care ever again. His wife died a year ago and he lives alone, with no friendly contacts. He cannot smoke because of the oxygen, and he cannot go fishing or leave his apartment to play poker any more. He asks that arrangements be made so that he is not readmitted and placed on the ventilator again.

Which of the following strategies is most likely to reassure the patient?

(A) Refer patient to a hospice with an inpatient unit.
(B) Order continuous positive airway pressure for home.
(C) Legally document a "do not resuscitate" directive.
(D) Refer patient to a hospice that can provide sedation at home.
(E) Evaluate patient for major depressive disorder.

ANSWER: D

A patient who faces dyspnea and suffocation cannot be served humanely without a ventilator unless the care team can provide sedation. A hospice that can provide home sedation would allow the patient to be confident that he will be comfortable at home until there is a final exacerbation. It would be wise to document the care plan and his role in shaping it; that documentation is usually sufficient without such legal requirements as a second witness or a notary. The patient could be evaluated for major depressive disorder, but his response to his situation is reasonable, and he is not so much withdrawn as isolated by illness. He might benefit from interventions to decrease his isolation, such as visits from hospice volunteers, nearby church or veterans organizations, and meals programs. Any consideration of more treatment, such as continuous positive airway pressure, should have been part of his ongoing evaluation; it would not be likely that additional treatment could offer major gains now. All hospice programs are required to have inpatient care available, which may be useful for him at a later point.

References
1. CMS. State Operations Manual. Appendix M – Guidance to Surveyors: Hospice (Rev. 1, 05-21-04). Section L 102 concerning statutory section 418.50 (b) Standard: Required Services, pp 16–17 at http://www.cms.hhs.gov/manuals/downloads/som107ap_m_hospice.pdf (accessed Nov 2009).
2. Lynn J, Goldstein NE. Advance care planning for fatal chronic illness: avoiding commonplace errors and unwarranted suffering. *Ann Intern Med.* 2003;138(10):812–820.
3. Quill TE, Byock IR; for ACP-ASIM End-of-Life Care Consensus Panel. Responding to intractable terminal suffering: the role of terminal sedation and voluntary refusal of food and fluids. *Ann Intern Med.* 2000;132(5):408–414.
4. The Hastings Center. *Guidelines for the Termination of Life-sustaining Treatment and the Care of the Dying.* Bloomington, IN; Indiana University Press; 1987 (updated guidelines anticipated 2010).

142. A 78-yr-old man comes to the office because he has pain in his left knee over the past month. History includes longstanding hypertension, type 2 diabetes mellitus, ischemic cardiomyopathy, and chronic kidney disease. He is on hydrochlorothiazide, metoprolol, lisinopril, atorvastatin, aspirin, and glipizide.

On examination, blood pressure is 132/80 mmHg, and pulse is 70 beats per minute. The left knee joint is tender on palpation, and effusion is evident. Celecoxib 200 mg q12h is prescribed.

After 12 days of therapy, the patient returns to the office because he has dyspnea, increased swelling in both legs, and fatigue. Blood pressure is increased to 178/102 mmHg. BUN is 71 mg/dL (baseline, 38 mg/dL) and serum creatinine concentration is 4.3 mg/dL (baseline, 2.1 mg/dL). Urinalysis shows low urine sodium, no cellular elements, and no proteinuria.

Which of the following is the most likely mechanism by which celecoxib caused acute renal failure in this patient?

(A) Drug-induced allergic interstitial nephritis
(B) Acute papillary necrosis with renal obstruction
(C) Drug-induced acute tubular necrosis
(D) Hemodynamic renal insufficiency
(E) Nephrotic syndrome

ANSWER: D

NSAIDs are a common cause of acute renal failure (SOE=A). NSAIDs (including cyclooxygenase-2 [COX-2] inhibitors) act to inhibit synthesis of renal cyclooxygenase and renal prostaglandin. Renal prostaglandins act as local vasodilators and modify the vasoconstrictor effects of angiotensin II and catecholamines. Thus, NSAIDs can produce an acute decline in glomerular filtration rate and renal plasma flow when given to patients with high angiotensin II and norepinephrine levels. This most often occurs with circulating volume depletion due to, for example, heart failure or cirrhosis. In these conditions, renal prostaglandin synthesis is upregulated to counteract the vasoconstrictive actions of angiotensin II and norepinephrine and to allow adequate renal plasma flow to support glomerular filtration. NSAIDs have little effect on renal function when given to patients with normal circulating volume; such patients have relatively low baseline levels of renal prostaglandin production. The patient in this case has ischemic cardiomyopathy and, thus, a significantly increased propensity for hemodynamically mediated acute renal failure. Initially, selective COX-2 inhibitors were thought to have a lower likelihood of causing acute renal failure; however, this has not proved to be the case, especially in older adults.

NSAIDs can lead to other renal abnormalities: they may increase blood pressure and antagonize the blood pressure-lowering effect of antihypertensive medications. NSAIDs can also lead to sodium retention, with resulting edema and exacerbation of heart failure (as in this case). Finally, NSAIDs can lead to acute tubulointerstitial nephritis, acute papillary necrosis, hyponatremia, hyperkalemia, acute ischemic renal insufficiency, and proteinuria. Caution and close monitoring of renal function are required for any patient on long-term NSAID therapy.

In this case, the clinical history included bland urine sediment, ie, there were no WBCs indicative of interstitial nephritis, no granular casts indicative of ischemic injury, and no proteinuria indicative of a nephrotic syndrome. The most likely explanation is that the COX-2 inhibitor led to hemodynamically mediated acute renal failure.

References

1. Cheng HF, Harris RC. Renal effects of non-steroidal anti-inflammatory drugs and selective cyclooxygenase-2 inhibitors. *Curr Pharmacol Des.* 2005;11(14):1795–1804.
2. Harris RC. COX-2 and the kidney. *J Cardiovasc Pharmacol.* 2006;47:S37–S42.

143. An 80-yr-old man uses a handheld magnifier to read medication labels and the newspaper. He has never been prescribed eyeglasses. History includes successful cataract surgery 8 yr ago. At a routine ophthalmology examination 6 mo ago, his vision was recorded as 20/40 in his right eye and 20/50 in his left eye for distance with no correction. Near vision was not recorded. He was told he had the "eyes of a 30-yr-old" and was scheduled to return in 1 yr.

Which of the following is the most likely cause of his inability to read without a magnifier?

(A) Early exudative (wet) macular degeneration
(B) Early nonexudative (dry) macular degeneration
(C) Glaucoma
(D) Opacification of the posterior capsule of his lens after cataract surgery
(E) Lack of eyeglasses

ANSWER: E

One of the most common causes of decreased vision in the United States is uncorrected refractive error (SOE=A). The patient had an excellent response to cataract surgery and can see at a distance. However, the ophthalmologist did not perform a refraction to determine if eyeglasses would improve his vision. Although there are intraocular lens implants that can provide for near and distant vision, they are not the lens of choice for all patients. This patient has good distant vision but did not receive eyeglasses to improve his near vision. He has "solved" the problem himself by using magnifiers. By providing him with a prescription for eyeglasses, he will likely be more independent, able to read more comfortably, and drive with better acuity.

Exudative and nonexudative macular degeneration affects near acuity and distant vision. An early sign of macular degeneration is central visual distortion or scotoma, which would also be apparent with distance. Some patients with early macular changes report that the door frame appears distorted or wavy. This patient was recently seen by his ophthalmologist, who gave the patient a good report.

Vision loss from glaucoma presents with peripheral field constriction. Near vision is not affected until the disease has progressed (SOE=A). Opacification of the posterior capsule develops after intraocular lens implantation; it affects distant as well as near vision.

References

1. *Age-Related Macular Degeneration, Preferred Practice Pattern.* San Francisco, CA: American Academy of Ophthalmology; 2006. Available at: http://one.aao.org/CE/PracticeGuidelines/PPP.aspx (accessed Nov 2009).
2. Lane SS. Posterior capsule opacification and YAG capsulotomy. *Am J Ophthalmol.* 2004;138(4):635–636.
3. Much JW, Liu C, Piltz-Seymour JR. Long-term survival of central visual field in end-stage glaucoma. *Ophthalmology.* 2008;115(7):1162–1166.

4. Prevent Blindness America. Vision Problems in the U.S. *Prevalence of Adult Vision Impairment and Age-Related Eye Disease in America.* 2008 Update. http://www.preventblindness.org/vpus/ (accessed Nov 2009).

144. A 75-yr-old woman comes to the office because she has burning pain and skin sensitivity to clothing on her left arm. She underwent surgical repair of a torn rotator cuff 4 mo ago, and she received 2 wk of outpatient rehabilitation after surgery.

On examination, vital signs are normal. The patient has good muscle strength in all directions at the shoulder. Passive range of motion of the shoulder and elbow is full but elicits pain. Slight edema is present from the elbow to the hand. There is some erythema of the hand and forearm, and the skin is sensitive to touch. There are no lesions on the hand or arm.

In addition to physical therapy, which of the following treatments is most effective?

(A) Intravenous regional sympathetic block with guanethidine
(B) Oral prednisolone
(C) Calcitonin
(D) Local anesthetic sympathetic blockade

ANSWER: B

This patient has a number of features common to complex regional pain syndrome (also known as reflex sympathetic dystrophy, shoulder-hand syndrome, and causalgia). The most disturbing symptom is pain, usually described as burning or deep and aggravated by movement. It does not follow a dermatomal distribution. Pain can be worsened by non-noxious stimuli (allodynia). The pain is usually accompanied by local edema and vasomotor changes. Early in the course, the skin is often erythematous and warm. Later, it may appear cyanotic, or mottled with livedo reticularis. Finally, the skin may become shiny and thin, and nails become brittle.

Physical therapy is helpful. In a study comparing physical therapy to occupational therapy and a control intervention of support offered by a social worker, physical therapy reduced pain and improved active mobility more than occupational therapy in patients with complex regional pain syndrome. Occupational therapy had a greater effect than the control intervention (SOE=B).

In a study comparing the effectiveness of different agents for complex regional pain syndrome, 83% of patients taking prednisolone and 17% of patients taking piroxicam improved significantly (SOE=B).

In a review of 7 randomized trials, intravenous regional sympathetic blocks did not appear to provide clinically significant improvement for patients with complex regional pain syndrome. In 4 trials, use of guanethidine did not have a significant effect on pain, and it was stopped prematurely in 1 trial because of the severity of adverse events (SOE=A).

Intranasal salmon calcitonin, 100 units q8h, combined with physical therapy was associated with decreased pain and improved mobility at 8 wk in a randomized, placebo-controlled trial with 66 patients. However, although the improvements were statistically significant, there was no clinically significant improvement in function (SOE=B).

The Cochrane Collaboration review of randomized trials of sympathetic blockade with local anesthetics in adults with complex regional pain syndrome showed no significant effect on obtaining at least 50% pain relief 30–120 min after blockade. Meta-analysis of longer-term relief was not possible because different studies evaluated different outcomes (SOE=B).

References

1. Cepeda MS, Carr DB, Lau J. Local anesthetic sympathetic blockade for complex regional pain syndrome. *Cochrane Database Syst Rev.* 2005 Oct 2005;(4):CD004598.
2. Kalita J, Vajpayee A, Misra UK. Comparison of prednisolone with piroxicam in complex regional pain syndrome following stroke: a randomized controlled trial. *QJM.* 2006;99(2):89–95.
3. Oerlemans HM, Oostendorp RA, de Boo T, et al. Pain and reduced mobility in complex regional pain syndrome I: outcome of a prospective randomised controlled clinical trial of adjuvant physical therapy versus occupational therapy. *Pain.* 1999;83(1):77.
4. Perez RS, Kwakkel G, Zuurmond WW, et al. Treatment of reflex sympathetic dystrophy (CRPS type 1): a research synthesis of 21 randomized clinical trials. *J Pain Symptom Manage.* 2001;21(6):511–526.
5. Sahin F, Yilmaz F, Kotevoglu N, et al. Efficacy of salmon calcitonin in complex regional pain syndrome (type 1) in addition to physical therapy. *Clin Rheum.* 2006;25(2):143–148.

145. A 79-yr-old woman comes for a follow-up office visit 2 wk after hospital discharge. She had been admitted for exacerbation of heart failure. She has atrial fibrillation, hypertension, systolic heart failure (New York Heart Association class III), and coronary artery disease. Medications include furosemide 20 mg q12h, potassium 10 mEq/d, lisinopril 10 mg/d, warfarin 2 mg/d, metoprolol 25 mg q12h, and since hospital discharge, spironolactone 12.5 mg/d.

On examination, the patient's weight is stable and she has returned to baseline function.

Laboratory tests:

	On hospital discharge	Today
Sodium (mEq/L)	137	139
Potassium (mEq/L)	4.7	5.3
BUN (mg/dL)	20	21
Creatinine (mg/dL)	1.1	1.3

Which of the following is the most appropriate next step?

(A) Discontinue spironolactone.
(B) Discontinue potassium supplement.
(C) Decrease lisinopril dosage.
(D) Increase lisinopril dosage.
(E) Change furosemide schedule to a single daily dose.

ANSWER: B

The increase in serum potassium is likely due to spironolactone. When spironolactone is introduced, serum potassium levels increase on average by about 0.3 mmol/L. Her potassium supplement should have been stopped when spironolactone was started. This woman is at particular risk of hyperkalemia with spironolactone because, in addition to potassium supplements, she takes an ACE inhibitor (lisinopril) and she has renal impairment.

Spironolactone use is associated with reduced mortality and fewer exacerbations of heart failure when used in patients with New York Heart Association class III or IV disease who were recently hospitalized for heart failure. Thus, it is an appropriate agent for this patient (SOE=A). Serum creatinine levels can increase by up to 20% with the use of aldosterone antagonists; this increase is not a reason to discontinue the spironolactone. In general, if the estimated creatinine clearance is <30 mL/min, spironolactone is not advised.

Discontinuing the potassium supplement will likely reduce the serum potassium level, obviating the need to decrease the dosage of lisinopril. ACE inhibitors improve survival and reduce morbidity in patients with left ventricular ejection fraction <40% (SOE=A). Although taking furosemide once daily may be more convenient, the highest priority is to stop the supplemental potassium.

Because the patient's weight is stable and her function has returned to baseline, there is no indication for increasing the lisinopril dosage.

References

1. Hunt SA, Abraham WT, Chin MH, et al. ACC/AHA 2005 guideline update for the diagnosis and management of chronic heart failure in the adult: A report of the American College of Cardiology/American Heart Association Task Force on Practice Guidelines (Writing Committee to Update the 2001 Guidelines for the Evaluation and Management of Heart Failure). *J Am Coll Cardiol.* 2005;46(6):1116–1143.
2. Jneid H, Moukarbel GV, Dawson B, et al. Combining neuroendocrine inhibitors in heart failure: reflections on safety and efficacy. *Am J Med.* 2007;120(12):1090.e1–8.

146. Which of the following should be undertaken *first* in an initial evaluation to determine if a new patient is at risk of falls?

(A) Check vision.
(B) Ask about previous falls.
(C) Examine feet.
(D) Check for arrhythmia.
(E) Perform a mental status examination.

ANSWER: B

Fall prevention is important to incorporate in the care of all older adults. Risk assessment and management reduce the incidence of falls, and in the primary care setting, can reduce the incidence of emergency treatment for fall injuries. The first step in assessing risk is to ask about previous falls (SOE=A). Patients who have fallen previously are at risk of future falls, especially if they have impaired mobility. Older adults often will not mention previous falls unless specifically asked about them. According to published guidelines, if a patient has fallen more than once in the past year, or has fallen once and has impaired gait or balance, fall risk should be fully assessed (SOE=C). The evaluation should identify factors that can be modified or eliminated to reduce fall risk. Modifiable factors include problems with balance and gait, use of more than four medications, postural hypotension, and home environmental hazards. Additional factors are sensory deficits, especially vision, and problems with feet and unsupportive footwear. Cardiac examination, including checking for arrhythmia, is indicated, especially if there are symptoms of lightheadedness or a history of syncope. Patients with dementia are at increased risk of falls, and a mental status screening test is an important part of the evaluation.

References

1. American Geriatric Society and British Geriatrics Society. *Clinical Practice Guideline for the Prevention of Falls in Older Persons.* New York: American Geriatrics Society; 2009 (http://www.americangeriatrics.org/).
2. Tinetti ME, Baker DI, King M, et al. Effect of dissemination of evidence in reducing injuries from falls. *N Engl J Med.* 2008;359(3):252–261.
3. Ganz DA, Bao Y, Shekelle PG, et al. Will my patient fall? *JAMA.* 2007;297(1):77–86.

147. Which of the following statements best characterizes nursing-home populations?

(A) The number of residents ≥65 yr old has increased since 1999.
(B) The proportion of residents ≥65 yr old has steadily increased.
(C) People ≥85 yr old are twice as likely to live in a nursing home as people 75–84 yr old.
(D) White residents have more impairments than black residents.
(E) Female residents have more impairments than male residents.

ANSWER: E

Women living in nursing homes need more assistance than men with ADLs. Women are more likely to need help with all ADLs; men are more likely to need no assistance. White residents have lower rates of dependence for each ADL than black residents or residents of other races.

In the United States in 2006, 1.62 million people ≥65 yr older (4.4%) lived in nursing homes or similar institutional settings. This rate has declined steadily since 1985, when 5.4% of people ≥65 yr old resided in nursing homes. The change was steepest in older age groups: the decline was 25% among those 65–74 yr old, and 37% among those ≥75 yr old. However, between 1985 and 1999, as the overall number of older people increased, the actual number of nursing-home residents ≥65 yr old increased. Since 1999, the number of adults living in nursing homes has declined back to the 1985 level.

The proportion of people living in nursing homes rises significantly with age: fewer than 2% are 65–74 yr old, 4.4% are 75–84 yr old, and 15.4% are ≥85 yr old. Depending on how support is defined, between 2% and 5% of older adults live in senior housing that provides at least one supportive service.

References

1. Administration on Aging. *A Profile of Older Americans: 2007.* Administration on Aging, U.S. Department of Health and Human Services. Washington, DC: U.S. Government Printing Office; 2007.
2. Federal Interagency Forum on Aging-Related Statistics. *Older Americans 2008: Key Indicators of Well-Being.* Federal Interagency Forum on Aging-Related Statistics. Washington, DC: U.S. Government Printing Office; 2008.

148. An 80-yr-old woman comes to the office for follow-up because a recent evaluation identified significant osteoporosis. She agrees to begin oral bisphosphonate therapy.

What is the most common adverse event of oral bisphosphonate therapy?

(A) Atrial fibrillation
(B) GI effects
(C) Osteogenic sarcoma
(D) Osteonecrosis of the jaw
(E) Thromboembolic disease

ANSWER: B

Bisphosphonate therapy is widely prescribed by geriatricians for management of osteoporosis. The importance of some serious, although rare, adverse events has tended to be overstated.

In a well-done systematic review, the most consistently noted adverse events associated with bisphosphonates were GI effects. Esophageal ulcers, as well as mild GI symptoms, such as acid reflux, appear to increase very slightly, but not statistically significantly over placebo with most bisphosphonates (SOE=A); however, the excess risk is probably minimal to nonexistent if administration instructions are strictly adhered to (SOE=B). The risk of more serious adverse events, such as perforations, ulcerations, and bleeding, was slightly increased with etidronate in a pooled analysis of 3 trials.

Among cardiac events, an increased risk of atrial fibrillation was found in one placebo-controlled trial of zoledronic acid. However, this finding was contradicted by the findings of another large trial published the same year. Another placebo-controlled trial suggested a possible increased risk of atrial fibrillation with alendronate.

There are many reported cases of osteonecrosis of the jaw in patients receiving intravenous bisphosphonates. The vast majority of cases are in patients who receive high doses of intravenous bisphosphonates for a cancer-related diagnosis; cases are much less common in patients being treated for osteoporosis. The risk posed by oral bisphosphonates is much less certain. Most patients who develop osteonecrosis of the jaw have had recent dental surgery, jaw trauma, or oral infection.

Osteosarcoma risk has been reported for teriparatide but not for bisphosphonates. Thromboembolic events are an issue for estrogens and selective estrogen-receptor modulators when used in treating osteoporosis, but not for bisphosphonates.

References

1. Black DM, Delmas PD, Eastell R, et al.Once-yearly zoledronic acid for treatment of postmenopausal osteoporosis. *N Engl J Med.* 2007;356(18):1809–1822.
2. Cummings SR, Schwartz AV, Black DM. Alendronate and atrial fibrillation. *N Engl J Med.* 2007;356(18):1895–1896.
3. Lyles KW, Coln-Emeric CS, Magaziner JS, et al. Zoledronic acid and clinical fractures and mortality after hip fracture. *N Engl J Med.* 2007;357(18):1799–1809.
4. MacLean C, Newberry S, Maglione M, et al. Systematic review: comparative effectiveness of treatments to prevent fractures in men and women with low bone density or osteoporosis. *Ann Intern Med.* 2008;148(3):197–213.
5. Strampel W, Emkey R, Civitelli R. Safety considerations with bisphosphonates for the treatment of osteoporosis. *Drug Safety.* 2007;30(9):755–763.

149. An 80-yr-old woman is admitted to the hospital with urosepsis. On examination, she weighs 60 kg (132 lb) and has a low-grade fever and increased respiratory rate. There is a consolidation in the right lower lobe. Laboratory results show normal electrolyte concentrations and a serum creatinine concentration of 1.8 mg/dL, which is her recent baseline value. She responds well to 2 days of intravenous antibiotics, and cultures reveal *Escherichia coli* sensitive to trimethoprim/sulfamethoxazole. Your pharmacist reminds you that this medication requires adjustment for patients with renal impairment.

Based on published equations, what is her estimated glomerular filtration rate (GFR)?

(A) >90 mL/min
(B) 60–90 mL/min
(C) 30–60 mL/min
(D) 10–30mL/min
(E) <10 mL/min

ANSWER: D

The most useful measure of kidney function is GFR (SOE=A). Other measures of kidney function, such as tubular function, acid-base and electrolyte excretion, and hormonal production, tend to run in parallel with GFR and are harder to measure. Serum creatinine alone may not give an accurate estimate of GFR in older adults. This is partly because of the decrease in lean muscle mass with aging and the concomitant decrease in creatinine production. The most common and clinically useful way to determine GFR in older adults is to use the serum creatinine concentration in one of several regression formulas. Currently, the Modification of Diet in Renal Disease (MDRD) formula for determining GFR is best validated in middle-aged people and is recommended by the National Kidney Foundation (SOE=A). This complex equation can be obtained by using an on-line calculator such as that found on www.nephron.com. Most laboratories also report this value with routine serum chemistries. This equation has not been validated in patients >70 yr old. An alternative equation is the Cockcroft-Gault formula, which also has not been validated in adults >80 yr old. The Cockcroft-Gault formula is:

GFR = (140 − age) × weight / 72 × serum creatinine (multiply by 0.85 for women)

Despite these shortfalls, these equations provide a prompt and reasonable estimate of GFR for clinical decision making. The formulas assume that the patient is in a steady state without a rapidly changing serum creatinine concentration.

For this patient with a serum creatinine concentration of 1.8 mg/dL, the Cockcroft-Gault estimated GFR is 23.6 mL/min. The MDRD is not validated in a person her age but would yield an estimated GFR of 29 mL/min. With either estimate, despite an only moderately increased serum creatinine, the GFR is extremely depressed and requires dosing adjustments to avoid complications. Thus, with older adults, normal kidney function cannot be assumed in the setting of apparently normal serum creatinine concentration. In situations in which a very accurate GFR determination is needed (eg, chemotherapy), a 24-hour creatinine clearance should be measured.

References

1. Levey AS, Bosch JP, Lewis JB, et al. A more accurate method to estimate glomerular filtration rate from serum creatinine: a new prediction equation. *Ann Intern Med*. 1999;130(6):461–479.
2. Rosner MH, Bolton WK. Renal function testing. *Am J Kidney Dis*. 2006;47(1):174–183.

150. A 70-yr-old woman has vaginal atrophy that has progressed since she stopped hormone therapy.

Which of the following is the most effective management strategy for this patient?

(A) Topical steroid cream
(B) Coal tar cream
(C) Aloe vera gel
(D) Second-generation antidepressants
(E) Vaginal estrogen tablets

ANSWER: E

About 20% of women have symptoms of atrophic vaginitis after menopause, and between 1% and 5% seek treatment. Unlike hot flashes, which abate, symptoms of atrophic vaginitis increase in severity over time. Oral or local estrogen preparations can improve symptoms, but vaginal irritation persists in 5%–10% of women. The use of oral estrogen (with progesterone if the patient has not had a hysterectomy) is not always necessary to obtain benefit. In an analysis of estrogenic preparations administered intravaginally in postmenopausal women with vaginal atrophy or vaginitis, local preparations were effective at lower estrogenic doses than oral preparations. Creams, tablets, pessaries, and the estradiol-releasing vaginal ring appeared to

have comparable efficacy in treating symptoms of vaginal atrophy (SOE=A). Patients seem to prefer tablets or the vaginal ring over creams. Few of these studies have follow-up data beyond 1 yr.

Topical steroid creams temporarily reduce inflammation but cause thinning of mucosa. Coal tar cream applied externally is effective for psoriasis but not for vaginal atrophy. There is only anecdotal evidence on use of aloe vera for vulvar itching. While aloe vera gel temporarily cools irritated skin, it neither provides long-term benefit to someone who needs estrogen, nor improves other symptoms, such as discharge. Second-generation antidepressants have been tried in patients with intractable itching associated with systemic disease. There are little data supporting its use at this time (SOE=D).

References

1. Bachmann G, Lobo RA, Gut R, et al. Efficacy of low-dose estradiol vaginal tablets in the treatment of atrophic vaginitis: a randomized controlled trial. *Obstet Gynecol*. 2008;111(1):67–76.
2. Castelo-Branco C, Cancelo MJ, Villero J, et al. Management of post-menopausal vaginal atrophy and atrophic vaginitis. *Maturitas*. 2005:52 Suppl 1:S46–52.
3. Sitruk-Ware R. New hormonal therapies and regimens in the postmenopause: routes of administration and timing of initiation. *Climacteric*. 2007;10(5):358–370.
4. Suckling J, Lethaby A, Kennedy R. Local oestrogen for vaginal atrophy in postmenopausal women. *Cochrane Database Syst Rev*. 2006;(4):CD001500.

151. A 68-yr-old woman comes to the office because she has shoulder pain that has deprived her of sleep for the past week. The pain also interferes with her responsibilities in caring for her young grandchildren. She has a 4-yr history of diabetes well controlled with oral hypoglycemic agents.

On examination, active motion of the shoulder is limited by pain. Passive motion is maintained. The lateral aspect of the shoulder is diffusely tender. Although the patient can support the weight of her arm against gravity, her arm drops when minimal resistance is added. Radiography of the shoulder is unremarkable.

Which of the following is the most appropriate next step?

(A) MRI of the shoulder
(B) Oral prednisone 10 mg/d
(C) Subacromial injection of corticosteroid with anesthetic followed by physical therapy
(D) Referral for surgical manipulation under anesthesia

ANSWER: C

Shoulder pain is common in older adults and can limit function and compromise self-care. Older adults are susceptible to rotator cuff injury with even minor trauma (eg, lifting groceries). Rotator cuff tendonitis causes shoulder pain that is worse between 60 and 120 degrees of abduction; it is often accompanied by subacromial bursitis, which causes a dull ache that precludes sleeping on the affected side. The tendonitis can be managed with injection of a corticosteroid mixed with an anesthetic into the subacromial space. Physical therapy should be started shortly after the injection to regain range of motion and strengthen periarticular muscles (SOE=B).

MRI can be used to evaluate the health of structures within the shoulder and for surgical repair of the rotator cuff. This patient's ability to abduct her arm against gravity, together with the lack of radiographic evidence of superior migration of the humeral head, suggests that the cuff is at least partially intact. Low-dose prednisone would be appropriate for patients with polymyalgia rheumatica, which presents with bilateral discomfort of the shoulder girdle, but not for those with rotator cuff injury.

Adhesive capsulitis results in painful loss of range of motion in all directions. It can result from stroke, trauma, untreated arthritis, or even minor injury, and it can develop in patients with diabetes without an inciting event. Manipulation under anesthesia to forceably increase range of motion is not appropriate. Physiotherapy with passive range of motion and stretching is recommended for adhesive capsulitis.

Reference

1. Burbank KM, Stevenson JH, Czarnecki GR, et al. Chronic shoulder pain: part II. Treatment. *Am Fam Physician.* 2008;77(4):493–497.

152. A 78-yr-old woman comes to the office because she has pain when she urinates. She has been seen three times for this problem in the last 3 mo. Each time she was told she had a urinary tract infection and was given a course of antibiotics. She has carefully followed the instructions for the antibiotics but has had no relief of symptoms.

Results of her last urinalysis:

WBCs	2 to 3 per high-power field
RBCs	0 to 2 per high-power field
Epithelial cells	Few
Nitrite	Negative
Leukocyte esterase	Negative

Which of the following should be done next?

(A) Send a clean-catch urine specimen for urinalysis and culture.
(B) Perform pelvic examination.
(C) Reassure the patient that she has asymptomatic bacteruria and that antibiotics are unlikely to help.
(D) Refer for cystoscopy.
(E) Order pelvic ultrasonography.

ANSWER: B

In this patient's previous visits, the urine specimen may not have been a clean catch, and positive cultures may represent contamination. After several rounds of antibiotics with no improvement in symptoms, the diagnosis of urinary tract infection should be suspect. Pelvic examination should be performed before additional laboratory work, ultrasonography, or referral for cystoscopy (SOE=D).

Urinary tract structures, deriving from the same embryologic origin as the genital tract, contain estrogen receptors and are estrogen dependent. The bladder, urethra, pelvic floor musculature, and endopelvic fascia are affected by a hypoestrogenic state, as is the vaginal epithelium with menopause. Possible consequences of urinary tract atrophy include urethral discomfort, frequency, hematuria, dysuria, and increased likelihood of urinary tract infection. Pelvic laxity and stress incontinence can also occur.

Diagnosis of vaginal atrophy is based on characteristic symptoms in the history and on findings of the physical examination. Classic findings include pale, dry vaginal epithelium that is smooth and shiny, with loss of most rugae. Laboratory tests are unnecessary and not diagnostic.

Unless contraindicated, systemic or local estrogen is the most effective treatment (SOE=A). Vaginal administration minimizes the degree of systemic absorption, although it can increase plasma levels of estrogen.

Local estrogen applications include low-dose creams, rings, and tablets. One strategy is low-dose vaginal estrogen cream 0.5 g/d for 3 wk, with twice-weekly administration thereafter. The estradiol ring (Estringe) delivers 6–9 mcg of estradiol to the vagina daily for 3 mo. The vaginal estrogen tablet (Vagifem) is usually recommended every day for 2 wk, then twice weekly. Progestins are not prescribed routinely for women treated with low-dose vaginal estrogen. In women with breast cancer, vaginal estrogen is not used for symptoms of urogenital atrophy unless recommended by the woman's oncologist.

Although asymptomatic bacteruria should not be treated with antibiotics, reassuring the patient will not address her urogenital symptoms.

References

1. Bachmann GA, Nevadunsky NS. Diagnosis and treatment of atrophic vaginitis. *Am Fam Physician.* 2000;61(10):3090–3096.
2. Castelo-Branco C, Cancelo MJ, Villero J, et al. Management of post-menopausal vaginal atrophy and atrophic vaginitis. *Maturitas.* 2005;52 Suppl 1:S46–52.
3. North American Menopause Society. The role of local vaginal estrogen for treatment of vaginal atrophy in postmenopausal women; 2007 position statement of The North American Menopause Society. *Menopause.* 2007;14:357–369.
4. Stamm WE. Estrogens and urinary-tract infection. *J Infect Dis.* 2007;195(5):623–624.
5. Weisberg E, Ayton R, Darling G, et al. Endometrial and vaginal effects of low-dose estradiol delivered by vaginal ring or vaginal tablet. *Climacteric.* 2005;8(1):83–92.

153. A 70-yr-old man comes to the office because he has difficulty walking, especially in the dark, and he is unable to read street signs during car rides because the environment appears to be "jumping up and down." History includes diabetes mellitus, peripheral neuropathy, and renal insufficiency. He was recently discharged after hospitalization for cellulitis in his legs, for which he received intravenous gentamicin and nafcillin. While he was hospitalized, he reported a continuous sense of imbalance, but he did not have vertigo. He did not notice any tinnitus, aural fullness, or hearing loss.

General physical examination is normal. However, gait is somewhat wide based and unsteady. A Romberg test is positive.

Which of the following is the most likely cause of his imbalance?

(A) Aminoglycoside ototoxicity
(B) Vestibular neuritis
(C) Benign paroxysmal positional vertigo
(D) Meniere disease
(E) Perilymph fistula

ANSWER: A

Gentamicin often causes isolated vestibular toxicity. In a study of 35 patients with aminoglycoside ototoxicity, 33 reported oscillopsia (having a sense of the environment "jumping" when in a moving car or when walking); only 3 noted a change in hearing.

There are no pre- or post-treatment pharmacologic interventions to attenuate aminoglycoside ototoxicity. Kidney function should be measured before beginning any potentially ototoxic medication. Major risk factors include impaired renal function, high drug serum concentrations, prior use of ototoxic medications, treatment course >14 days, preexisting sensorineural hearing loss, and age >65 yr old. Patients should be referred for vestibular rehabilitation, which includes learning compensatory strategies for loss of vestibular input. Patients with peripheral neuropathy generally have more difficulty compensating for bilateral vestibular loss.

Vestibular neuritis typically presents with subacute onset of spontaneous vertigo. In benign paroxysmal positional vertigo, episodes are brief and associated with positional change only. Meniere disease presents with aural fullness, hearing loss, tinnitus, and vertigo. Perilymph fistula typically presents with hearing loss and episodic vertigo.

References

1. Herdman SJ. Vestibular rehabilitation. *Neurotology.* 2006;12(4):151–168.
2. Ishiyama G, Ishiyama A, Kerber K, et al. Gentamicin ototoxicity: clinical features and the effect on the human vestibulo-ocular reflex. *Acta Otolaryngol.* 2006;126(10):1057–1061.
3. Rizzi MD, Hirose K. Aminoglycoside ototoxicity. *Curr Opinion Otolaryngol Head Neck Surg.* 2007;15(5):352–357.

154. A 90-yr-old man is brought to the emergency department by his family because he has had an abrupt change in behavior. The patient moved into his daughter and son-in-law's house a few months ago, because he was no longer able to manage living alone. A few days ago, he became aggressive and angry, and hit his son-in-law for no apparent reason. He has also become incontinent in the last few days. He has multiple bruises, which the family suspects are from falling. History includes moderate dementia and benign prostatic hyperplasia.

On examination, blood pressure is 160/90 mmHg; all other vital signs are normal. He is demanding to be released from "prison" and is aggressive with the staff. The physical examination is unremarkable. Although he is uncooperative with the neurologic examination, he appears to be moving all extremities well.

Which of the following is the most appropriate next step?

(A) Bladder scan
(B) Lumbar puncture
(C) Electroencephalography
(D) CT of the brain
(E) Basic metabolic panel, CBC, and pulse oximetry

ANSWER: E

This patient demonstrates an acute change in his cognition and behavior from his baseline deficits. Increased confusion, new falls, and new incontinence all suggest a new underlying illness or medication adverse event. The index of suspicion for delirium in this situation should be high: an acute change in mental status may be the only sign of a serious acute illness. Even when the physical examination is unremarkable, metabolic abnormalities should be pursued, including measuring serum chemistries, renal function, glucose, and oxygen saturation. Urinalysis is indicated, as well as review of all prescribed and OTC medications.

The most common causes of acute confusion are medical illness, metabolic disturbance, and medications. Stroke, hemorrhage, meningitis, and encephalitis are much less common, and should be considered after more likely causes are excluded. Thus, lumbar puncture is not part of the routine evaluation for delirium. Many OTC medications with strong anticholinergic properties (eg, diphen-hydramine) are easily accessible and often misperceived by patients as safer than prescription drugs, yet can cause delirium.

In an older man with benign prostatic hyperplasia, urinary retention can manifest itself as a change in mental status. However, medical illness, metabolic abnormalities, and medications are more common causes of delirium.

Electroencephalography can demonstrate a pattern consistent with delirium but will not provide a diagnostic rationale for its cause, unless seizures are strongly suspected. CT of the brain, to exclude intracranial or subdural hemorrhages, structural lesions (meningiomas or metastatic brain tumors), or strokes, may be indicated if the patient's laboratory and other tests are unremarkable.

References
1. Inouye SK. Delirium in older persons. *N Engl J Med.* 2006;354(11):1157–1165.
2. Voyer P, Cole MG, McCusker J, et al. Prevalence and symptoms of delirium superimposed on dementia. *Clin Nurs Res.* 2006;15(1):46–66.

155. A 67-yr-old woman comes to the office for a routine visit. Her chief concern is chronic constipation. She would like to know if dietary fiber would be helpful. She worries about the increased risk of cardiovascular disease and diabetes as she ages, and she would like to avoid medications if possible. She walks one-half mile twice weekly and is slowly trying to increase her level of exercise. Her diet consists mostly of processed foods and red meat. History includes borderline dyslipidemia. She is on no medications and has no history of vascular disease, diabetes, or hypertension.

On examination, weight is 72.6 kg (160 lb; body mass index, 28 kg/m^2). Physical examination is otherwise unremarkable. Total cholesterol level is 190 mg/dL, triglycerides are 115 mg/dL, and low-density lipoprotein level is 122 mg/dL. Thyroid function studies are normal.

In response to her questions about dietary fiber, which of the following is true?

(A) Increasing soluble fiber is an effective remedy for constipation.
(B) Commercial dietary fiber supplements inhibit absorption of several vitamins and minerals.
(C) Increasing insoluble fiber is unlikely to reduce heart disease risk.
(D) Some forms of soluble fiber can increase risk of heart disease or diabetes.

ANSWER: C

Dietary fibers are the carbohydrate components of plant cell walls that are resistant to digestion by intestinal enzymes. There are two general categories: water-insoluble fibers and water-soluble fibers. Although both types are present in all plant foods, the ratio and absolute amount of each varying according to a plant's characteristics. Dietary sources of *insoluble* fiber include vegetables such as green beans and dark green leafy vegetables, fruit skins and root vegetable skins, whole-wheat products, wheat oat, corn bran, seeds, and nuts. Dietary sources of *soluble* fiber include oat/oat bran, dried beans and peas, nuts, barley, flax seed, fruits such as oranges and apples, and vegetables such as carrots.

The beneficial effects are somewhat different for each type of fiber. Both types lower the energy density of the diet. The added bulk also offers short-term satiety, which helps control appetite and prevent overeating. Water-insoluble fiber possesses passive water-attracting properties that help to increase fecal bulk, soften the feces, and shorten intestinal transit time; it is these properties that make insoluble fiber an effective remedy for constipation (SOE=A). As a further benefit, water-insoluble fiber has the effect of lowering intraluminal pressure within the colon, which can help to prevent formation of colonic diverticula. There is no evidence that including insoluble fiber will decrease heart disease.

There is no evidence that dietary fiber, whether contained within plant foods or supplied as commercial dietary fiber supplements, inhibits absorption of vitamins or minerals. The most widely marketed dietary fiber supplements are composed predominantly of soluble fibers that are fermentable. This includes psyllium-based fiber supplements (eg, Metamucil, which is 66% soluble fiber) and guar gum– or wheat dextrin–based fiber supplements (eg, Benefiber, which is 100% soluble fiber). Fermentable dietary fibers are metabolized by the colonic flora, yielding various breakdown products such as fatty acids that can increase absorption of minerals, especially calcium and magnesium. Some plant foods can reduce the absorption of minerals and vitamins like calcium, zinc, vitamin C, and magnesium, but this is caused by the presence of phytate, not by fiber.

On average, North Americans consume <50% of the dietary fiber recommended for optimal health by many professional health organizations. Evidence is growing that increasing the amount of fiber, especially water-soluble fiber, in their diets would offer Americans important benefits by lowering cholesterol levels and preventing heart disease. A diet high in water-soluble fiber appears to be effective in lowering the postprandial surge in serum glucose, which can be beneficial in the prevention and treatment of diabetes (SOE=A). Studies indicate that soluble fiber, when combined with a low-fat, low-cholesterol diet, can lower total blood cholesterol by 4%–6% and low-density lipoprotein cholesterol by 4%–8% more than a low-fat diet alone. The greatest decreases are attainable when initial blood cholesterol concentrations are increased. Some studies demonstrate an inverse association between total dietary fiber intake and rate of fatal and nonfatal myocardial infarctions, suggesting the possible importance of fiber in cardiovascular disease prevention (SOE=A). Most of the effects of soluble fibers were demonstrated using fiber concentrates. Comparable amounts of fiber can be obtained from food sources if the diet is carefully formulated.

References

1. Galisteo M, Duarte J, Zarzuelo A. Effects of dietary fibers on disturbances clustered in the metabolic syndrome. *J Nutr Biochem*. 2008;19(2):71–84.
2. Petchetti L, Frishman WH, Petrillo R, et al. Nutriceuticals in cardiovascular disease: psyllium. *Cardiol Rev*. 2007;15(3):116–122.
3. Roy CC, Kien CL, Bouthillier L, et al. Short-chain fatty acids: ready for prime time? *Nutr Clin Pract*. 2006;21(4):351–366.
4. Theuwissen E, Mensink RP. Water-soluble dietary fibers and cardiovascular disease. *Physiol Behav*. 2008;94(2):285–292.
5. Weickert MO, Pfeiffer AF. Metabolic effects of dietary fiber consumption and prevention of diabetes. *J Nutr*. 2008;138(3):439–442.

156. The Seventh Report of the Joint National Committee on Prevention, Detection, Evaluation, and Treatment of High Blood Pressure (JNC7) recommends which of the following for the initial treatment for hypertension in older adults?

(A) ACE inhibitor
(B) Thiazide diuretic
(C) Calcium channel blocker
(D) β-Blocker
(E) Angiotensin-receptor blocker

ANSWER: B

JNC7 guidelines state that thiazide diuretics, either in combination or alone, should be the initial treatment for hypertension in most patients (SOE=A). However, thiazide diuretics are not necessarily the first choice for patients with other conditions. JNC7 identifies compelling indications for the use of medications other than hydrochlorothiazide for initial management of hypertension. ACE inhibitors and β-blockers are recommended for initial treatment of hypertension in asymptomatic patients with impaired left ventricular systolic function. ACE inhibitors or angiotensin-receptor blockers are recommended for patients with hypertension and early chronic kidney disease. Calcium channel blockers are recommended in patients with diabetes or a high risk of coronary disease (SOE=A). In each of these diseases, clinical trials have demonstrated benefit of specific classes of antihypertensive agents.

Reference

1. Chobanian AV, Bakris GL, Black HR, et al; National Heart, Lung and Blood Institute Joint National Committee on Prevention, Detection, Evaluation, and Treatment of High Blood Pressure; National High Blood Pressure Education Program Coordinating Committee. The Seventh Report of the Joint National Committee on Prevention, Detection, Evaluation, and Treatment of High Blood Pressure: the JNC 7 report. *JAMA.* 2003;289(19):2560–2572.

157. An 86-yr-old woman with dementia and heart failure has difficulty getting to the bathroom and is increasingly incontinent. She can no longer prepare food for herself or take medications reliably. She lives in the city with her son, who is away from home during the day. He is no longer comfortable leaving his mother alone, but neither he nor his mother wants her to move to a nursing home. The patient qualifies for Medicare and Medicaid.

If available, which of the following is the most appropriate recommendation?

(A) Enrollment in a social health maintenance organization (HMO)
(B) Admission to a nearby nursing home
(C) Referral to Program of All-inclusive Care of the Elderly (PACE)
(D) Hiring a full-time nurse to care for the patient at home
(E) Referral to state Department of Aging for assessment

ANSWER: C

PACE is a managed-care program developed to address the needs of older adults who have a level of disability that makes them eligible for nursing-home care. It was modeled after the innovative program in San Francisco, On Lok, which focused on caring for Asian Americans in their home community. PACE services are provided by an interdisciplinary team comprising primary care physicians; nurses; social workers; physical, occupational, and recreational therapists; pharmacists; dieticians; home care coordinators; PACE center managers; personal care attendants; and drivers. Daily services are commonly provided at an adult day healthcare center, and multidisciplinary care is highly coordinated. Enrollment in PACE is associated with higher patient satisfaction, improved health status and function, fewer nursing-home admissions, improved quality of life, and lower mortality than usual care (SOE=B). PACE is a comprehensive managed-care program that is paid for through Medicare and Medicaid funds and by the participant's own contributions. Unfortunately, the program is available only in selected, primarily urban environments.

The social HMO was also developed with the intent of keeping older adults in the community. It is a capitated program for frail Medicare recipients with complex medical needs. A social HMO provides the full range of Medicare benefits offered by standard HMOs plus additional services that include care coordination, chronic care benefits covering short-term nursing-home care, and home- and community-based services. Evaluations indicate mixed results regarding cost and effectiveness of social HMOs in caring for frail older adults (SOE=C).

The patient and her son do not want her to be admitted to a nursing home, although Medicaid would cover the costs of this long-term care. Hiring a full-time nurse to care for the patient at home would not be covered by either Medicare or Medicaid and would be very expensive. Referral to the state Department of Aging for assessment may result in more home support than is usually available from the Medicaid program, but full-day care by any type of care provider would not likely be covered. Of the options, only PACE would provide the comprehensive care coordination best suited for this patient.

References

1. Chatterji P, Burstein NR, Kidder D, et al. *Evaluation of the Program for All-Inclusive Care for the Elderly (PACE) Demonstration: The Impact of PACE on Participant Outcomes.* Cambridge, MA: ABT Associates Inc.; 1998.
2. Mukamel DB, Temkin-Greener H, Delavan R, et al. Program characteristics and enrollees' outcomes in the program for all-inclusive care for the elderly (PACE). *Milbank Quarterly.* 2007;85(3):499–531.
3. Thompson TG. Evaluation results for the social/health maintenance organization II demonstration. Washington, DC: Department of Health and Human Services; 2002.

158. Which of the following is the most reliable screen for hearing impairment?

(A)   Screening version of the Hearing Handicap Inventory for the Elderly (HHIE–S)
(B)   Abbreviated Profile of Hearing Aid Benefit
(C)   Tinnitus Handicap Questionnaire
(D)   Whisper test

ANSWER: A

Medicare offers a one-time preventive examination. Two self-report measures, the screening version of the (HHIE–S) and the Dizziness Handicap Inventory, are recommended for use by physicians. The (HHIE–S) is widely used to assess hearing handicap, ie, hearing loss that interferes with performing ADLs. The (HHIE–S) consists of 10 questions regarding hearing difficulty in various situations: half of the questions cover self-reported emotional consequences of hearing loss, and half cover self-reported activity limitations and restrictions. The screen is quick and easy to administer and inexpensive. It has high reliability and validity, as well as adequate sensitivity and specificity. Patients who score >8 should be referred to an audiologist to evaluate hearing and to determine the need for medical or nonmedical interventions.

An alternative screening tool is a hand-held otoscope (AudioScope), which generates pure tones at 500, 1000, 2000, and 4000 Hz and at two intensity levels, 25 or 40 dB. Outcome on the (HHIE–S) predicts need for hearing aids, whereas the AudioScope screen predicts level of hearing impairment.

The Tinnitus Handicap Questionnaire assesses self-reported handicapping effects of tinnitus. It can be used before and after treatment to measure effectiveness of therapy for tinnitus. The Abbreviated Profile of Hearing

Aid Benefit is often used to assess outcomes with hearing aids. It quantifies the self-reported disabling effects of hearing impairment and assesses ease of communication, reverberation, speech understanding in the presence of background noise, and aversiveness to sound.

The whisper test, in which the tester whispers words at a measured distance from the patient's ear, is not as accurate a screen for hearing loss as the HHIE–S.

References

1. Bagai A, Thavendiranathan P, Detsky A. Does this patient have hearing impairment? *JAMA.* 2006; 295(4):416–428.
2. Danhauer J, Celani K, Johnson C. Use of hearing and balance screening survey with local primary care physicians. *Am J Audiol.* 2008;17(1):3–13.
3. Johnson C, Danhauer J, Koch L, et al. Hearing and balance screening and referrals for Medicare patients: a national survey of primary care physicians. *J Am Acad Audiol.* 2008;19(2):171–190.

159. A 75-yr-old man returns for a routine clinic visit after a year's hiatus. During this time he cared for his wife of 50 yr, who had Alzheimer's dementia, with help from family and a home hospice program. His wife died 4 mo ago. His medical history includes hypertension, which is well controlled on hydrochlorothiazide. He is independent in IADLs, except for relying on his son to provide transportation and help with finances.

He has no specific complaints, but on questioning states he thinks about his wife frequently and yearns for their life together as it was in the past, before she became so ill. He still finds her death difficult to accept and often wakes up expecting her to be in the bed with him. In the immediate weeks after her death he was unable to sleep or eat as usual, but this has improved somewhat. His children visit frequently. As he talks about his wife, he cries. The physical examination is otherwise unremarkable.

Which of the following is the most likely diagnosis?

(A)   Caregiver burnout
(B)   Grief
(C)   Complicated grief
(D)   Depression
(E)   Delirium

ANSWER: B

This patient is experiencing grief, or bereavement. The time course and symptoms of grief experienced by older adults vary widely and are culturally dependent. Caregivers may experience anticipatory grief as they contemplate separation from their loved one. Bereavement after the passing of the loved one can include the symptoms of major depressive disorder. The diagnosis of major depressive disorder in the setting of grief is difficult, and requires persistence of symptoms over time, interference with daily functioning, and loss of capacity for pleasure.

Complicated grief is more common when a caregiver is not prepared for death of the loved one. In complicated grief, the person experiences persistent yearning for the loved one as well as traumatic stress symptoms such as numbness, disbelief, and bitterness. These symptoms must be present at least 6 mo and significantly interfere with daily function to diagnose complicated grief. Although traditional psychotherapy and tricyclic antidepressants have not been found as effective for treatment of complicated grief, recommendations for treatment include combined traumatic grief therapy and SSRIs. While the patient does express disbelief in the loss of his wife, he does not meet criteria for complicated grief.

Caregivers, particularly of dementia patients, may experience an emotional, psychological, physical, and emotional "load" of caring for patients. Caregiver burnout is a term used to describe severe fatigue, exhaustion, and negative mental health symptoms related to providing care. Several scales, such as the Zarit Burden Interview, quantify caregiver stress and measure outcomes in interventions designed to reduce caregiver burden. In this case, the patient is no longer providing care.

The patient does not meet criteria for the diagnosis of major depressive disorder: depressed mood/anhedonia for at least 2 wk and concomitant symptoms (sleep changes, lack of interest in usual activities, guilt, lack of energy, decreased concentration, appetite changes, psychomotor retardation or agitations, and suicidal thoughts).

The diagnosis of delirium requires altered attention, in addition to changes in cognition that are not due to dementia or depression. The patient does not have an attention deficit or cognitive changes noted on examination.

References

1. Etters L, Goodall D, Harrison BE. Caregiver burden among dementia patient caregivers: a review of the literature. *J Am Acad Nurse Pract.* 2008;20(8):423–428.
2. Fiske A, Wetherell JL, Gatz M. Depression in older adults. *Annu Rev Clin Psychol.* 2009;5:363–389.
3. Holland JM, Currier JM, Gallagher-Thomson D. Outcomes from the Resources for Enhancing Alzheimer's Caregiver Health (REACH) program for bereaved caregivers. *Psychol Aging.* 2009;24(1):190–202.
4. Schulz R, Boerner K, Shear K, et al. Predictors of complicated grief among dementia caregivers: a prospective study of bereavement. *Am J Geriatr Psychiatry.* 2006;14(8):650–658.
5. Schultz R, Hebert R, Boerner K. Bereavement after caregiving. *Geriatrics.* 2008;63(1):20–22.

160. An 80-yr-old woman is admitted to the hospital with altered mental status. It is her third admission in 3 mo. She lives with her son, who is her healthcare proxy. He shops for the household and helps her with her medications. History includes diabetes mellitus, atrial fibrillation, macular degeneration, and osteoarthritis. Medications include warfarin, insulin glargine, lisinopril, and metoprolol. After her last hospitalization, the patient received 2 wk of home healthcare services; the nurses reported that the son purchased foods inconsistent with a diabetic diet despite receiving nutrition counseling.

On examination, the patient is lethargic and oriented only to her name. Vital signs are within normal limits. Blood glucose concentration is >400 mg/dL by fingerstick measure. Hemoglobin A_{1c} level is 9%, and INR is 1.

The patient's mental status improves with administration of insulin and intravenous fluids. She reports that her son went on vacation for 1 wk, and she was unable to administer her own medications. The inpatient team wants to discharge the patient to a skilled-nursing facility for short-term rehabilitation, but she states that she wants to return home.

Which of the following is the most appropriate next step in caring for this patient?

(A) Notify Adult Protective Services.
(B) Administer the Mini–Mental State Examination.
(C) Assess her capacity to understand the risks and benefits of her living situation.
(D) Discharge her to her home with home healthcare services for 4 wk.
(E) Contact the patient's healthcare proxy (her son) to obtain permission to discharge her to a skilled-nursing facility

ANSWER: C

The most appropriate next step in this patient's management is to assess her capacity to understand the risks and benefits of returning home (SOE=D). The first step in assessment is to establish whether the patient is willing to accept interventions. If she is unwilling, then the physician must determine whether she has the capacity to refuse interventions. The determination must be made within the context of a particular situation or decision, in this case the patient's ability to participate in discharge planning. The inpatient medical team favors discharge to a skilled-nursing facility for short-term rehabilitation, but the patient is refusing this option in favor of returning home. For this patient, establishing capacity requires that she demonstrate the following: expressing a choice, understanding the relevant information regarding her discharge options, appreciating her situation and its consequences, and having the ability to reason about her options. If the patient has decision-making capacity with respect to discharge planning and if her stated preference is not the result of undue influence or coercion, she has the right to return home despite the inpatient medical team's concerns about the safety of her home environment. The medical team must respect the patient's right to autonomy. They can offer services and pursue interventions that will increase oversight of the home, eg, referral to Adult Protective Services (APS), implementation of home healthcare services, and communication with the patient's primary doctor to ensure timely follow-up. In contrast, if the patient is not able to demonstrate decision-making capacity for discharge planning, then the inpatient team should present the options to her healthcare proxy.

APS provide services to older or disabled adults who are in danger of mistreatment or neglect, are unable to protect themselves, and have no one to assist them. A referral to APS would not be indicated while the patient remains in the hospital. If the patient were discharged home, a referral to APS would be appropriate to provide additional monitoring. After the referral is made, APS would attempt to visit the patient at home to assess whether there is abuse or neglect. If the patient has decision-making capacity, APS would only be able to inform her about available social or health services; APS cannot order the patient to agree to additional services. If the patient does not have decision-making capacity and is a victim of neglect or abuse, APS can petition the court to appoint a guardian who may be granted power over the patient and his or her property.

The Mini–Mental State Examination can provide useful information to the physician who is evaluating the patient's decision-making capacity, but it is not equivalent to a capacity assessment. For example, a patient with a Mini–Mental State Examination score consistent with dementia may still have capacity to complete a healthcare proxy form or make other healthcare decisions. Discharging the patient home with home care services may be an option after the patient's capacity has been assessed. Communication with the patient's son is appropriate because he is the patient's healthcare proxy, but he cannot make discharge decisions for the patient unless she lacks capacity to make decisions herself.

References
1. Appelbaum PS. Assessment of patients' competence to consent to treatment. *N Engl J Med.* 2007;357(18):1834–1840.
2. Lachs MS, Pillemer K. Elder abuse. *Lancet.* 2004;364(9441);1263–1272.
3. Teaster PB, Dugar TA, Mendiondo M, et al. The 2004 Survey of Adult Protective Services: Abuse of Adults 60 Years of Age and Older. Washington, DC: The National Center on Elder Abuse; 2006.

161. What percent of people ≥65 yr old report a functional limitation, ie, an inability to perform an ADL or an IADL?

(A) 23%
(B) 35%
(C) 42%
(D) 51%
(E) 60%

ANSWER: C

In 2005, 42% of adults ≥65 yr old reported a functional limitation in an ADL or an IADL. This is a decrease from 1992, when 49% of adults in this age group had functional impairment. ADLs include bathing, dressing, eating, getting in and out of a chair, walking, and using the toilet. IADLs include using the telephone, doing light or heavy housework, preparing meals, shopping, and managing money. Twelve percent had difficulty with one or more IADLs; the remaining 30% had impairment in one or more ADLs.

Women are more likely than men to have functional impairment: 47% of women and 35% of men ≥65 yr old report difficulties. Functional impairment increases with age. For example, 5% of adults 65–74 yr old have difficulty with dressing; the proportion increases to 25% for adults ≥85 yr old. Similarly, of adults who have difficulty walking, 17% are 65–74 yr old, whereas 46% are ≥85 yr old.

References

1. Administration on Aging. *A Profile of Older Americans: 2007.* Administration on Aging, U.S. Department of Health and Human Services. Washington, DC: U.S. Government Printing Office; 2007.
2. Federal Interagency Forum on Aging-Related Statistics. *Older Americans 2008: Key Indicators of Well-Being.* Federal Interagency Forum on Aging-Related Statistics. Washington, DC: U.S. Government Printing Office; 2008.

162. Personality disorders are present in 10%–18% of adults of all ages in the community, and affect healthcare use and health outcomes.

Which of the following best describes the rate of personality disorder in older adults compared with rates in the general population?

(A) Rates are much lower (1%–3%).
(B) Rates are slightly lower (5%–10%).
(C) Rates are slightly higher (18%–20%).
(D) Rates are much higher (24%–32%).

ANSWER: B

Personality disorder refers to patterns of culturally non-normative inner experiences, traits, and behaviors that are associated with impaired social or occupational functioning or subjective distress. The disorder comprises a variety of behaviors: some people may be self-aggrandizing, hypersensitive to criticism, and unable to empathize with others; others may be aloof, solitary, and indifferent; still others may be submissive, uncomfortable when alone, and excessively dependent.

Personality disorders persist into late life. They are present in 5%–10% of community-dwelling older adults (SOE=B), a somewhat lower prevalence than that of mixed-age adult populations. Recent data from the National Comorbidity Survey Replication suggest that age differences are primarily due to lower rates of cluster B personality disorders (histrionic, borderline, narcissistic, and antisocial personalities) in older adults than in younger adults. Similarly, the National Epidemiologic Survey found lower prevalence rates for specific personality disorders in older than in younger nonclinical groups, and an overall prevalence rate of 15% for "any personality disorder" in the sample. Several studies have found that age differences in prevalence rates vary by type of personality disorder and are most marked for borderline, antisocial, and schizotypal personalities when evaluated in cross-sectional studies.

Prevalence estimates of personality disorder in older adults are higher than or comparable to prevalence rates of Axis I disorders, such as major affective disorder, alcohol abuse/dependence, and dementia (10%). Much higher rates of personality disorder are observed only in clinical samples of older adults, with rates ranging from 10% to 63% (average across studies of 42%) reported (SOE=B). Depressed older adults with personality disorder have slower responses to or less successful outcomes after standardized treatment (SOE=B) than depressed older adults without personality disorder.

References

1. Balsis S, Gleason ME, Woods CM, et al. An item response theory analysis of DSM-IV personality disorder criteria across younger and older age groups. *Psychol Aging.* 2007;22(1):171–185.
2. Grant BF, Hasin DS, Stinson FS, et al. Prevalence, correlates, and disability of personality disorders in the United States: results from the National Epidemiologic Survey on Alcohol and Related Conditions. *J Clin Psychiatry.* 2004;65(7):948–958.
3. Hahn SR, Kroenke K, Spitzer RL, et al. The difficult patient: prevalence, psychopathology, and functional impairment. *J Gen Intern Med.* 1996;11(1):1–8.
4. Lenzenweger MF, Lane MC, Loranger AW, et al. DSM-IV personality disorders in the National Comorbidity Study Replication. *Biol Psychiatry.* 2007;62(6):553–564.

163. An 84-yr-old nursing-home resident is evaluated because she has been sleeping more over the last few days. At the beginning of the visit, the patient is still sleeping in bed in her nightgown; this is unusual for her. Staff reports that she recently seems less likely to recognize familiar people. The patient has no complaints and is distracted by the birds chirping outside her window. History includes stroke with persistent left hemiplegia, hypertension, dyslipidemia, diabetes, and mild dementia. Her hypertensive medications were recently adjusted by her cardiologist to improve blood pressure control. On examination, vital signs are unremarkable. She is disoriented to place and time. Her neurologic examination is otherwise unchanged from previous evaluations.

Which of the following is the most likely cause of her cognitive and behavioral changes?

(A) Progressive dementia
(B) Major depressive disorder
(C) Delirium
(D) New stroke

ANSWER: C

The key element in this patient's presentation is the acute change in her cognition and behavior. The most plausible explanation for her group of symptoms is delirium: an acute change in mental status (behavior and cognition), altered level of consciousness, and inattention. Delirium is often under-recognized in community-living, cognitively intact adults (SOE=B); it is even more difficult to detect in nursing-home residents with preexisting cognitive deficits. Nurses who interact with patients on a regular basis are most likely to identify cognitive and behavioral changes in their patients quickly. Recognition of delirium is essential—it is often the only symptom of an occult acute medical problem. Any suspicion of delirium must be followed with complete history and physical examination and targeted laboratory and radiologic tests.

The changes in the patient's behavior and cognition are too pronounced and acute to be due to progression of dementia, unless the patient has had a stroke or trauma that is not apparent in the neurologic examination. Dementia is most often slowly progressive, without sudden changes. Inattention is usually seen in advanced dementia or in dementias with Lewy bodies, neither of which is present in this case. Major depressive disorder can cause behavior changes but does not usually cause the degree of lethargy or inattention seen in this patient. Depression also would present more gradually.

Given the lack of additional changes in this patient's neurologic examination, it is premature to assume that her delirium is due to stroke or trauma. Although stroke or trauma can present with delirium, more likely causes are acute medical illness, medication toxicity, and metabolic disturbances.

References

1. Fick D, Hodo D, Lawrence F, et al. Recognizing delirium superimposed on dementia: assessing nurses' knowledge using case vignettes. *J Geront Nurs.* 2007:33(2):40–47.
2. Inouye SK. Delirium in older persons. *N Engl J Med.* 2006:354(11):1157–1165.
3. Voyer P, Cole MG, McCusker J, et al. Prevalence and symptoms of delirium superimposed on dementia. *Clin Nurs Res.* 2006:15(1):46–66.

164. A 72-yr-old woman comes to the office because she has pain at the site of a maxillary tooth extraction performed 8 mo earlier. She has a history of metastatic breast cancer and has been receiving intravenous bisphosphonate for the past 12 mo.

On examination, the extraction socket has not healed, and the gingival tissue is open, with bone protruding from the site. The area is erythematous, and some purulent drainage is apparent.

Which of the following is the most likely diagnosis?

(A) Metastatic cancer to the maxilla
(B) Osteomyelitis of the maxilla
(C) Periodontitis
(D) Osteonecrosis of the jaw
(E) Incomplete tooth extraction with residual root

ANSWER: D

Bisphosphonate-related osteonecrosis of the jaw is a devastating complication of bisphosphonate therapy used for bone cancer lesions or osteoporosis. The American Association of Oral and Maxillofacial Surgeons define this complication clinically as "exposed bone in the maxillofacial region that has persisted for more than 8 wk in patients with current or previous treatment, without a history of radiation therapy to the jaw." It is most commonly seen after tooth extraction but can also develop with periodontal disease or trauma to the oral cavity, or spontaneously.

Bisphosphonate-related osteonecrosis of the jaw can produce pain, swelling, infection, fistulae, and jaw fracture.

Breast cancer is unlikely to metastasize to the maxilla. Although the lesion has signs of secondary infection, the underlying pathophysiology is necrotic bone rather than infection. In cases of infected bisphosphonate-related osteonecrosis of the jaw, oral antibiotics and antibacterial mouth rinses are usually adequate to treat the infection, without biopsy (SOE=B).

Normal healing of the extraction socket produces soft-tissue healing within 1 mo and bony healing by 6 mo. Although healing can be slower in older patients, especially if they have diabetes, an extraction socket should not remain open for >6 mo, unless there is underlying pathology.

Periodontitis is unlikely because it is present only when teeth are present, not in the area of a prior extraction.

Incomplete tooth extraction with residual root is unlikely because this does not usually present with extruding bone from the socket. In addition, residual root can be easily excluded with a radiograph.

References

1. AAOMS 2007 American Association of Oral and Maxillofacial Surgeons Position Paper on Bisphosphonate-Related Osteonecrosis of the Jaws. *J Oral Maxillofac Surg.* 65(3):369–376.
2. Eckert AW, Maurer P, Meyer L, et al. Bisphosphonate-related jaw necrosis—severe complication in maxillofacial surgery. *Cancer Treat Rev.* 2007;33(1):58–63.
3. Migliorati CA, Siegel MA, Elting LS. Bisphosphonate-associated osteonecrosis: a long-term complication of bisphosphonate treatment. *Lancet Oncol.* 2006;7(6):508–514.
4. Marx RE, Sawatari Y, Fortin M, et al. Bisphosphonate-induced exposed bone (osteonecrosis/osteopetrosis) of the jaws: risk factors, recognition, prevention, and treatment. *J Oral Maxillofac Surg.* 2005;63(11):1567–1575.

165. An 81-yr-old woman comes to the office to establish care. She was brought by her daughter, with whom she has been living since the recent death of her husband. She is a former smoker and drinks socially on occasion. History includes osteoarthritis of the hip and knees, hypertension, and incontinence, which has recently worsened and limits her comfort with venturing outside of home. She had a stroke several years ago that left her with some right-sided weakness, for which she uses a cane. Medications include ibuprofen, glucosamine, hydrochlorothiazide, aspirin, a multivitamin, and since her husband's death, fluoxetine. She is allergic to lisinopril.

On examination, weight is 90.7 kg (200 lb) and height is 1.65 m (65 in) (body mass index, 33.4 kg/m^2). Blood pressure is 126/78 mmHg and pulse is 70 beats per minute and regular. She has a left carotid bruit, slight weakness and rigidity in her right arm and leg with associated gait abnormality, and bilaterally decreased dorsalis pedis and posterior tibial pulses. Both feet have slight edema. She scores 29/30 on the Mini–Mental State Examination, and 11/15 on the Geriatric Depression Scale.

Laboratory results:

Fasting glucose	165 mg/dL
Hemoglobin A_{1c}	7.5 g/dL
Total cholesterol	215 mg/dL
High-density lipoprotein	35 mg/dL
Low-density lipoprotein (calculated)	140 mg/dL
Triglycerides	200 mg/dL
Potassium	5.0 mEq/dL
Creatinine	1.3 mg/dL

Fasting glucose level 2 days later is 158 mg/dL. Urinalysis is positive for microalbuminuria.

Which of the following medications is most likely to decrease her cardiovascular risk?

(A) Glipizide
(B) Metformin
(C) Rosiglitazone
(D) Valsartan
(E) Simvastatin

ANSWER: E

Given this patient's history of stroke and evidence of peripheral vascular disease, the most immediate threat to her health and independence is her substantial risk of further macrovascular complications. She already takes low-dose aspirin daily. Secondary prevention of further cardiovascular disease by targeting her dyslipidemia is the most immediate priority, with a goal of reducing her low-density lipoprotein level to ≤100 mg/dL. This can be most reliably and safely approached with a statin, which can also modestly increase her high-density lipoprotein level (SOE=A).

Addition of valsartan can protect against further deterioration in renal function, but angiotensin-receptor blockers have not been shown to affect mortality in patients with diabetes (SOE=A). Hence, the addition of valsartan is of lower priority than the addition of simvastatin. ACE inhibitors decrease mortality in diabetic patients with microalbuminuria and preexisting heart disease (SOE=A), but this patient is allergic to lisinopril.

The patient's moderate fasting glucose and hemoglobin A_{1c} levels do not necessitate immediate intervention, especially given the more immediate risks of vascular complications from dyslipidemia. Aggressive management of increased blood glucose concentrations (especially focused on reducing hemoglobin A_{1c} level to ≤6 g/dL) is appropriate for a patient with type 1 diabetes in whom microvascular complications might be prevented. In this patient, however, the risk of hypoglycemia would be substantial with aggressive hypoglycemic therapy. In the ACCORD (Action to Control Cardiovascular Risk in Diabetes) study, cardiovascular and total mortality increased among patients who received aggressive hypoglycemic therapy, causing premature termination of that arm of the trial (SOE=A).

For a less aggressive approach to managing this patient's increased blood glucose concentrations, metformin would likely be the first choice, especially because she may benefit from an associated reduction in weight (with careful attention to her renal function). Glipizide might be effective if metformin were not tolerated or proved ineffective. Rosiglitazone, however, is contraindicated even in the presence of this patient's clear insulin insensitivity, because of her history of heart failure and dependence on thiazide diuretics, and in light of the adverse cardiovascular and mortality outcomes associated with its use in recent controlled trials and previous smaller studies (SOE=A).

References
1. Colhoun HM, Betteridge DJ, Durrington PN, et al. Primary prevention of cardiovascular disease with atorvastatin in type 2 diabetes in the Collaborative Atorvastatin Diabetes Study (CARDS): multicentre randomised placebo-controlled trial. *Lancet.* 2004;364(9435):685–696.
2. Gaede P, Lund-Andersen H, Parving HH, et al. Effect of a multifactorial intervention on mortality in type 2 diabetes. *N Engl J Med.* 2008;358(6):580–591.
3. Gerstein HC, Riddle MC, Kendall DM, et al. Glycemia treatment strategies in the Action to Control Cardiovascular Risk in Diabetes (ACCORD) trial. *Am J Cardiol.* 2007;99(12A):34i–43i.
4. Heart Protection Study Collaborative Group. MRC/BHF Heart Protection Study of cholesterol lowering with simvastatin in 20,536 high-risk individuals: a randomized placebo-controlled trial. *Lancet.* 2002;360(9326):7–22.
5. Strippoli GF, Craig M, Deeks JJ, et al. Effects of angiotensin converting enzyme inhibitors and angiotensin II receptor antagonists on mortality and renal outcomes in diabetic nephropathy: systematic review. *BMJ.* 2004;329(7470):828.

166. A 72-yr-old woman is brought in to the office by her daughter because of worsening lethargy and personality change over the last 2 mo with no other symptoms. She has had to retire from teaching because of episodes of confusion and irritability. About 2 mo ago, she was involved in a minor car accident but had no apparent injuries. Physical examination, including the neurologic examination, is normal.

Which test is most likely to confirm the diagnosis?

(A) Thyrotropin concentration
(B) Vitamin B_{12} concentration
(C) Electroencephalography
(D) Geriatric Depression Scale
(E) CT of the head

ANSWER: E

Subdural hematoma is usually due to head trauma and can be seen after deceleration in a motor vehicle accident. Symptoms can include confusion, personality changes, headache, and lethargy. The temporal association of this patient's decline with a history of car accident should raise suspicion for a subdural hematoma. Patients with chronic subdural hematomas are often thought to have dementia, depression, or drug intoxication. While this patient's symptoms are consistent with hypothyroidism, she has no other symptoms of hypothyroidism and no other findings on examination that suggest hypothyroidism. Vitamin B_{12} deficiency is less likely because of the absence of neurologic findings, such as decreased sensation. An electroencephalogram might show nonspecific findings, but any abnormalities would indicate the need for CNS imaging. While this patient might be depressed or have an abnormal score on the Geriatric Depression Scale, this would not obviate the need to search for a cause for new-onset confusion in a patient with a history of trauma.

References

1. Roger EP, Butler J, Benzel EC. Neurosurgery in the elderly: brain tumors and subdural hematomas. *Clin Geriatr Med.* 2006;22(30):623–624.
2. Schebesch KM, Woertegen C, Rothoerl RD, et al. Cognitive decline as an important sign for an operable cause of dementia: chronic subdural hematomas. *Zentralbl Neurochir.* 2008;69(2):61–64.

167. A 72-yr-old man comes to the office because he has anejaculatory orgasms. Over the last 3 yr, he has not consistently ejaculated with orgasm, and he has had no ejaculations for 3 mo. For the past 5 yr, he has taken tamsulosin 0.4 mg/d for lower urinary tract symptoms associated with benign prostatic hyperplasia. He has had no pelvic trauma, pain, or change in his lower urinary tract symptoms. He is monogamous and has intercourse once or twice a week with his wife of 40 yr.

Digital rectal examination reveals an asymmetric prostate of approximately 25 mL, with a hard nodule in the left lower lobe. The remainder of the examination is normal. Urinalysis is normal. His prostate-specific antigen (PSA) level is 9.5 ng/mL.

Which of the following is the most appropriate next step?

(A) Referral to a urologist
(B) Bone scan
(C) CT of the pelvis
(D) MRI of the pelvis
(E) Measurement of free PSA

ANSWER: A

Based on his physical examination and PSA level, this patient most likely has prostate cancer. In a patient with a remaining life expectancy of >5 yr, the next step is transrectal ultrasound-guided biopsy (SOE=C). The optimal treatment for prostate cancer in men of this age has not yet been determined, so treatment decisions are usually based on patient preference and estimated remaining life expectancy.

The patient's anejaculatory orgasms most likely represent retrograde ejaculation due to either benign prostatic hyperplasia or tamsulosin therapy and are not directly related to the current findings. A bone scan is reserved for detecting metastasis in the presence of known disease and is unlikely to be informative in patients with a PSA level <10 ng/mL. CT or MRI of the pelvis is reserved for identifying local spread or evaluating patients in whom the suspicion of cancer is high despite negative biopsy findings. A high proportional free PSA level will not exclude prostate cancer with a high enough level of certainty given this patient's symptoms and physical findings.

References

1. Hellstrom WJ, Sikka SC. Effects of acute treatment with tamsulosin versus alfuzosin on ejaculatory function in normal volunteers. *J Urol.* 2006;176(4 Pt 1):1529–1533.
2. Lee R, Localio AR, Armstrong K, et al. A meta-analysis of the performance characteristics of the free prostate specific antigen test. *Urology.* 2006;67(4):762–768.
3. Lin K, Lipsitz R, Miller T, et al; U.S. Preventive Services Task Force. Benefits and harms of prostate-specific antigen screening for prostate cancer: an evidence update for the U.S. Preventive Services Task Force. *Ann Intern Med.* 2008;149(3):192–199.

168. An 86-yr-old established patient is being treated for hypertension, heart failure, and atrial fibrillation. He was discharged 2 wk ago from a rehabilitation nursing facility that he entered after hospitalization for a stroke and aspiration pneumonia. Home healthcare orders were written and billed a few days ago. Today the home health nurse calls the office because she is concerned about the patient's functional decline and poor oral intake, and thinks that he is "just not doing well." The nurse wonders about depression, notes that the patient is on several new medications, and is not sure if his wife can handle caregiving.

The nurse reports that the patient's blood pressure is 145/80 mmHg, pulse is 80 beats per minute and irregularly irregular, respiratory rate is 18 breaths per minute, and temperature is 36.6°C (97.8°F). She requests a physician house call today because the patient is unable to travel.

Which of the following is true regarding Medicare physician payment regulations that would affect billing for a house call in this situation?

(A) House calls on the same day as a home health nurse visit are prohibited.
(B) Maximal payment for this house call would be about $100.
(C) Charging for a house call would be "double-dipping" because of recent billing for care certification.
(D) The patient does not have a diagnosis or reason to justify a house call.
(E) Prolonged service codes could be added to the bill if needed.

ANSWER: E

There is widespread misunderstanding that house calls (home visits) on the same day as home health agency visits are not permitted or are denied payment by Medicare. This is not true. Because of concern about inappropriate practice patterns in some regions of the country, some Medicare carriers require documentation in the provider's clinical note that the medical home visit did not duplicate the home health agency visit.

The Medicare fee schedule for home visits ranges up to about $150 for the most complex established patient visit (Current Procedural Terminology [CPT] 99350). Payment for home visits can be augmented by billing for prolonged services if the visit extends >30 min beyond the typical face-to-face time for the selected service code as published by CPT.

Billing for home care certification is independent of direct face-to-face services. While payment may be denied if care certification and a direct care service are billed on the same date, there is no prohibition against billing for both services during the same period. Medicare initiated payment for home care certification to encourage more active engagement of physicians in home health care.

Accepted diagnoses for a home visit cover a wide range of medical conditions, which in this case could include stroke, pneumonia, atrial fibrillation, hypertension, or failure to thrive.

It is good practice to document the reason that the patient was seen at home rather than in the office; some Medicare carriers have issued and require Local Coverage Determinations as part of the documentation in case of an audit.

References
1. Physician Services. Centers for Medicare and Medicaid Services. United States Department of Health and Human Services. http://www.cms.hhs.gov/center/physician.asp (accessed Nov 2009).
2. Beebe M, Dalton JA, Espronceda M, et al. Current Procedural Terminology, 2009. Chicago, IL: American Medical Association; 2009.

169. An 88-yr-old man comes to the clinic for the first time in 18 mo, accompanied by his son. The patient states that he has no active medical problems. He has lived alone since his wife's death 10 yr ago. He is not sexually active and does not smoke or drink alcohol. The son states that his father has lost weight, is less active socially than he used to be, has little energy or endurance, and spends most of his time reading or watching television. On detailed questioning, the patient indicates that he often skips meals but otherwise feels his appetite is unchanged. He does all his own cooking. His son notes that when his dad comes to his house on weekends, he eats well. The patient indicates that he does not have problems sleeping, swallowing, or voiding. He has had no change in bowel habits, no incontinence, and no depressive symptoms. History includes early-stage prostate cancer, for which he had a prostatectomy 8 yr ago; at follow-up 1 yr ago, his urologist told him there was no evidence of recurrence. Screening colonoscopy done 2 yr ago was normal. The patient takes a daily multivitamin.

On examination, the patient weighs 62.6 kg (138 lb; body mass index, 22 kg/m^2), which, according to medical records, is 13% less than he weighed 18 mo ago. The rest of his physical examination is normal. His score on the Mini–Mental State Examination is 29/30; his score on the Yesavage Geriatric Depression Scale–Short Form is 2/15. Fecal guaiac is negative. Urinalysis, CBC, electrolytes, vitamin B$_{12}$, and liver, renal, and thyroid function tests are normal. Prostate-specific antigen is undetectable. ECG reveals normal sinus rhythm, and chest radiography is normal.

Which of the following is the most appropriate next step?

(A) CT of the chest, abdomen, and pelvis
(B) Upper and lower endoscopy
(C) Upper GI series with small-bowel follow-through
(D) Complete radiographic bone survey
(E) No further diagnostic testing

ANSWER: E

Involuntary weight loss in older adults is always cause for concern. It is often a harbinger of subsequent adverse clinical events, including death. The risk of death increases in direct proportion to the amount and rate of the weight loss. As a general rule, loss of >5% body weight within 1 mo or >10% in 6 mo should prompt a careful evaluation. However, even lesser amounts of weight loss can be clinically significant. Among community-dwelling older adults, weight loss of 5% over 3 yr is associated with increased mortality.

In older patients, potential causes of involuntary weight loss are often readily identifiable by history and physical examination alone. When this is not the case, more thorough diagnostic evaluation is warranted, using the same basic, focused panel of tests as was obtained for this patient. Additional tests are ordered only as required to investigate abnormalities identified in the initial screen. If the initial screen is unrevealing, a period of "watchful waiting" is appropriate, rather than more extensive undirected testing (SOE=B). In the case presented, the initial evaluation did not identify any abnormalities that would warrant further diagnostic testing. Addressing the patient's known risk factors for weight loss, such as social isolation and low level of physical activity, would probably benefit him more than additional tests.

Use of CT of the chest, abdomen, and pelvis is controversial when the initial diagnostic evaluation is normal in older adults with weight loss (SOE=D). Although several studies have demonstrated that such an approach will sometimes identify unrecognized malignancy or other serious disease, there is no evidence that this information results in improved patient outcome. Such testing is also associated with a high probability of false-positive results that can lead to further, potentially harmful diagnostic testing. Substituting MRI for CT can decrease the risk of contrast-induced pathology but does not improve diagnostic accuracy. Similar concerns pertain to the use of endoscopy or barium studies. Because this patient has no evidence of metastatic cancer, a bone survey is not warranted.

References

1. Bouras EP, Lange SM, Scolapio JS. Rational approach to patients with unintentional weight loss. *Mayo Clin Proc.* 2001;76(9):923–929.

2. Hernandez JL, Riancho JA, Matorras P, et al. Clinical evaluation for cancer in patients with involuntary weight loss without specific symptoms. *Am J Med.* 2003;114(8):631–637.

3. Lankisch P, Gerzmann M, Gerzmann JF, et al. Unintentional weight loss: diagnosis and prognosis. The first prospective follow-up study from a secondary referral centre. *J Intern Med.* 2001;249(1):41–46.

4. Locher JL, Roth DL, Ritchie CS, et al. Body mass index, weight loss, and mortality in community-dwelling older adults. *J Gerontol A Biol Sci Med Sci.* 2007;62(12):1389–1392.

5. Metalidis C, Knockaert DC, Bobbaers H, et al. Involuntary weight loss. Does a negative baseline evaluation provide adequate reassurance? *Eur J Intern Med.* 2008;19(5):345–349.

170. An 82-yr-old woman who lives alone in an apartment is found by the building manager wandering in the basement, apparently lost. She knows her name and the building address but is not sure when she left her apartment. She cannot say what time of day it is now, although she has a watch. She seems intermittently agitated. The building manager notifies her family.

Her daughter finds that her mother has been incontinent of urine. She thinks that her mother has a fever and, unable to reach the mother's physician, takes her to the emergency department. Once there, the mother demands that no one speak with her daughter, whom the mother says abuses her. The mother also verbally (but not physically) refuses to cooperate with the examination and tests, and says that she wants to go home. She knows where she is and the time of day, and she can recall three words after diversionary discussion. She can do simple math (ie, add and subtract). She is easily distracted and cannot stay with a task for more than a few minutes. She refuses to let the emergency department staff call her personal physician, saying that he is "in cahoots with" her daughter.

Which of the following is the most appropriate course?

(A) Videotape her behavior to document the need to treat her against her will.
(B) Ask the daughter to produce evidence that she has durable power of attorney or, if there is no legal document, that she is the next of kin.
(C) Continue evaluation as possible, obtain history from personal physician, and document the emergency conditions.
(D) Sedate the patient to proceed with the examination.

ANSWER: C

The patient is delirious, although improving and fairly stable. The delirium is likely related to an acute illness (such as infection), medication, or metabolic disorder; other possible causes include a small stroke. The patient should be protected from hurting herself when she is not fully capable of making her own decisions. There is little reason to suspect that the daughter is not an appropriate next of kin, because she was called by the building manager, came to her mother's rescue, is identified by the mother as her daughter, and is trying to help. It would make sense to ask about durable power of attorney and, if one exists, to obtain it to guide longer-term treatment. However, the emergency department physician is required only to exercise reasonable judgment as to the competence of the patient to make her own choices and the appropriateness of the apparent surrogate. Videotaping the situation and keeping that videotape on file against future claims would add costs and delays without addressing any immediate need. A violent delirious patient may require sedation, but doing so would complicate diagnosis, monitoring, and return to mental clarity. Because the patient is stable or improving and is manageable, sedation or tranquilizers should be avoided.

References

1. American College of Emergency Physicians. Code of Ethics for Emergency Physicians. http://www.acep.org/practres.aspx?id=29144 (accessed Nov 2009).
2. Appelbaum PS. Clinical Practice: Assessment of patients' competence to consent to treatment. *N Engl J Med.* 2007;357(18):1834–1840.
3. Inouye SK. Delirium in older persons. *N Engl J Med.* 2006;354(11):1157–1165.

171. An 86-yr-old man comes to the office for a routine visit. He is in good health and has never been screened for colon cancer.

Which of the following should you recommend?

(A) Colonoscopy
(B) Fecal DNA test
(C) Flexible sigmoidoscopy
(D) Air-contrast barium enema
(E) No testing

ANSWER: E

Fecal tests for colon cancer (such as tests for occult blood and DNA tests) are designed to detect colorectal cancer and some polyps, whereas structural tests (eg, colonoscopy, flexible sigmoidoscopy, double-contrast barium enema, and CT colonography) can detect both cancers and adenomatous polyps. However, colonoscopy and flexible sigmoidoscopy (to a lesser degree) entail possible serious complications. High-risk individuals—a personal or family history of colorectal cancer, adenomas, inflammatory bowel disease, or high-risk genetic syndromes—should have screening colonoscopy.

New fecal tests have been developed to improve the sensitivity of the fecal guaiac test, which can be <50%; sensitivity increases with annual screening. The new tests include fecal immunochemical tests and fecal DNA tests. However, the effect of screening on clinical outcomes with these tests is not known, and appropriate testing intervals have not been determined.

The U.S. Preventive Services Task Force (USPSTF) recommends screening for colorectal cancer using high-sensitivity fecal occult blood testing, sigmoidoscopy, or colonoscopy in adults 50–75 yr old (SOE=A). The USPSTF recommends against routine screening for colorectal cancer in adults 76–85 yr old. The likelihood that detection and early intervention will yield a mortality benefit declines after age 75 because of the long average time between adenoma development and cancer diagnosis, and the likelihood of competing mortality risks from comorbid conditions. There may be considerations that support colorectal cancer screening in individual patients of this age (SOE=B). Clinicians should discuss screening decisions with patients and include information on test quality and availability.

The USPSTF recommends against screening for colorectal cancer in adults >85 yr old (SOE=A). The USPSTF concludes that evidence at present is insufficient to assess the benefits and harms of CT colonography and fecal DNA testing as screening modalities for colorectal cancer (SOE=C). CT colonography also presents concerns regarding cumulative radiation exposure when used as a screening modality.

References

1. Levi Z, Rozen P, Hazazi R, et al. A quantitative immunochemical fecal occult blood test for colorectal neoplasia. *Ann Intern Med.* 2007;146(4):244–255.
2. Lieberman DA. Screening for colorectal cancer. *N Engl J Med.* 2009;361(12):1179–1187.
3. U.S. Preventive Services Task Force. Screening for Colorectal Cancer. http://www.ahrq.gov/CLINIC/uspstf/uspscolo.htm (accessed Nov 2009).
4. Whitlock EP, Lin JS, Liles E, et al. Screening for colorectal cancer: a targeted, updated systematic review for the U.S. Preventive Services Task Force. *Ann Intern Med.* 2008;149(9):638–658.
5. Zauber AG, Lansdorp-Vogelaar I, Knudsen AB, et al. Evaluating test strategies for colorectal cancer screening: a decision analysis for the U.S. Preventive Services Task Force. *Ann Intern Med.* 2008;149(9):659–669.

172. A 72-yr-old man comes to the office because he has increased difficulty with urination, including poor stream, straining to void, and occasional urinary incontinence. History includes benign prostatic hyperplasia, dyslipidemia, type 2 diabetes mellitus, and painful peripheral neuropathy; past medical history is significant for transient ischemic attack. Medications include clopidogrel 75 mg/d, doxazosin 2 mg at bedtime, glipizide 10 mg/d, atorvastatin 20 mg/d, and gabapentin 400 mg q8h. The patient's peripheral neuropathy has been difficult to manage. Further increase of gabapentin is not possible because it causes him dizziness. Nortriptyline 25 mg at bedtime was started 2 wk ago, and the patient reports decreased pain.

On examination, the patient's prostate is not enlarged, nor is his bladder palpable. Urinalysis is normal.

Which of the following should be done next to manage this patient's voiding difficulties?

(A) Increase doxazosin.
(B) Discontinue nortriptyline.
(C) Begin tolterodine.
(D) Obtain postvoid residual level.
(E) Obtain prostate-specific antigen level.

ANSWER: D

Although this patient's benign prostatic hyperplasia may be progressing, the recent addition of nortriptyline warrants excluding urinary retention due to introduction of a new medication. This is best accomplished through ultrasonography or straight catheterization assessment of postvoid residual. Medications with anticholinergic effects, such as nortriptyline, can cause urinary retention by inhibiting contraction of bladder smooth muscle. Although nortriptyline has less anticholinergic activity than amitriptyline, it can cause urinary retention in susceptible individuals. Because nortriptyline[OL] has provided some pain relief in this patient, it should not be discontinued until the postvoid residual is accurately measured. If the residual is normal, it is unlikely that nortriptyline is contributing to his urinary symptoms.

The patient is on a low dosage of doxazosin for benign prostatic hyperplasia; increasing the dosage is a reasonable option to manage his symptoms after drug-induced urinary retention is excluded (SOE=A).

Tolterodine has anticholinergic activity and is used to treat symptoms of overactive bladder (eg, urinary frequency, urgency, urge incontinence). If this patient has urinary retention, tolterodine-related urinary retention could worsen incontinence. Adding anticholinergic bladder medication (eg, tolterodine) to α-adrenergic blocker therapy can improve symptoms in men with benign prostatic hyperplasia and symptoms of overactive bladder (SOE=A). Tolterodine could be considered after both α-blocker therapy has been maximized and postvoid residual has been excluded. Measuring the level of prostate-specific antigen is unlikely to assist in management of this patient's voiding symptoms.

References

1. Gibbs CF, Johnson TM 2nd, Ouslander JG. Office management of geriatric urinary incontinence. *Am J Med.* 2007;120(3):211–220.
2. Kaplan SA, Roehrborn CG, Rovner ES, et al. Tolterodine and tamsulosin for treatment of men with lower urinary tract symptoms and overactive bladder: a randomized controlled trial. *JAMA.* 2006;296(19):2319–2328.
3. Rosenberg MT, Staskin DR, Kaplan SA, et al. A practical guide to the evaluation and treatment of male lower urinary tract symptoms in the primary care setting. *Int J Clin Pract.* 2007;61(9):1535–1546.

OL Not approved by the U.S. Food and Drug Administration for this use.

173. A 78-yr-old man comes to the office because he recently fell for no apparent reason. He has had cognitive problems for 5 yr. At first, friends noticed that he often seemed inattentive and was easily distractible. He began having trouble navigating to the location of his poker game, held at a different person's house each month. His family noticed that he was intermittently confused and often talked of seeing different friends (deceased) at his house. He is no longer able to organize his social calendar or prepare a tax return, which he previously did with ease. The family believes that recently his memory has begun "failing" as well. The history suggests dementia with Lewy bodies.

Which of the following statements is most accurate about dementia with Lewy bodies?

(A) Clinical suspicion is increased if parkinsonism was present ≥2 yr before the dementia.
(B) A history of exposure to neuroleptic agents with no adverse event excludes the diagnosis.
(C) Occipital lobe hypermetabolism is seen on positron emission tomography (PET).
(D) Associated visual hallucinations are usually complex and vivid.

ANSWER: D

Diagnostic criteria for dementia with Lewy bodies are subdivided into central, core, suggestive, and supportive features. The central feature, dementia, is required, although memory impairment is often less conspicuous than deficits in attention, executive function, and visuospatial ability, especially early in the disease course. Core features consist of fluctuating cognition, recurrent visual hallucinations, and spontaneous parkinsonism. Suggestive features consist of rapid-eye movement (REM) sleep behavior disorder, severe neuroleptic sensitivity, and low dopamine-transporter uptake in the basal ganglia observed on single-proton emission CT or PET. Supportive features, such as syncope, delusions, or autonomic dysfunction, are common but do not have diagnostic specificity. Diagnosis usually specifies degree of certainty by denoting "probable" or "possible" dementia with Lewy bodies. The central feature (dementia) must always be present. If one core feature is present, the diagnosis is "possible dementia with Lewy bodies"; 2 or more core features suffice for a diagnosis of probable dementia with Lewy bodies. Probable Lewy body dementia should not be diagnosed on the basis of suggestive features alone, even if all three are present. If one or more suggestive features accompany at least one core feature, probable Lewy body dementia can be diagnosed. In the absence of any core feature, a single suggestive feature suffices for a diagnosis of possible dementia with Lewy bodies.

The criteria make formal note of the temporal sequence of symptoms, specifying that parkinsonism should occur after or concurrent with the onset of dementia to warrant the diagnosis of dementia with Lewy bodies. If parkinsonism is well established by the time dementia occurs, then the diagnosis is Parkinson's disease dementia. A gap of at least 1 yr between onset of dementia and parkinsonism is recommended to facilitate distinction between dementia with Lewy bodies and Parkinson's disease dementia.

Visual hallucinations in dementia with Lewy bodies are often complex, detailed, and vivid. The hallucinations tend to be recurrent, and patients often retain a degree of insight into their unreality. The degree of insight can be helpful in deciding whether to initiate antipsychotic therapy, which can cause clinical deterioration in a patient with Lewy body dementia.

Occipital lobe hypometabolism on PET can be a marker for dementia with Lewy bodies and is a supportive feature for the diagnosis. Neuroleptic sensitivity is suggestive of dementia with Lewy bodies. It refers to the clinical deterioration that is seen in approximately 50% of patients with dementia with Lewy bodies who are exposed to neuroleptics and have a history of severe neuroleptic reaction. Because 50% of patients with dementia with Lewy bodies do not react adversely, past neuroleptic use without adverse event does not exclude the diagnosis. Sensitivity reactions are characterized by acute onset or exacerbation of parkinsonism and impaired consciousness. Because these reactions can have high morbidity and mortality, deliberate pharmacologic challenge with a neuroleptic agent should never be contemplated as a diagnostic strategy.

References
1. Emre M, Aarsland D, Brown R, et al. Clinical diagnostic criteria for dementia associated with Parkinson's disease. *Mov Disord*. 2007;22(12):1689–1707.

2. McKeith IG, Dickson DW, Lowe J, et al. Diagnosis and management of dementia with Lewy bodies: Third report of the DLB Consortium. *Neurology*. 2005;65(12):1863–1872.

174. An 89-yr-old man is admitted to a nursing home for rehabilitation after being hospitalized for pneumonia. He is anxious and fidgety. He is widowed and lives in the community. History includes hypertension, benign prostatic hyperplasia, major depressive disorder, and chronic back pain. Medications on transfer from the hospital to the nursing home include metoprolol, oxybutynin, paroxetine, acetaminophen with codeine, and amitriptyline.

Which of the following medications is *least* likely to contribute to delirium?

(A) Amitriptyline
(B) Acetaminophen with codeine
(C) Oxybutynin
(D) Paroxetine
(E) Metoprolol

ANSWER: E

All of these medications have some anticholinergic properties, but the metoprolol has the least potential impact on mental status (SOE=B). Amitriptyline, codeine, and oxybutynin have strong anticholinergic properties, are associated with delirium, and should be avoided. Both amitriptyline and codeine also have active metabolites, which can result in accumulation of drug and metabolite in the system, especially during times of stress and illness. Similarly, paroxetine has significant anticholinergic effects in older adults.

Although the pathophysiology of delirium is unknown and may be multifactorial, there is consensus that suppression of cholinergic neurons contributes to delirium (SOE=C). Older adults with impaired cholinergic systems, such as those with Alzheimer's dementia, are more susceptible to delirium. Thus, anticholinergic medications should be avoided in older adults, especially when they are most susceptible to delirium, such as while hospitalized.

In some studies, delirium symptoms and severity have been associated with serum anticholinergic activity level; other studies have not shown a clear association. Adjustments to medications with anticholinergic properties can reduce the serum anticholinergic activity level and reduce delirium symptoms (SOE=B). If delirium develops, the medication regimen should be reviewed to eliminate or reduce agents with anticholinergic properties.

References

1. Flacker JM, Cummings V, Mach JR Jr, et al. The association of serum anticholinergic activity with delirium in elderly medical patients. *Am J Geriatr Psych*. 1998;6(1):31–41.
2. Han L, McCusker J, Cole M, et al. Use of medications with anticholinergic effect predicts clinical severity of delirium symptoms in older medical inpatients. *Arch Intern Med*. 2001;161(8):1099–1105.
3. Kiely DK, Jones RN, Bergmann MA, et al. Association between psychomotor activity delirium subtypes and mortality among newly admitted post-acute facility patients. *J Gerontol Biol Sci Med Sci*. 2007;62(2):174–179.

175. A 69-yr-old man comes to the office to establish care. His wife is being treated for osteoporosis and she wants know whether her husband should also undergo a screening assessment.

Which of the following is the strongest risk factor for osteoporosis in men?

(A) Androgen deprivation therapy
(B) Low dietary intake of vitamin D
(C) Respiratory disease
(D) Thyroid replacement therapy
(E) Type 2 diabetes mellitus

ANSWER: A

Osteoporosis is a problem in older men, but data on screening guidelines are still being accrued. Literature review indicates that the most important risk factors for osteoporotic fractures in men are age ≥70 yr old and low body weight (body mass index <25 kg/m^2 or weight <70 kg [154 lb]) (SOE=A). Other risk factors include weight loss, physical inactivity, corticosteroid use, previous osteoporotic fracture, and androgen deprivation therapy (SOE=A). Androgen deprivation therapy (pharmacologic or by orchiectomy) is a strong predictor of both osteoporosis and fracture.

Multiple other risk factors for osteoporosis in men have been reported, but the strength of the association is inconclusive in most cases. Some of the other reported risk factors include cigarette smoking, alcohol use, vitamin D and calcium intake, respiratory disease, thyroid replacement therapy, and type 2 diabetes mellitus. These possible risk factors have plausible physiologic rationales, and some are supported by data on osteoporosis and fractures in women or inconsistent data in men.

References

1. Kanis JA, Borgstrom F, De Laet C, et al. Assessment of fracture risk. *Osteoporosis Int.* 2005;16(6):581–589.

2. Liu H, Paige N, Goldzweig C, et al. Screening for osteoporosis in men: a systematic review for an American College of Physicians Guideline. *Ann Intern Med.* 2008;148(9): 685–701.

3. Qaseem A, Snow V, Shekelle P, et al. for the Clinical Efficacy Assessment Subcommittee of the American College of Physicians. Screening for osteoporosis in men: a clinical practice guideline from the American College of Physicians. *Ann Intern Med.* 2008;148(9):680–684.

176. An 86-yr-old woman is brought to the office by her home health attendant for an urgent visit. The patient has Alzheimer's dementia and rheumatoid arthritis. Her daughter lives in another city and has privately hired a 24-hour home attendant because her mother requires total assistance with toileting and bathing. She can ambulate slowly with a rolling walker but is primarily homebound because of her arthritis. The attendant asks that the patient be given a prescription for a sleeping pill because neither of them has slept through the night for the past week. She reports that the patient has been asking to go to the bathroom every 2 hours and has had multiple incidents of urinary incontinence when she could not reach the bathroom in time. The patient refuses to wear a diaper. The patient has also begun calling out for her deceased husband at night. The attendant reports limiting the patient's fluid intake after lunch to try to decrease the patient's need to urinate at night. Last night, she gave the patient diphenhydramine to help her sleep.

Which of the following is the most appropriate initial step for determining whether the patient is being mistreated?

(A) Interview patient and caregiver separately.
(B) Administer the Mini–Mental State Examination.
(C) Order a complete urinalysis and urine culture.
(D) Begin a second-generation antipsychotic agent.
(E) Begin an anticholinergic agent.

ANSWER: A

Interviewing the patient and caregiver separately is the most appropriate and critical first step in caring for this patient (SOE=D). Several factors suggest the possibility of mistreatment: 1) there is a single primary caregiver (ie, the home health attendant); 2)

the patient's dementia, functional impairment, and urinary incontinence increase her dependence on the caregiver; and 3) the patient has behavioral difficulties (nighttime hallucinations). These factors have led to an imbalance between the patient's needs and the attendant's ability to meet those needs. The physician should recognize the imbalance and screen for mistreatment by interviewing the patient and caregiver separately.

Victims of mistreatment can be reluctant to reveal abuse or neglect because of shame, fear of retaliation, or desire to keep the family structure intact. Talking with the patient alone can demonstrate the physician's desire to create a safe and confidential environment for disclosure. Separate interviews also allow the physician to detect and document discrepancies in the histories provided, such as the patient and caregiver reporting different reasons for a suspicious injury, or inconsistencies between caregiver reports and objective findings, such as a caregiver's report that medications are being provided consistently in the presence of subtherapeutic drug levels.

Appropriate general inquiries about the patient's home environment, functional status, and relationships with caregivers include: "What is your home like? Do you need help getting to the bathroom? Tell me about your relationship with your son." The physician can then progress to more directed questions as suggested by the American Medical Association and others. Questions that might be appropriate for this patient include: "Are you afraid of anyone in your home? Has anyone ever threatened you? Are you alone a lot? Has anyone ever failed to help you when you were unable to help yourself? Do you have to wait a long time for food or medicine?"

The presence of cognitive impairment should not preclude a private interview with the patient. Techniques such as repeating the patient's responses, using simple, clear language, and speaking slowly can be helpful when communicating with an older adult with sensory or cognitive deficits.

When interviewing caregivers, the physician should maintain an empathetic and nonjudgmental attitude. Questions that might be appropriate for this patient's home health attendant include: "How long have you been working with the patient? What are your responsibilities? How are you coping with your responsibilities?" In this case, it may be appropriate to encourage the patient's daughter to hire additional caregivers, and to educate the home attendant about the importance of fluid intake, the risks of diphenhydramine, and the etiology and course of delirium.

Evaluating the patient's cognitive status (with the Mini–Mental State Examination or comparable screening tool) is critical because it can help determine the patient's decision-making capacity. However, the first step in assessing for mistreatment would be to interview the patient and the attendant separately.

Urinalysis and urine culture to exclude urinary tract infection as the cause of the patient's incontinence and delirium are indicated but would not be the initial step in management. Prescription of antipsychotic or anticholinergic medications would not be appropriate without first excluding urinary tract infection, discouraging use of diphenhydramine, and introducing nonpharmacologic behavioral techniques.

References

1. Lachs MS, Pillemer K. Elder abuse. *Lancet.* 2004;364(9441):1263–1272.
2. Liao S. Elder mistreatment. http://pier.acponline.org/eldermistreatment. In: PIER [online database]. Philadelphia, PA: American College of Physicians; 2003.
3. Mahnaz A, Lachs MS. Elder abuse and neglect: what physicians can and should do. *Cleve Clin J Med.* 2002;69(10):801–808.

177. An 85-yr-old African-American woman with Alzheimer's disease is admitted to a nursing facility for rehabilitation. She is deconditioned after recent hospitalization for community-acquired pneumonia. The nursing home assesses patients on admission for risk of developing pressure ulcers.

Which of the following has been validated for risk assessment of pressure ulcers in nonwhite populations?

(A) Norton scale
(B) Gosnell scale
(C) Waterlow scale
(D) Care Dependency Scale
(E) Braden scale

ANSWER: E

Assessment of pressure ulcers is more difficult in darkly pigmented skin. In 1997, the National Pressure Ulcer Advisory Panel revised the definition of stage I ulcers because of difficulty in distinguishing nonblanching erythema in nonwhite populations (SOE=C). To date, only the Braden scale has been validated

in nonwhite populations (SOE=B). A cutoff score of 18 provides good validity for predicting the risk of pressure ulcers in black adults ≥75 yr old.

The Norton scale was first described in the early 1960s and is still widely used. It has been modified to increase its accuracy but is not validated for nonwhite populations. There are >40 scales described in the literature to predict risk of pressure ulcers, including the Gosnell and Waterlow scales and the Care Dependency Scale (SOE=C). Like the modified Norton scale, these scales have not yet been validated for nonwhite populations.

References

1. Anthony D, Parboteeah S, Saleh M, et al. Norton, Waterlow and Braden scores: a review of the literature and a comparison between the scores and clinical judgment. *J Clin Nurs.* 2008;17(5):646–653.
2. Pancorbo-Hidalgo PL, Garcia-Fernandez FP, Lopez-Medina IM, et al. Risk assessment scales for pressure ulcer prevention: a systematic review. *J Adv Nurs.* 2006;54(1):94–110.
3. Vanderwee K, Grypdonck M, Defloor T. Non-blanchable erythema as an indicator for the need for pressure ulcer prevention: a randomized-controlled trial. *J Clin Nurs.* 2007;16(2):325–335.

178. A 65-yr-old woman comes to the office because she has constant burning of the tongue and palate, most pronounced when she wakes up in the morning. During the day she also experiences taste alteration, such as a bitter taste. Her medical history is unremarkable; her only medications are aspirin 81 mg and a multivitamin daily. On physical examination, the oropharynx is normal.

Which of the following is the most likely diagnosis?

(A) Xerostomia
(B) Candidiasis
(C) Geographic tongue
(D) Burning mouth syndrome
(E) Salicylate adverse event

ANSWER: D

Burning mouth syndrome involves the interaction of several biologic and psychologic systems. It is characterized by a burning sensation or other dysesthesia of the oral mucosa (glossodynia or glossalgia), without accompanying abnormal clinical or laboratory findings. Burning mouth syndrome is more prevalent among older adults and women, especially postmenopausal women, with an overall female-to-male ratio of 7:1. The prevalence in the United States is approximately 0.7%, with numbers in Europe as high as 7%. In most cases, there is no detectable cause.

The oral mucosal pain is often accompanied by subjective complaints of dysgeusia (ie, taste alteration) and xerostomia, despite normal salivary function. The sensations commonly involve the anterior two-thirds of the tongue, the hard palate, the lips, and to a lesser extent gingival tissue. Rarely, symptoms involve the mouth floor or soft palate. Various local and systemic conditions are associated with burning mouth syndrome, such as food or drug allergy, diabetes, menopause, oral lichen planus, and denture use. Deficiency of iron or vitamin B_{12} has also been pursued as a cause. Several investigators have noted an association between glossodynia and generalized anxiety and depression.

The most common treatment for burning mouth syndrome is a topical rinse, such as capsaicin, doxepin, or lidocaine (SOE=D). Systemic medications that have been tried include first- and third-generation antidepressants, anticonvulsants, opioids, and benzodiazepines.

Fungal infection, which can contribute to the burning sensation, must be considered. A normal examination makes this unlikely, and most patients with burning mouth syndrome test negative for candidiasis.

Geographic tongue is usually asymptomatic. When it is symptomatic, it causes pain while eating and does not cause taste alteration.

Salicylates do not cause a burning sensation, and xerostomia is more often associated with a dry sensation or difficulty swallowing.

References

1. Carbone M, Pentenero M, Carrozzo M, et al. Lack of efficacy of alpha-lipoic acid in burning mouth syndrome: a double-blind, randomized, placebo-controlled study. *Eur J Pain.* 2009;13(5):492–496.
2. Felice F, Gombos F, Esposito V, et al. Burning mouth syndrome (BMS): evaluation of thyroid and taste. *Med Oral Patol Oral Cir Bucal.* 2006;11:E22–25.
3. Maltsman-Tseikhin A, Moricca P, et al. Burning mouth syndrome: will better understanding yield better management? *Pain Pract.* 2007;7(2):151–162.
4. Patton LL, Siegel MA, Benoliel R, et al. Management of burning mouth syndrome: systematic review and management recommendations. *Oral Surg Oral Med Oral Pathol Oral Radiol Endod.* 2007;103 Suppl:S39.e1–13.

179. An 81-yr-old woman recently admitted to a nursing facility is frequently incontinent of urine. History includes Alzheimer's disease and lumbosacral stenosis. Medications include calcium, vitamin D, and acetaminophen. The patient's family states that her incontinence has remained essentially unchanged for the past 6 mo. The patient is unable to give a detailed history and denies bladder problems. Observations by the nursing staff suggest a diagnosis of overactive bladder with urge incontinence.

On examination, there is no evidence of severe atrophic vaginitis, pelvic prolapse, or fecal impaction. Catheterization within a few minutes of an episode of incontinence reveals residual volume of 40 mL. Urinalysis of the specimen obtained by catheterization shows 3+ bacteria and 6 WBCs per high-power field; the culture grows >100,000 colony-forming units of *Escherichia coli*, sensitive to cephalexin.

Which of the following is the most appropriate next step?

(A) Oxybutynin 2.5 mg q8h
(B) Long-acting tolterodine 4 mg/d
(C) Cephalexin
(D) Prompted-voiding program
(E) Urodynamic testing

ANSWER: D

The most appropriate intervention for this patient would be a trial of prompted voiding. Between 25% and 40% of nursing-home patients respond well to this behavioral protocol, and responsiveness can generally be determined after a trial of 3 to 5 days (SOE=A). Some patients benefit from the addition of a bladder relaxant such as oxybutynin or tolterodine, but because of potential adverse events, these medications should be used as an adjunct to a toileting program (SOE=A). Bladder relaxants have anticholinergic adverse events and may worsen cognitive impairment or precipitate delirium in patients with dementia (SOE=A). These agents should be used only in selected patients who have bothersome overactive bladder symptoms, who do not respond to a toileting program alone, and who demonstrate both tolerance of and responsiveness to the medication. In chronically incontinent nursing-home patients with stable symptoms who have no other signs of infection, eradicating bacteriuria does not reduce the severity of incontinence, even if there is pyuria (SOE=A). Moreover, treating asymptomatic bacteriuria is not recommended in the nursing home. Urodynamic testing is not contraindicated, even in frail nursing-home patients, but the results would not change the initial approach to management (SOE=C).

References
1. Fink HA, Taylor BC, Tacklind JW, et al. Treatment interventions in nursing home residents with urinary incontinence: a systematic review of randomized trials. *Mayo Clin Proc.* 2008;83(12):1332–1343.
2. Nicolle LE. Asymptomatic bacteriuria: review and discussion of the IDSA Guidelines. *Int J Antimicrobial Agents.* 2006;28 Suppl 1:S42–48.

180. An 84-yr-old man comes to the office because he has pain in his lower back and right buttock. The pain has progressively worsened over the past year. It is most pronounced when he stands or walks for a prolonged period, and is often relieved when he sits. The pain is most severe when he first stands after sitting and when he tries to get in or out of an automobile. He has difficulty climbing stairs.

On examination, there is mild symmetric immobility of the lumbar spine. The straight-leg raise test is normal bilaterally. He has full strength of the proximal and distal muscles of both lower legs. There is 30° abduction, 45° external rotation, and 10° internal rotation of the left hip; and 10° abduction, 20° external rotation, and no internal rotation of the right hip. When the patient walks, he limps favoring his right leg.

Which of the following is the most appropriate next step?

(A)   Radiography of the lumbar spine
(B)   MRI of the lumbar spine
(C)   Nerve conduction studies of the right lower leg
(D)   Radiography of the right hip
(E)   Bone scan

ANSWER: D

Hip disease is the great masquerader in musculoskeletal conditions. It classically causes pain in the groin, but it can present with pain in the thigh, lateral hip, buttock, and knee. Differentiation of hip from back disease is often difficult in patients with buttock and lateral hip pain. Pain when changing from supine to sitting position and with bending or stooping suggests the back as the cause of buttock pain. Hip disease is suggested if there is significant pain when a patient first gets out of a chair or bed or when there is difficulty ascending stairs, because hip flexion is the most important action when climbing. The patient should be assessed while he or she is walking. A limp is characteristic of hip disease and is rarely seen in back disease in the absence of sciatica.

For this patient, the most appropriate next step in the evaluation would be plain radiography of the right hip (SOE=D). The normal straight-leg raise test and absence of weakness of the proximal and distal leg muscles make back disease less likely. The presence of a limp especially suggests the hip as the cause of the pain, as do decreased range of motion of the right hip and relatively normal range of the left. In a study that compared hip with spine disease as a cause of back and leg pain, features that best predicted hip disease were groin pain, limp, and limited internal rotation of the hip. Therefore, radiography and MRI of the lumbar spine are not indicated.

The absence of sciatica makes lumbosacral radiculopathy less likely as the cause of this patient's pain, making nerve conduction studies of the right lower leg a less useful diagnostic study in this patient. A bone scan in this patient would probably show increased uptake at the hips and other joints, consistent with degenerative joint disease. However, this finding is nonspecific and would be of little use in the evaluation of this patient.

References
1. Brown MD, Gomez-Marin O, Brookfield KF, et al. Differential diagnosis of hip disease versus spine disease. *Clin Orthop Relat Res.* 2004;419:280–284.
2. Mengiardi B, Pfirmann CW, Hodler J. Hip pain in adults: MR imaging appearance of common causes. *Eur Radiol.* 2007;17(7):1746–1762.

181. A 75-yr-old woman is brought to the emergency department because she has right lower-quadrant pain that has gradually increased in intensity over 36 hours, with associated nausea and diarrhea. She reports no relieving or exacerbating factors, and is otherwise healthy.

On examination, she appears uncomfortable. Temperature is 36.9°C (98.4°F), blood pressure is 140/85 mmHg, pulse is 94 beats per minute, and respiratory rate is 16 breaths per minute. She has right lower-quadrant abdominal tenderness with no guarding or rebound. Bowel sounds are depressed. CBC is normal (WBC is 9/μL with no left shift). Urinalysis demonstrates pyuria. Plain radiograph of the abdomen demonstrates nonspecific changes.

Which of the following is the best next step?

(A) Barium enema
(B) Urine culture
(C) CT of the abdomen and pelvis
(D) Ultrasound of the abdomen
(E) Urgent sigmoidoscopy

ANSWER: C

Appendicitis accounts for approximately 5% of acute abdominal cases in older adults. Less than one-third of older adults have the classic presentation of epigastric abdominal pain that ultimately radiates to the right lowerquadrant, with associated anorexia, nausea, vomiting, fever, and leukocytosis. Many other factors make diagnosis difficult: obtaining an adequate history may be difficult, and altered pain perception can interfere with the patient's ability to describe and report pain. Up to one-third of patients are reported to have delayed seeking care. Fever and leukocytosis are absent in up to 20% of patients. Misleading clinical features such as urinary frequency and pyuria suggest cystitis and, in about 10% of patients, diarrhea suggests gastroenteritis. Because 50% of patients do not receive a correct diagnosis on admission to the emergency department, medical care can be delayed, which accounts for the relatively high rates of perforation, with associated postoperative complications and mortality, among older patients. Whenever a patient has right lower-quadrant pain and tenderness, appendicitis must remain high on the list of diagnostic possibilities.

In most settings, CT of the abdomen is the test of choice to diagnose acute appendicitis in adults. Although graded-compression ultrasonography is used preferentially to diagnose appendicitis in some settings, CT performs better in head-to-head comparisons (SOE=A). CT is particularly effective for diagnosis of abdominal pain in older adults, in whom multiple intra-abdominal pathologies can present quite similarly.

Serial examinations are inappropriate because doing so would delay definitive diagnosis and treatment, which would increase the risk of perforation. The use of analgesics in patients presenting with abdominal pain has been controversial because of the concern that analgesics can impair diagnostic accuracy; however, randomized trials have not supported that contention (SOE=B).

References
1. Amoli HA, Golozar A, Keshavarzi S, et al. Morphine analgesia in patients with acute appendicitis: a randomised double-blind clinical trial. *Emerg Med J.* 2008;25(9):586–589.
2. Laurell H, Hansson LE, Gunnarsson U. Acute abdominal pain among elderly patients. *Gerontol.* 2006;52(6):339–344.
3. Martinez JP, Mattu A. Abdominal pain in the elderly. *Emerg Med Clinics NA.* 2006;24(2):371–388.
4. Storm-Dickerson TL, Horattas MC. What have we learned over the past 20 years about appendicitis in the elderly? *Am J Surg.* 2003;185(3):198–201.

182. A 77-yr-old man is evaluated on admission to a nursing facility. He has uncontrolled type 2 diabetes mellitus, hypertension, and asthma. The patient is missing several teeth on both upper and lower jaws; he wears upper and lower partial dentures. The patient has no history of smoking or drinking. Captopril 12.5 mg q12h, glyburide 10 mg/d, and a steroid inhaler are prescribed. He is referred for dental evaluation.

Which of the following is most likely to be found?

(A) Periodontal disease
(B) Aphthous ulcer
(C) Squamous cell carcinoma
(D) Osteonecrosis of the jaw

ANSWER: A

Certain systemic conditions, such as poorly controlled diabetes, are associated with periodontal disease (SOE=B). Possible causative factors include reduced polymorphonuclear leukocyte function, abnormalities in collagen metabolism, and formation of advanced glycation end products, which adversely affect collagen stability and vascular integrity.

Because between 40% and 80% of patients with diabetes have dry mouth, salivary gland dysfunction is likely. Patients with diabetes are predisposed to fungal infections and caries, possibly because of increased salivary glucose levels and xerostomia. In addition, oral fungal infections, especially with *Candida albicans*, are more common in patients who wear dentures.

This patient is least likely to have squamous cell carcinoma. Because he has no history of smoking, his risk of getting oral cancer is low. Further, no association has been reported between oral cancer and diabetes.

Recurrent aphthous ulcers are among the most common oral mucosal lesions physicians and dentists observe. Although their cause is still unknown, several predisposing factors are known to contribute to their development, most commonly inflammatory bowel diseases, vitamin deficiency, and food allergies. Diabetes is not known to be one of the common risk factors.

The most common risk factors for developing osteonecrosis of the jaw are trauma, radiotherapy, chemotherapy, steroid therapy, and bisphosphonate therapy.

References

1. Akintoye SO, Greenberg MS. Recurrent aphthous stomatitis. *Dent Clin North Am.* 2005;49(1):31–47, vii-viii.
2. Demmer RT, Jacobs DR Jr, Desvarieux M. Periodontal disease and incident type 2 diabetes: results from the First National Health and Nutrition Examination Survey and its epidemiologic follow-up study. *Diabetes Care.* 2008;31(7):1373–1379.
3. Gutta R, Louis PJ. Bisphosphonates and osteonecrosis of the jaws: science and rationale. *Oral Surg Oral Med Oral Pathol Oral Radiol Endod.* 2007;104(2):186–193.
4. Mealey BL, Rose LF. Diabetes mellitus and inflammatory periodontal diseases. *Curr Opin Endocrinol Diabetes Obes.* 2008;15(2):135–141.
5. Williams RC, Barnett AH, Claffey N, et al. The potential impact of periodontal disease on general health: a consensus view. *Curr Med Res Opin.* 2008;24(6):1635–1643.

183. A 65-yr-old man is brought to the office by his wife because he has recently been falling frequently and becoming more irritable and forgetful.

On examination, blood pressure is 110/70 mmHg. He has poor upward gaze, masked facies, and nuchal rigidity.

Which of the following is most likely to be observed on physical examination?

(A) Resting tremor
(B) Autonomic dysfunction
(C) Depression
(D) Axial rigidity
(E) Bradykinesia

ANSWER: D

Progressive supranuclear palsy (PSP) is marked by supranuclear gaze palsy with progressive voluntary gaze impairment and marked rigidity. Onset is usually during the late 50s and early 60s, followed by rapid deterioration to death. Besides a supranuclear gaze palsy, other features that distinguish PSP from Parkinson's disease are striking axial rigidity and a less prominent tremor. Falling and gait disturbance are frequent manifestations of PSP. Multiple system atrophy consists of three overlapping parkinsonian syndromes (ie, olivopontocerebellar atrophy, Shy-Drager syndrome, and striatonigral degeneration). These syndromes are characterized by components of Parkinson's disease and autonomic symptoms, cerebellar signs, and possibly upper motor neuron signs and severe dysarthria and stridor.

The National Institute of Neurological Disorders and the Society for Progressive Supranuclear Palsy has proposed clinical diagnostic criteria based on neuropathologic cases. The inclusion criteria include gradual progression, onset after age 40, vertical supranuclear ophthalmoplegia, and prominent postural instability with falls within 1 yr of symptom onset (SOE=C).

References

1. Burn DJ, Lees AJ. Progressive supranuclear palsy: where are we now? *Lancet Neurol.* 2002;1(6):359–369.
2. Christine CW, Aminoff MJ. Clinical differentiation of parkinsonian syndromes: prognostic and therapeutic relevance. *Am J Med.* 2004;117(6):412–417.
3. Olanow CW, Stern MB, Sethi K. The scientific and clinical basis for the treatment of Parkinson disease. *Neurology.* 2009;72(21 Suppl 4):S1–136.
4. Rao G, Fisch L, Srinivasan S, et al. Does this patient have Parkinson disease? *JAMA.* 2003;289(3):347–353.

184. A 71-yr-old woman is frequently admitted to the hospital for complications associated with diabetes, coronary artery disease, and COPD. She routinely sees an endocrinologist, cardiologist, and pulmonary specialist, but each physician works in a different practice. She is regularly frustrated by medication changes by one doctor that are not communicated in a timely fashion to the others. She has recently read an article about the patient-centered medical home and wishes to know if that is available to her.

Which of the following is true of a patient-centered medical home?

(A) Physician services are routinely provided in the patient's home.
(B) Resources are available to refurbish and make homes more suitable for frail older adults.
(C) Physicians receive capitated payments under a Medicare Advantage or Medicare managed-care program.
(D) Physicians provide patient care working with healthcare teams with emphasis on patient self-management.

ANSWER: D

The idea of a patient-centered medical home is increasingly pursued by organizations representing primary care physicians. The American Academy of Pediatrics introduced the concept in 1967 and initially referred to a central location for archiving a child's medical record. The concept has since expanded to incorporate accessible, continuous, comprehensive, family-centered, coordinated, compassionate, and culturally effective care. Participating practices usually must undergo structural and organizational changes. Care is not usually provided to patients in their own homes. The practice can assess patient homes for safety but would be unlikely to provide resources for renovations. The concept of the medical home does not require capitated payment. For the program to be widely implemented, payment reform to support primary care physicians in developing this model may be necessary. Medicare waiver programs are underway. The National Committee for Quality Assurance recommends that the patient-centered medical home include the following: access and connection, patient tracking and registry functions, care management, patient

self-management support, electronic prescribing, test tracking, referral tracking, performance reporting and improvement, and advanced electronic communications.

References

1. American Academy of Family Physicians, American Academy of Pediatrics, American College of Physicians, American Osteopathic Association. *The Joint Principles of the Patient Centered Medical Home.* February 2007. http://www.medicalhomeinfo.org/Joint%20Statement.pdf (accessed Nov 2009).
2. Goroll AH, Berenson RA, Schoenbaum SC, et al. Fundamental reform of payment for adult primary care: comprehensive payment for comprehensive care. *J Gen Intern Med.* 2007;22(3):410–415.
3. National Committee for Quality Assurance (NCQA). Physician practice connection—patient-centered medical home; 2008. http://www.ncqa.org/tabid/631/Default.aspx (accessed Nov 2009).

185. In response to a recent newspaper article that criticized its care of frail older adults with multiple medical problems, a health system considers using a care management and information technology program called Care Management Plus. This program was developed by Intermountain Health Care in Salt Lake City, Utah.

Which of the following best describes the Care Management Plus program?

(A) It depends on multiple subspecialty consultations to increase the level of care for patients with chronic illness.
(B) It advocates strict adherence to standard disease-oriented protocols.
(C) It reduces the incidence of death and hospitalization among older adults with diabetes.
(D) It reduces physician income in a fee-for-service system.

ANSWER: C

In the Care Management Plus model, primary care physicians refer patients to a care manager (either a nurse or social worker), instead of referring them for subspecialty consultations. The care managers assess the patient's needs, help to create a care plan, and then help implement that plan. This can involve providing patient education, facilitating medication management, linking to community resources, using the electronic medical record for follow-up with other providers, checking on patients, and evaluating health outcomes.

Although disease-oriented protocols and outcome measures are used, the care management plans are individualized for each patient. In an outcome study of older adults with diabetes, this model was associated with a 20% reduction in death and a 24% reduction in hospitalizations, saving Medicare up to $274,000 per clinic (SOE=B). A subsequent study demonstrated an 8%–12% improvement in productivity for physicians who sent patients to a care manager compared with those who did not. The improvement in productivity, which translated into an additional $99,000 in clinic revenue, demonstrates that this model can be cost-effective, even in the Medicare fee-for-service system.

References

1. Dorr DA, Wilcox A, Donnelly SM, et al. Impact of generalist care manager on patients with diabetes. *Health Serv Res.* 2005;40(5 Pt 1):1400–1421.
2. Dorr DA, Wilcox A, Burns L, et al. Implementing a multidisease chronic care model in primary care using people and technology. *Dis Manag.* 2006;9(1):1–15.
3. Dorr DA, Wilcox A, McDonnell KJ, et al. Productivity enhancement for primary care providers using multicondition care management. *Am J Manag Care.* 2007;13(1):22–28.

186. An 80-yr-old man comes to the office because he has had a left frontal headache and blurry vision for 2 wk. In addition, he has been feeling more tired, and his jaw aches when he eats. He denies nausea, vomiting, neck stiffness, or visual loss. On examination, there is no nuchal rigidity or temporal tenderness. His pupils are round, equal in size, and reactive to light. Visual acuity, visual fields, fundoscopic examination, and extraocular movements are normal.

Which of the following is most likely to confirm the diagnosis?

(A) CT of the head
(B) Temporal artery biopsy
(C) Slit-lamp examination
(D) Tonometry
(E) Cerebral angiography

ANSWER: B

Temporal (giant cell) arteritis is a vasculitis that affects the large- and medium-size blood vessels. Criteria that distinguish giant cell arteritis from other types of vasculitis include age >50 yr old, localized headache, tenderness or decreased pulse of the temporal artery, RBC sedimentation rate >50 mm/h, and a biopsy positive for necrotizing arteritis.

The presence of 3 criteria has a sensitivity of 93% and specificity of 91.2%. Other common symptoms include fever, fatigue, weight loss, jaw claudication, and visual loss.

If temporal arteritis is suspected, temporal artery biopsy is indicated. In a meta-analysis of 21 studies, biopsy was positive in 39% of patients with suspected temporal arteritis. In this meta-analysis, the features associated with an increased likelihood of temporal arteritis were jaw claudication (positive likelihood ratio 4.2) and diplopia (positive likelihood ratio 3.4). Normal sedimentation rate was associated with a decreased likelihood of temporal arteritis (negative likelihood ratio 0.2) (SOE=A).

References

1. Salvarani C, Cantini F, Hunder G. Polymyalgia rheumatica and giant cell arteritis. *Lancet.* 2008;372(9634):234–245.
2. Smetana GW, Shmerling RH. Does this patient have temporal arteritis? *JAMA.* 2002;287(1):91–101.

187. A 67-yr-old woman comes to the clinic because she has dizziness, headaches, and insomnia. Her symptoms fluctuate daily, have persisted for >1 yr, and have prompted repeated medical visits. Since her retirement 2 yr ago, she takes care of her grandchildren; when her symptoms are severe, she confines herself to home and cannot fulfill her usual family responsibilities. In previous evaluations, there was no focal neurologic deficit; MRI excluded acoustic neuroma; and thyrotropin, CBC, and comprehensive metabolic panel were all normal. Meclizine, zolpidem, and acetaminophen were prescribed but provided little benefit. When directly asked, she admits feeling stressed and annoyed by mounting family responsibilities but asserts that she is most distressed by the headaches and dizziness. She does not ruminate about these concerns, enjoys socializing with friends, participates in her usual hobbies, and has noted no changes in appetite, concentration, or energy.

Which of the following is the most likely diagnosis?

(A) Hypochondriasis
(B) Somatization disorder
(C) Undifferentiated somatoform disorder
(D) Major depressive disorder

ANSWER: C

Undifferentiated somatoform disorder is characterized by one or more physical complaints lasting >6 mo and associated with significant distress or impairment in functioning. Physical symptoms and functional impairment either cannot be explained by a known medical condition, or are in excess of what would be expected based on medical findings. As with many other somatoform disorders, symptoms are not manufactured; psychologic factors are presumed to play a strong role in the onset and persistence of the physical problems. Undifferentiated somatoform disorder is among the most common somatoform disorders in late life. In this case, the patient's acknowledged stress and resentment in the context of family responsibilities are temporally associated with the onset of her physical symptoms, and her unintentional "sick role" behavior appears to relieve her of expectations that she will routinely provide child care for her grandchildren.

Hypochondriasis is a somatoform disorder in which a person's fears of having a serious disease persist despite medical evaluation and reassurance, often leading to repeated medical visits. It is based on a misinterpretation of bodily symptoms, leading to ruminations about the disease. Somatization disorder is another somatoform disorder strongly associated with psychologic factors, in which physical complaints are in excess of what would be expected based on medical findings. However, it is characterized by early onset (before age 30) and chronic history, and it involves multiple organ systems: at least 4 sites of pain; 2 GI symptoms; 1 sexual; and 1 pseudoneurologic symptom other than pain. This patient does not ruminate excessively or express fears of having a serious illness, as in hypochondriasis, or exhibit the early onset and multiple system involvement seen in somatization disorder.

Major depressive disorder in late life can be aggravated by somatic preoccupations. Although this patient reports distress and insomnia, she does not display depressed mood, anhedonia, or neurovegetative symptoms nearly every day as seen in major depressive disorder. When somatic preoccupation or hypochondriac symptoms appear in the context of late-life major depressive disorder and persist after treatment with antidepressants and/or psychotherapy, they can predict early recurrence of depressive symptoms (SOE=B).

References

1. Agronin ME. Somatoform disorders. In: Blazer DG, Steffens DC, eds. *The American Psychiatric Publishing Textbook of Geriatric Psychiatry*. 4th ed. Washington, DC: American Psychiatric Publishing Inc; 2009.
2. Dombrovski AY, Mulsant BH, Houck PR, et al. Residual symptoms and recurrence during maintenance treatment of late-life depression. *J Affective Dis.* 2007;103(1–3):77–82.
3. Wijeratne C, Brodaty H, Hickie I. The neglect of somatoform disorders by old age psychiatry: some explanations and suggestions for future research. *Int J Geriatr Psychiatry.* 2003;8:812–819.

188. A 70-yr-old man comes to the office to establish care. He is generally healthy and has always had normal blood pressure. Family history includes diabetes mellitus and hypertension; his father died of a stroke and his mother of cancer. He eats a low-sodium, low-fat diet.

On examination, blood pressure is 150/90 mmHg without postural change. Cardiac examination is normal, and there is no evidence of hypertensive retinopathy or peripheral vascular disease. Laboratory studies (including creatinine concentration of 0.8 mg/dL) and electrocardiography are normal.

At a repeat check 1 mo later, blood pressure is 154/92 mmHg without postural change. He reports that a reading taken with a friend's blood pressure cuff was 134/80 mmHg.

Which of the following is the most appropriate next step in managing this patient's increased blood pressure?

(A) Repeat blood pressure measurement in 1 mo.
(B) Obtain 24-hour ambulatory blood pressure record.
(C) Refer to a dietitian for dietary counseling.
(D) Recommend a regular exercise regimen.
(E) Begin hydrochlorothiazide.

ANSWER: B

This patient's blood pressure is increased during examination. Because he has no history of hypertension and no evidence of end-organ damage, anxiety related to the office visit (ie, "white-coat" hypertension) should be considered. Ambulatory blood pressure monitoring (ABPM) can be useful for assessing both hypertension and hypotension. According to guidelines from the *Joint National Committee on Prevention, Detection, Evaluation, and Treatment of High Blood Pressure (JNC7)*, ABPM is warranted for evaluation of white-coat hypertension, hypertension that is resistant to pharmacotherapy, hypotensive symptoms during treatment for hypertension, episodic hypertension, and autonomic dysfunction (SOE=A). ABPM is a better predictor of cardiovascular events than office-based blood pressure readings (SOE=B). In addition, it allows for nighttime measurement of blood pressure, which may be more predictive of mortality. Blood pressure should decrease at night by at least 10% ("nocturnal dipping"); patients who do not exhibit this decrease may have an increased risk of cardiovascular and renal disease.

The patient has already returned for repeat measurement; another visit is not likely to reveal new information (SOE=D). Because the patient already follows a low-sodium and low-fat diet, referral to a dietitian is unlikely to be helpful (SOE=D). While there are many benefits to prescribing exercise, ABPM is the next best step to confirm or refute the diagnosis of hypertension (SOE=D).

References

1. Hansen TW, Jeppesen J, Rasmussen S, et al. Ambulatory blood pressure and mortality: a population-based study. *Hypertension*. 2005;45(4):499–504.
2. Pickering TG, Shimbo D, Haas D. Ambulatory blood-pressure monitoring. *N Engl J Med*. 2006;354(22):2368–2374.
3. Staessen JA, Thijs L, Fagard R. Predicting cardiovascular risk using conventional vs ambulatory blood pressure in older patients with systolic hypertension. Systolic Hypertension in Europe Trial Investigators. *JAMA*. 1999;282(6):539–546.

189. A 72-yr-old man comes to the office for evaluation of dyspnea that has progressed slowly over 6 yr. He has COPD and has used albuterol as needed for 6 yr. He has a daily nonproductive cough and wheezes intermittently. He can no longer participate in activities such as golf. Six months ago he had an exacerbation of COPD requiring prednisone. He has never been hospitalized or gone to the emergency room. He quit smoking 3 mo ago.

On examination, temperature is 36°C (96.8°F), blood pressure is 145/85 mmHg, heart rate is 96 beats per minute, and respiratory rate is 22 breaths per minute. There is no accessory muscle use. Bibasilar crackles are audible, and exhalation is slightly prolonged. Cardiac examination is normal. There is trace ankle edema but no cyanosis or clubbing.

Oxygen saturation on room air is 93%. Chest radiography displays hyperinflated lungs.

Pulmonary function tests:

FVC	85% of predicted
FEV_1	60% of predicted
FEV_1/FVC ratio	60%

After treatment with a bronchodilator, FEV_1 increases by 11% and FVC increases by 10%.

In addition to continuing albuterol as needed, which of the following is the most appropriate treatment at this time?

(A) Albuterol q6h
(B) Ipratropium bromide q6h
(C) Albuterol/ipratropium bromide q6h
(D) Tiotropium q24h
(E) Inhaled corticosteroids q12h

ANSWER: D

Bronchodilator medications are central to the symptomatic management of COPD. Inhaled is preferred over oral administration because it has similar efficacy and fewer adverse events. Bronchodilators are given either as needed for relief of persistent or worsening symptoms, or on a regular basis to prevent or reduce symptoms. For patients with mild COPD, short-acting bronchodilators are recommended as needed (SOE=A). Choices include short-acting β_2-agonists such as albuterol, short-acting anticholinergic agents such as ipratropium bromide, or albuterol and ipratropium bromide combined as a single agent. For patients with symptomatic COPD that is of moderate severity or worse, regular treatment with a long-acting bronchodilator is recommended (SOE=A). Choices include the long-acting anticholinergic agent tiotropium and the long-acting β_2-agonists formoterol and salmeterol. Combining bronchodilators with different mechanisms and durations of action can increase the degree of bronchodilation with fewer adverse events than increasing the dosage of a single bronchodilator (SOE=A). Inhaled corticosteroids decrease exacerbations and improve health status. They are typically reserved for patients with severe COPD and repeated exacerbations (SOE=A). The combination of an inhaled corticosteroid with a long-acting bronchodilator is more effective than the individual components in reducing exacerbations, improving lung function and health status, and slowing decline in lung function (SOE=A).

This patient's FEV$_1$ (60% of predicted) indicates moderate COPD. Regular treatment with a long-acting bronchodilator such as tiotropium is recommended and preferred over the short-acting bronchodilators albuterol, ipratropium bromide, and combination albuterol/ipratropium bromide. Inhaled corticosteroids are reserved for patients with frequent exacerbations of severe COPD (SOE=A).

References

1. Celli BR, MacNee W; HTS/ERS Task Force. Standards for the diagnosis and treatment of patients with COPD: a summary of the ATS/ERS position paper. *Eur Respir J.* 2004;23(6):932–946.
2. Global Initiative for Chronic Obstructive Lung Disease. *Global Strategy for the Diagnosis, Management, and Prevention of Chronic Obstructive Pulmonary Disease—Updated 2007.* Bethesda, MD: National Institutes of Health, National Heart, Lung and Blood Institute; 2007. Available at: http://www.goldcopd.com (accessed Nov 2009).
3. Wilt TJ, Niewoehner D, MacDonald R, et al. Management of stable chronic obstructive pulmonary disease: a systematic review for a clinical practice guideline. *Ann Intern Med.* 2007;147(9):639–653.

190. A 90-yr-old resident of an assisted-living facility is evaluated because over the past 2 wks she has become withdrawn and no longer greets friends, her clothes and hair are now messy, and she no longer ambulates with confidence. She is independent in most IADLs. History includes dry macular degeneration diagnosed 10 yr earlier. She visited a vision rehabilitation center a few years ago and received devices and strategies to cope with her vision loss.

Physical findings are essentially unchanged from previous examinations. She is referred to an ophthalmologist.

Which of the following is most likely to be causing the changes in this patient?

(A) Branch retinal artery occlusion
(B) Acute angle-closure glaucoma
(C) Chronic open-angle glaucoma
(D) Progression of macular degeneration
(E) Vitreous hemorrhage

ANSWER: D

Progression of macular degeneration has caused a decline in this patient's visual acuity and affected her function. Very possibly she believes that nothing more can be done for her vision and she may be depressed. As macular degeneration progresses, patients often become withdrawn and quality of life deteriorates. It is important for patients and their families to recognize that dry macular degeneration can progress to wet macular degeneration. If there is any change in vision, the patient would benefit from seeing an ophthalmologist immediately for appropriate interventions (SOE=B).

Branch retinal artery occlusion is manifested by sudden loss of vision in one eye: a segment of the visual field is lost, sometimes involving central vision. Patients can be unaware at first, especially when vision in the unaffected eye is spared. Nonembolic causes, such as vasospasms and coagulopathies, can be responsible, but more frequently the cause is an embolism. Emboli are reported to be visible on funduscopic evaluation in 62% of cases. Most often the temporal vessels are involved, at the bifurcation of the vessel. Predisposing factors include atherosclerosis, coronary artery disease, hypertension, and dyslipidemia. Patients with central retinal artery occlusion who present with an acuity of 20/40 or better may be able to maintain good vision with early, aggressive treatment. Of patients presenting with visual acuity of 20/100 or worse, improvement to 20/40 or better is likely in only 14% (SOE=A).

Chronic open-angle glaucoma most often presents with slowly progressive peripheral visual field loss caused by optic nerve damage from chronic glaucoma. The loss is often asymmetric and rarely sudden. In the present case, the patient's change in behavior suggests a central loss more than a peripheral field loss.

Acute angle-closure glaucoma can be associated with corneal edema, halos around lights, blurred vision, redness of the eye, headache, eye pain, and sometimes nausea and vomiting. Intraocular pressure is high. Often the anterior chamber of the eye (the area between the cornea and iris lens plane) is shallow (SOE=A). Early intervention is needed to preserve vision. It is unlikely that symptoms of acute angle-closure glaucoma would go unnoticed for 2 wk, or that an affected individual would not seek help.

References

1. American Academy of Ophthalmology. *Primary Open-Angle Glaucoma, Preferred Practice Pattern.* San Francisco, CA: American Academy of Ophthalmology; 2005. Available at: www.aao.org/ppp (accessed Jul 2009).

2. Mason JO 3d, Shah AA, Vail RS, et al. Branch retinal artery occlusion: visual prognosis. *Am J Ophthalmol.* 2008;146(3):455–457.

3. Rosenberg EA, Sperazza LC. The visually impaired patient. *Am Fam Physician.* 2008;77(10):1431–1436.

4. Sahel JA, Bandello F, Augustin A, et al. for the MICMAC Study Group. Health-related quality of life and utility in patients with age-related macular degeneration. *Arch Ophthalmol.* 2007;125(7):945–951.

5. Wong T, Chakravarthy U, Klein R, et al. The natural history and prognosis of neovascular age-related macular degeneration: a systematic review of the literature and meta-analysis. *Ophthalmology.* 2008;115(1):116–126.

191. A 79-yr-old woman presents with a lump on the right upper quadrant of her left breast. Mammography reveals a 1.3-cm spiculated lesion. Biopsy reveals a high-grade, poorly differentiated, infiltrating ductal carcinoma of the breast, with negative margins and no evidence of lymphovascular invasion. She is concerned that breast conservation treatment (ie, lumpectomy or partial mastectomy) and postoperative radiotherapy would not be "as good as" a full mastectomy.

Which of the following statements is true?

(A) Breast conservation treatment is the standard of care for all patients with early disease.

(B) Breast conservation treatment is associated with the same quality of life as mastectomy.

(C) Overall survival and disease-free survival are worse for breast conservation treatment than mastectomy.

(D) Older patients are more likely to be offered breast conservation therapy than younger patients.

ANSWER: A

Breast conservation treatment consists of breast-conserving surgery (ie, lumpectomy or partial mastectomy) and postoperative radiotherapy. It is recommended as the standard of care for patients of all ages with early stage breast cancer and has been shown in large randomized trials to have efficacy similar to that of mastectomy (SOE=A). It has also been shown to be associated with a better quality of life than mastectomy in patients ≥70 yr old (SOE=A). Furthermore, most older women prefer breast conservation to mastectomy but are less likely to receive such treatment.

Many factors must be considered when deciding the optimal treatment regimen for older women, including estimated life expectancy, medical comorbidites, functional status, goals of care, and ability to travel to a radiation oncology facility.

References

1. de Haes JC, Curran D, Aaronson NK, et al. Quality of life in breast cancer patients aged over 70 years, participating in the EORTC 10850 randomised clinical trial. *Eur J Cancer.* 2003;39(7):945–951.

2. Giordano SH, Hortobagyi GN, Kau SW, et al. Breast cancer treatment guidelines in older women. *J Clin Oncol.* 2005;23(4):783–791.

3. Hurria A, Leung D, Trainor K, et al. Factors influencing treatment patterns of breast cancer patients age 75 and older. *Crit Rev Oncol Hematol.* 2003;46(2):121–126.

4. Wildiers H, Kunkler I, Biganzoli L, et al. Management of breast cancer in elderly individuals: recommendations of the International Society of Geriatric Oncology. *Lancet Oncol.* 2007;8(12):1101–1115.

192. Which of the following statements regarding treatment for major depressive disorder is true?

(A) Most older adults with the diagnosis are treated by a psychiatrist.

(B) In older adults on an effective dosage of antidepressants, the response rate is close to 80% after 8 wk.

(C) Risk of recurrence or relapse is higher in patients who did not reach full remission.

(D) Augmentation with a second agent is not appropriate after a partial response to one antidepressant.

(E) Psychosocial interventions have little impact on rate of remission or risk of recurrence.

ANSWER: C

The stigma associated with mental illness and the scarcity of psychiatrists in most rural areas are significant barriers to treatment of major depressive disorder. Most older adults with major depressive disorder present to their primary care doctor with multiple somatic symptoms, anxiety, poor sleep, or concerns about decline in cognitive performance. Because of the nonspecific nature of the symptoms, the inability of many patients to voice sadness, and the limited time available to primary care doctors to address multiple medical problems and medications, major depressive disorder is often overlooked. Patients are often treated with anxiolytic or sleep agents, and symptoms are likely to worsen. Even with correct diagnosis, patients are rarely referred to a psychiatrist. For patients without suicidal thoughts or psychosis, referral to a psychiatrist is often unnecessary;

second-generation antidepressant medications and nonpharmacologic interventions can be effectively prescribed by primary care doctors.

Often these medications are prescribed at inappropriately low dosages, or for too short a time. All antidepressant medications require a trial of 8 wk at full therapeutic dosage before their efficacy in a particular patient can be evaluated; the best evidence indicates that a significant percentage of nonresponders or partial responders will achieve remission if the trial is continued until week 12. However, even under the best conditions, the response rate is unlikely to exceed 60% (in many trials it can be as low as 40%, barely reaching statistical significance), particularly at 8 wk. In some trials, it approached 80% after ≥12 wk.

In many trials, a significant reduction in symptoms is considered as a response to treatment. However, partial response is associated with a high risk of relapse and recurrence (SOE=A). Full remission is a return to a fully euthymic mood with no residual symptoms. Remission is associated with a higher level of psychosocial function, significantly lower risk of relapse or recurrence, and overall improvement in quality of life indicators. Remission is rarely achieved with a single medication. Results of the STAR-D trial support the practice of switching interventions for patients in whom the initial agent failed, or dosage augmentation for patients who have a partial response to treatment (SOE=A). The morbidity and mortality associated with untreated major depressive disorder are significant, and most of the medications currently used as first- and second-line treatment are well tolerated, even in combination. Several studies provide evidence in support of psychosocial interventions to improve response to medications, improve functioning, and decrease risk of relapse or recurrence.

References

1. Nelson JC, Delucchi K, Schneider L. Efficacy of second generation antidepressants in late-life depression: a meta-analysis of the evidence. *Am J Geriatr Psychiatry*. 2008;16(7):558–567.
2. Reynolds CF, Dew MA, Pollock B, et al. Maintenance treatment of major depression in old age. *N Engl J Med*. 2006;354(11):1130–1138.
3. Trivedi MH, Rush AJ, Wisniewski SR, et al. Evaluation of outcome with citalopram for depression using measurement-based care in Star*D: implication for clinical practice. *Am J Psychiatry*. 2006;163(1):28–40.
4. Trivedi MH, Fava M, Wisniewski SR, et al; STAR*D Study Team. Medication augmentation after the failure of SSRI for depression. *N Engl J Med*. 2006;354(12):1243–1252.

193. An 80-yr-old woman comes to the office because she has been dizzy. When asked for specifics, she is vague, but states that she often feels unsteady when walking. She has also felt lightheaded a few times when getting up in the morning. She has had no falls. History includes hypertension, type 2 diabetes mellitus, dyslipidemia, and anxiety. Medications are hydrochlorothiazide, lisinopril, aspirin, metformin, simvastatin, and trazodone.

On examination, blood pressure is 125/82 mmHg and pulse is 80 beats per minute with no orthostatic changes. Her gait is slightly wide but otherwise normal. There is evidence of mild peripheral neuropathy. Her score on the Geriatric Depression Scale is 3/15.

Which of the following is the most likely cause of her dizziness?

(A) Anxiety
(B) Somatization disorder
(C) Medication adverse event
(D) Multifactorial triggers

ANSWER: D

Complaints of dizziness are often vague, and its diagnosis and treatment can be frustrating for both patients and practitioners. Dizziness in older adults may be thought of as a geriatric syndrome that is often caused by several underlying risk factors. In one study, 56% of older adults who described dizziness had multiple different sensations, and 74% had multiple different triggers. In many of these adults, no obvious, single diagnosis could be made. Characteristics associated with "dizziness syndrome" included anxiety, depressive symptoms, impaired hearing, use of 5 or more medications, postural hypotension, impaired balance, and past myocardial infarction. Authors of the study suggested that a strategy to reduce several factors might be an effective approach for many older adults with dizziness.

A multifactorial origin of dizziness is most likely in this patient, because her sensations of dizziness vary and have no obvious cause on physical examination. Although it would be reasonable to look at different interventions to address her dizziness, including adjusting antihypertensive medications and initiating physical therapy, there is no proof that such an approach improves outcome (SOE=C).

References

1. Tinetti ME, Williams CS, Gill TM. Dizziness among older adults: a possible geriatric syndrome. *Ann Intern Med.* 2000;132(5):337–344.
2. Drachman, DA. Occam's razor, geriatric syndromes, and the dizzy patient. *Ann Intern Med.* 2000;132(5):403–405.

194. A 92-yr-old woman has several stage I and II pressure ulcers on her buttocks and heels 1 wk after treatment for a urinary tract infection and dehydration. She lives in a nursing home and has advanced dementia.

Which of the following is the best tool for monitoring the healing of her pressure ulcers?

(A) Braden scale
(B) Bates-Jensen Wound Assessment Tool
(C) Norton scale
(D) Waterlow scale
(E) Cubbin-Jackson scale

ANSWER: B

The Bates-Jensen Wound Assessment Tool, also called the Pressure Sore Status Tool, is a validated instrument for assessing the healing of pressure ulcers (SOE=B). Developed in 1992 and revised in 2001, it assigns a numeric score for each of the following wound characteristics: size, depth, edges, undermining, necrotic tissue type, necrotic tissue amount, exudate type, exudate amount, surrounding skin color, peripheral tissue edema, peripheral tissue induration, granulation tissue, and epithelization. Location and shape of the wound are noted but not scored. The Bates-Jensen Wound Assessment Tool is not a risk-assessment tool; it is used once a pressure ulcer has developed. The pressure ulcer should be scored at baseline, and then at regular intervals to evaluate response to treatment. Another validated, but less time-consuming, tool for assessing healing is the Pressure Ulcer Scale for Healing (PUSH), which focuses on size of ulcer, amount of exudate, and tissue type.

The Braden, Norton, Waterlow, and Cubbin-Jackson scales are used to assess the risk of developing a pressure ulcer. The most widely used tools to assess the risk of developing a pressure ulcer are the Braden and Norton scales. The Braden scale is valid and

reliable and provides the best estimate of risk. It rates sensory perception, moisture, mobility, nutrition, friction, and shear. A score of ≤18 on the Braden scale indicates increased risk of development of pressure ulcers. The Norton risk scale assesses mental state, physical condition, activity, mobility, and incontinence. The Waterlow scale has high sensitivity but low specificity, resulting in unnecessary prevention measures. The Cubbin-Jackson scale for skin risk assessment has been used in 2 studies specifically designed for patients in intensive care units.

References

1. National Pressure Ulcer Advisory Panel. *PUSH Tool 3.0*, available free at http://www.npuap.org (accessed Nov 2009).
2. Pancorbo-Hidalgo P, Garcia-Fernandez F. Risk assessment scales for pressure ulcer prevention: a systematic review. *J Adv Nurs.* 2006;54(1):94–110.
3. Sussman C, Bates-Jensen B. *Wound Care: A Collaborative Practice Manual.* Gaithersburg, MD: Aspen Publications; 2007:157–158.

195. A previously active 75-yr-old man with benign prostatic hyperplasia undergoes transurethral resection of the prostate. He has no other chronic conditions and takes no medications. His hospitalization is prolonged because of several postoperative complications, and he is transferred to a rehabilitation unit to regain strength. On discharge to home, his walking speed is 0.4 m/sec. He notes that he feels exhausted most of the time.

For which of the following is he at increased risk in the next year?

(A) Death
(B) New diagnosis of cancer
(C) Permanent placement in nursing home
(D) Recurrence of symptoms from benign prostatic hyperplasia
(E) Parkinson's disease

ANSWER: A

While this previously active and healthy man did not show signs of clinical frailty before hospitalization, he has decreased physical reserves (eg, slow gait, exhaustion) after an acute stressor, hospitalization for transurethral resection of the prostate. Frailty places him at risk of poor outcomes: increased mortality, decreased function, falls, and hospitalization. Poor health outcomes in individuals with frailty have been demonstrated in population studies from the Cardiovascular Health Study and the Women's Health and Aging Studies (SOE=A).

Frailty has not been associated with subsequent development of specific diseases or nursing-home placement.

References

1. Bandeen-Roche K, Xue QL, Ferrucci L, et al. Phenotype of frailty: characterization in the women's health and aging studies. *J Gerontol A Biol Sci Med Sci*. 2006;61(3):262–266.
2. Fried LP, Tangen CM, Walston J, et al. Frailty in older adults: evidence for a phenotype. *J Gerontol A Biol Sci Med Sci*. 2001;56(3):M146–156.

196. A 78-yr-old man comes to the office because he has fatigue and weakness that have progressed over the past 6 mo. He is an avid golfer but is now unable to complete his usual round of golf. History includes dyslipidemia and gouty arthritis well controlled for 10 yr. Medications include atorvastatin, colchicine, and allopurinol.

On examination, there is hyperpigmentation over his face and neck, but no rash. He has weakness of the neck flexors, and he cannot rise from a chair without using his arms. Reflexes are diminished in both legs.

Which of the following will most likely yield the correct diagnosis?

(A) Electromyography and nerve conduction studies
(B) MRI using a fat-suppression sequence
(C) Sural nerve biopsy
(D) Muscle biopsy using a percutaneous needle
(E) Open muscle biopsy

ANSWER: E

Generalized muscle weakness that is most prominent in the proximal muscle groups, in addition to fatigue, suggests that this patient has myositis (inflammatory muscle disease). Open muscle biopsy remains the gold standard for differentiating myositis from drug-induced and other myopathies, dermatomyositis, polymyositis, and inclusion-body myositis (SOE=C).

Initial diagnostic efforts should focus on excluding conditions that can result in muscle weakness. The list of potentially myotoxic medications is lengthy. Statins can have effects ranging from asymptomatic increase in creatine phosphokinase to painful myopathy to rhabdomyolysis. Colchicine can cause myopathy as well as peripheral neuropathy. Metabolic diseases (eg, hypothyroidism, vitamin D deficiency) should also be excluded.

Electrodiagnostic testing will exclude neuropathy but will not distinguish inclusion-body myositis from drug-induced myopathies that exhibit overlying neuropathy. Needle insertion for electromyography can cause tissue damage that may influence muscle morphology and complicate interpretation. MRI using fat-suppression sequences can demonstrate inflammation and may be useful in selecting which muscle to biopsy but does not provide a definitive diagnosis. Sural nerve biopsy is most useful in the evaluation of mononeuritis multiplex due to suspected vasculitis, but it is not useful in evaluating cases of myositis or myopathy without nerve involvement. Percutaneous needle biopsy does not permit accurate assessment of muscle morphology.

References

1. Ahn SC. Neuromuscular complications of statins. *Phys Med Rehabil Clin N Am*. 2008;19(1):47–59.
2. Greenberg SA. Inflammatory myopathies: evaluation and management. *Semin Neurol*. 2008;28(2):241–249.
3. Jackson CE. A clinical approach to muscle diseases. *Semin Neurol*. 2008;28(2):228–240.
4. Tiwari A, Bansal V, Chugh A, et al. Statins and myotoxicity: a therapeutic limitation. *Expert Opin Drug Saf*. 2006;5(5):651–666.

197. An 85-yr-old man with Alzheimer's disease who lives in a nursing facility has become minimally reactive over the past year to his family's efforts to engage him in conversation. Nursing staff report that he seems sad at times, rarely initiates conversation, and is occasionally suspicious of other residents and staff. The occupational therapist is no longer able to engage him in therapy. Appetite, weight, and sleep are unchanged.

Physical and laboratory evaluations do not identify new medical problems.

Which of the following is the most likely explanation for this patient's behavior?

(A) Apathy
(B) Psychosis
(C) Major depressive disorder
(D) Frontal lobe syndrome

ANSWER: A

The most common neuropsychiatric symptom in patients with dementia is dysregulation of mood, which encompasses both depressive symptoms and apathy (SOE=A). Apathy is the only behavioral symptom that has been shown to affect both ADLs and IADLs, beyond the level of cognitive impairment. There is little evidence to support use of a specific agent to treat dementia-related apathy.

Depressive symptoms, seen in up to 50% of patients with dementia, can be differentiated from apathy by the presence of sad mood and psychic distress. There does not seem to be a direct relationship between presence of major depressive disorder and severity of dementia. Major depressive disorder is often unrecognized in patients with dementia, but it may be responsive to psychotropic intervention.

Psychosis in dementia is usually manifested by delusions and hallucinations. Frequently, delusions include beliefs that others are stealing the patient's (misplaced) belongings, and paranoid ideation with persecutory themes, such as food being poisoned or spousal infidelity.

Disinhibition, indifference to the impact of one's behavior on others, and coarsening of personality out of proportion to the extent of memory impairment are manifestations of frontotemporal dementia or injury to the frontal lobes. These behaviors can also be seen in vascular dementia or in Alzheimer's disease, as Alzheimer's progresses in the brain from the temporal and parietal areas to the frontal cortex. However, the irritability, sadness, and paucity of interaction described in this case are more compatible with the apathy of advanced Alzheimer's disease than with a frontal lobe syndrome.

There appears to be a cumulative increase in the incidence of psychotic symptoms with disease progression: in patients with Alzheimer's disease, prevalence of psychoses is 20% at year 1 and 51% by year 4 (SOE=B). Psychotropic and environmental strategies can help reduce psychotic symptoms.

Verbal aggression (screaming, cursing) is common. Disruptive vocalizations, especially those with affective themes or sounds, have been associated with occult depression. Physical aggression (eg, hitting, biting, scratching, grabbing) is typically more evident among male patients, younger patients, and depressed or psychotic patients. Aggression is common during patient care activities, especially toileting and bathing. Adjusting the environment is usually the first-line intervention for mild cases; psychopharmacologic management is reserved for more severe or persistent cases. Antipsychotic agents may be more effective in treating aggression than other behavioral or psychotic symptoms in dementia.

Aberrant motor behaviors in patients with dementia include wandering, pacing, banging, and rummaging. Typically, psychotropic medication does not ameliorate—and can even aggravate—motor behavior, but environmental strategies may be effective. Federal nursing home legislation prohibits prescription of antipsychotic agents for wandering and related behaviors.

Often the behavioral disturbances described above do not occur in isolation; >50% of patients exhibit more than two behavioral disturbances. There are symptom clusters: for example, dementia patients with paranoid delusions are most likely to show higher levels of agitation, wandering, and angry or hostile outbursts. Age and gender are associated with different symptoms as well. For example, older men are more likely to demonstrate psychosis and aggression than women or younger men. Older women are most likely to demonstrate delusions. In general, the presence of behavioral problems is associated with faster progression of dementia and more rapid mortality.

References

1. Lyketsos CG, Lopez O, Jones B, et al. Prevalence of neuropsychiatric symptoms in dementia and mild cognitive impairment: results from the cardiovascular health study. *JAMA.* 2002;288(12):1475–1483.
2. Onor ML, Saina M, Trevisioi M, et al. Clinical experience with risperidone in the treatment of behavioral and psychological symptoms of dementia. *Prog Neuropsychopharmacol Biol Psychiatry.* 2007;31(1):205–209.
3. Paulsen JS, Salmon DP, Thal LJ, et al. Incidence and risk factors for hallucinations and delusions in patients with probable AD. *Neurology.* 2000;54(10):1965–1971.
4. Steinberg M, Shao H, Zandi P, et al. Point and 5-year period prevalence of neuropsychiatric symptoms in dementia: the Cache County Study. *Int J Geriatr Psychiatry.* 2008;23(2):170–177.

198. An 82-yr-old man comes to the office for preoperative evaluation before elective hip replacement. He cannot walk 2 blocks without incapacitating hip pain. He has no chest pain or dyspnea, and there is no history of myocardial infarction, stroke, or diabetes mellitus. He has hypertension and dyslipidemia. Medications are atenolol 50 mg/d and lovastatin 20 mg/d.

On physical examination, blood pressure is 140/70 mmHg and heart rate is 76 beats per minute and regular. On auscultation, chest and lungs are clear; there is a 2/6 systolic ejection murmur, and there is no third or fourth heart sound. There is no edema, and pulses are intact. ECG shows normal sinus rhythm with left ventricular hypertrophy.

Which of the following is indicated as part of his preoperative evaluation?

(A) Stress echocardiography
(B) Nuclear stress test
(C) Coronary angiography
(D) Measurement of creatinine
(E) Measurement of brain natriuretic peptide

ANSWER: D

This patient has poor functional capacity (<4 metabolic equivalents) and is scheduled for elective noncardiac surgery. The need for additional preoperative testing is based on the number of clinical risk factors and the type of surgery planned. In patients with no clinical risk factors, no additional testing is required. In patients with 1 or 2 clinical risk factors and controlled heart rate, cardiac stress testing is at the discretion of the physician. In patients with ≥3 clinical risk factors, stress testing is recommended before vascular surgery and is optional before intermediate-risk surgery (SOE=B).

According to the Revised Cardiac Risk Index, clinical risk factors include a history of ischemic heart disease, heart failure, cerebrovascular disease (ie, history of transient ischemic attack or stroke), diabetes mellitus, and renal insufficiency (preoperative serum creatinine >2 mg/dL). This patient's creatinine concentration must be obtained to calculate his risk factor score. If the concentration is <2 mg/dL, his score would be 0 because he has no other clinical risk factors. Therefore, no cardiac evaluation would be indicated. If his creatinine concentration is >2 mg/dL, his score would be 1 and further cardiac noninvasive evaluation would be optional. He

is on a β-blocker and his heart rate is controlled. His β-blocker should be continued perioperatively. Any patient on a β-blocker preoperatively should be continued on β-blockers in the perioperative period (SOE=A).

Measurement of brain natriuretic peptide would not be useful in this patient with no signs or symptoms of heart failure.

Reference

1. Fleisher LA, Beckman JA, Brown KA, et al. ACC/AHA 2007 guidelines on perioperative cardio-vascular evaluation and care for noncardiac surgery: a report of the American College of Cardiology/ American Heart Association Task Force on Practice Guidelines (Writing Committee to Revise the 2002 Guidelines on Perioperative Cardiovascular Evaluation for Noncardiac Surgery). *J Am Coll Cardiol.* 2007;50(17):e159–241.

199. A 75-yr-old woman comes to the office because she has had repeated episodes of profound dizziness and syncope, along with at least 2 episodes in which she found herself on the floor but was unaware of how she fell. Each episode has been preceded by a prodrome during which she feels warm and is diaphoretic and progressively lightheaded. The episodes are most likely to occur when she has been standing for a long time, such as during church services. History includes hypertension, for which she takes hydrochlorothiazide daily.

On physical examination, blood pressure is 142/84 mmHg while supine and 110/70 mmHg while upright; heart rate is 76 beats per minute while supine and 80 beats per minute while upright. There is no jugular venous distension or carotid bruit. Lungs are clear. Carotid upstroke is normal with a II/VI systolic murmur at the base; the second heart sound is intact, and there is no gallop.

Which of the following is the most appropriate next step?

(A) Stop hydrochlorothiazide.
(B) Begin oral midodrine 5 mg three times daily (about 4 hours apart, not too close to bedtime).
(C) Begin fludrocortisone 0.1 mg q12h.
(D) Obtain tilt-table test.

ANSWER: A

Physical examination of this patient reveals orthostatic hypotension, an important cause of syncope in older adults. When a standing position is assumed, gravity induces pooling of blood in the lower extremities. Blood pressure is normally maintained by vasoconstriction and increased heart rate when circulatory volume is decreased. The incidence and prevalence of orthostatic hypotension in older adults are affected by numerous age-related changes in cardiovascular structure and function, such as impaired baroreflex function, diastolic dysfunction, higher prevalence of disorders that directly or indirectly impair autonomic function, common use of vasoactive medications, and impaired salt and water balance.

The most commonly accepted definition of orthostatic hypotension is a decrease of >20 mmHg in systolic blood pressure or >10 mmHg in diastolic blood pressure on standing. In most patients with orthostatic hypotension, the drop in blood pressure is detected within 2 min of assuming an upright posture. Some patients, however, have delayed orthostatic intolerance, and blood pressure falls progressively over 15–45 min. This dysautonomic response to upright posture can be detected during a tilt-table test. In this particular patient, the diagnosis of orthostatic hypotension is apparent on physical examination, which eliminates the need for the tilt-table test.

Initial treatments for orthostatic hypotension include withdrawal of potentially exacerbating medications; accordingly, stopping hydrochlorothiazide is the best option in this patient (SOE=B). If necessary, physiologic interventions should be introduced next (eg, compressive devices such as stockings or abdominal bands, counterpressure maneuvers like squatting or leg crossing). Pharmacologic therapy (eg, fludrocortisone and midodrine) should be used only if other measures fail. Patients should be 1) reassured that the problem can be controlled; 2) taught to avoid predisposing factors and triggering events, such as volume depletion and prolonged upright posture; and 3) taught maneuvers to abort an episode of orthostasis. In older adults, supine hypertension can coexist with and be exacerbated by treatment of orthostatic hypotension. Some degree of supine hypertension may have to be tolerated to minimize the short-term risk of orthostasis and associated falls.

References

1. Gupta V, Lipsitz LA. Orthostatic hypotension in the elderly: diagnosis and treatment. *Am J Med.* 2007;120(10):841–847.
2. Henry R, Rowe J, O'Mahony D. Haemodynamic analysis of efficacy of compression hosiery in elderly fallers with orthostatic hypotension. *Lancet.* 1999;354(9172):45–46.
3. Podoleanu C, Maggi R, Brignole M, et al. Lower limb and abdominal compression bandages prevent progressive orthostatic hypotension in elderly persons: a randomized single-blind controlled study. *J Am Coll Cardiol.* 2006;48(7):1425–1432.

200. An 80-yr-old woman comes to the office because she recently has had difficulty eating and swallowing solid food. She notes that when she prepares to swallow, the food scrapes her cheeks and the roof of her mouth. History includes hypertension, diabetes mellitus, kidney stones, and major depressive disorder. Medications include hydrochlorothiazide, metformin, and fluoxetine. For the first time in many years, a recent dental examination revealed several cavities, which were located at the roots of the teeth.

Which of the following is the most likely explanation for these oral problems?

(A) Usual aging
(B) Salivary ductal stones
(C) Adverse effect of metformin
(D) Adverse effect of hydrochlorothiazide and fluoxetine
(E) Immune dysfunction

ANSWER: D

This patient's difficulty eating and swallowing solid foods in the context of new dental cavities is most consistent with xerostomia, or decreased saliva. Saliva has several functions: it is a protective cleanser with antibacterial activity, a buffer that inhibits demineralization, a lubricant, and a transport medium to taste sensors. These functions are seriously altered in xerostomia. Signs and symptoms of xerostomia include oral dryness or burning, changes in tongue surface or taste, dysphasia, cheilosis, difficulty with speech, and development of root caries. Many conditions and treatments contribute to xerostomia, such as radiation or chemotherapy; psychologic, endocrine, and nutritional disorders; and adverse effect of medication (>200 commonly used medications can cause xerostomia). Antihypertensive medications (especially diuretics) and antidepressants (especially first-generation SSRIs) reduce saliva flow. Metformin is not known to decrease salivary flow. Immune diseases, such as Sjögren syndrome, and diabetes can increase cavities but are not likely to produce xerostomia.

While older adults are likely to have a decreased amount of active glandular tissue, salivary flow does not decrease significantly with age. The causes of salivary stones (sialoliths) are largely unknown; theories include autoimmune and inflammatory causes. Kidney stones are unrelated to salivary stones. Salivary stones do not usually cause xerostomia; they usually affect only one gland (commonly the submandibular gland) on only one side, so saliva is still present in the other major and minor salivary glands.

Treatment for patients with xerostomia includes scrupulous oral hygiene with a soft toothbrush, fluoride rinses, reduced alcohol consumption, frequent intake of water, saliva substitutes, and avoidance of highly acidic foods (SOE=B).

References

1. Masters KJ. Pilocarpine treatment of xerostomia induced by psychoactive medications. *Am J Psychiatry*. 2005;162(5):1023.
2. Moore PA, Guggenheimer J. Medication-induced hyposalivation: etiology, diagnosis, and treatment. *Compend Contin Educ Dent*. 2008;29(1):50–55.
3. Murray Thomson W, Chalmers JM, John Spencer A, et al. A longitudinal study of medication exposure and xerostomia among older people. *Gerodontology*. 2006;23(4):205–213.

201. An 86-yr-old nursing-home resident is discharged to a medical floor after 2 days in the intensive care unit, to which she had been admitted because of progressive respiratory distress. While in the intensive care unit, she pulled out her intravenous lines, removed oxygen tubing, and was violent with staff. Her behavior improved after she received as-needed doses of risperidone, and risperidone 0.5 mg q12h was begun. History includes COPD, diastolic heart failure, mild dementia, transient ischemic attacks, type 2 diabetes mellitus, and hypertension.

Which of the following is the best approach with regard to this patient's antipsychotic medication?

(A) Continue risperidone indefinitely.
(B) Taper risperidone.
(C) Discontinue risperidone and begin lorazepam.
(D) Discontinue risperidone and begin haloperidol.
(E) Discontinue risperidone and use restraints as needed.

ANSWER: B

The patient demonstrated signs of delirium in the intensive care unit. In this setting, the use of antipsychotic agents to control agitation and violent behavior is appropriate, because the healthcare staff is at risk of harm and the patient's behavior is interfering with lifesaving interventions (SOE=C). However, because this patient did not require risperidone before hospitalization, it should be tapered gradually over the next few days, and she likely can be discharged without antipsychotics (SOE=B). If the patient is discharged on an antipsychotic agent, it may be continued indefinitely, with potential for unnecessary adverse events.

Lorazepam is associated with higher mortality among critically ill patients with delirium than antipsychotic agents (SOE=B). It can be useful for agitated patients who do not respond to antipsychotic agents and need sedation to allow lifesaving interventions. Benzodiazepines are indicated for specific conditions such as alcohol- or GABA-withdrawal delirium, or delirium related to seizures (SOE=C).

Haloperidol is often used in critically ill patients with respiratory distress, because it has less impact on respiratory drive than do benzodiazepines. However, because the patient has responded well to risperidone, it is not prudent to change medications at this stage. Using restraints may not only exacerbate this patient's delirium but can also precipitate respiratory distress.

References

1. Ely EW, Stephens RK, Jackson JC, et al. Current opinions regarding the importance, diagnosis, and management of delirium in the intensive care unit: a survey of 912 healthcare professionals. *Crit Care Med*. 2004;32:106–112.
2. Jacobi J, Fraser GL, Coursin DB, et al. Clinical practice guidelines for the sustained use of sedatives and analgesics in the critically ill adult. *Crit Care Med*. 2002;30(1):119–141.
3. Pandharipande P, Ely EW. Sedative and analgesic medications: risk factors for delirium and sleep disturbances in the critically ill. *Crit Care Clin*. 2006;22(2):313–327.

202. In a community hospital in a large urban area, the rate of delirium for patients on the orthopedic service is higher than the rate for similar patients at other hospitals in the city. The hospital decides to implement a delirium reduction program based on the Hospital Elder Life Program (HELP) and published trials.

Based on previously published data, a delirium reduction program is most likely to be successful if it targets which of the following risk factors?

(A) Polypharmacy, cognitive impairment, hearing or vision impairment, diabetes mellitus, and previous history of postoperative delirium
(B) Inattention, polypharmacy, constipation, immobility, and hearing or vision impairment
(C) Cognitive impairment, sleep deprivation, immobility, vision or hearing impairment, and dehydration
(D) Cognitive impairment, polypharmacy, constipation, pressure ulcers, urinary incontinence, and orthostatic hypotension

ANSWER: C

A clinical trial published in 1999 demonstrated that a multicomponent delirium reduction program (The Hospital Elder Life Program) could significantly reduce the incidence and severity of delirium among hospitalized older adults (SOE=A). The original program instituted protocols that targeted the following conditions: cognitive impairment, sleep deprivation, immobility, vision or hearing impairment, and dehydration. Although polypharmacy, previous postoperative delirium, diabetes mellitus, constipation, pressure ulcers, urinary incontinence, and orthostatic hypotension are common among frail hospitalized older adults and can be associated with delirium, they were not identified specifically as factors that could be modified to reduce delirium.

Inattention is a cardinal feature of delirium, but not a risk factor for delirium. However, screening patients for delirium with a tool such as the Confusion Assessment Method, which includes inattention as a key element, is important when implementing a quality-improvement intervention to recognize and reduce delirium.

References
1. Bradley EH, Webster TR, Baker D, et al. After adoption: sustaining the innovation. A case study of disseminating the Hospital Elder Life Program. *J Am Geriatr Soc.* 2005;53(9):1455–1461.
2. Inouye SK, Baker DI, Fugal P, et al. Dissemination of the Hospital Elder Life Program: implementation, adaptation, and successes. *J Am Geriatr Soc.* 2006;54(10):1492–1499.
3. Inouye SK, Bogardus ST, Charpentier PA, et al. A multicomponent intervention to prevent delirium in hospitalized older patients. *N Engl J Med.* 1999;340(9):669–676.

203. An 84-yr-old nursing home resident with progressive Alzheimer's disease is evaluated because he displays aggressive sexual behavior. His behavior has deteriorated over the past month; he now grabs female staff and patients and displays his genitals. Most recently he was found trying to get into bed with a female resident. Despite positive behavioral efforts and staff training for consistency in approach, his aggressive behavior continues. He was discharged from two other residential facilities for comparable behavior. Medical history is not contributory. Treatment with risperidone 0.5 mg q12h has helped his agitation and combativeness, but not his sexual acting out.

Which of the following is the most appropriate next step for treating this patient?

(A) Prescribe a dopaminergic agonist.
(B) Prescribe an SSRI.
(C) Prescribe medroxyprogesterone acetate.
(D) Prescribe a benzodiazepine.

ANSWER: C

Dementia is usually associated with reduced sexual drive, but increased libido can occur. The incidence of sexually inappropriate behavior in Alzheimer's disease ranges from 2% to 25% and may be influenced by disease severity. The greatest concern regards resident and staff safety. If behavioral interventions have not succeeded and constant supervision is not possible, hormonal intervention (medroxyprogesterone acetate, estrogen, antiandrogens, or gonadotropin-releasing hormone agonists) aimed at reducing testosterone or raising estrogen should be considered. Although this is not approved for this purpose by the FDA, such an approach is the most successful alternative at present for reducing inappropriate sexual behavior (SOE=C).

Use of dopaminergic agents is associated with increase in libido (SOE=C). If a patient is taking a dopaminergic agent, the medication should be switched to a different class of agents if possible. Benzodiazepine therapy alters sexual drive, but it is not the first choice because it is associated with worsening cognitive function and falls in older adults.

If this were of more recent onset, assessment for potential delirium would be appropriate. Transfer to another facility is not in the best interests of the patient and has not solved the problem in the past.

SSRI treatment is associated with loss of libido and erectile dysfunction but is not the first choice for disinhibited sexual behavior resulting from dementia.

References

1. Dhikav V, Anand K, Aggarwal N. Grossly disinhibited sexual behavior in dementia of Alzheimer's type. *Arch Sex Behav.* 2007;36(2):133–134.
2. Stewart JT. Optimizing antilibidinal treatment with medroxyprogesterone acetate. *J Am Geriatr Med.* 2005;53(2):359–360.
3. Zeiss AM, Davies HD, Tinklenberg JR. An observational study of sexual behavior in demented male patients. *J Gerontol A Biol Sci Med Sci.* 1996;51(6):M325–M329.

204. An 85-yr-old man comes to the office to discuss the recurrence of anxiety attacks, of which he has a chronic history. He describes periods of intense fear and anxiety that last from 30 min to several hours and that are accompanied by physical and autonomic symptoms. He does not drink, has no history of alcohol or drug abuse, and has no other psychiatric issues. History includes hypertension, osteoarthritis, and urinary retention related to prostatic hyperplasia. He was diagnosed with panic disorder as an adult and took diazepam for the panic attacks, although not for the past 20 yr. He is interested in restarting treatment with diazepam.

Physical examination and laboratory evaluation (thyrotropin, CBC, metabolic profile) indicate nothing likely to cause new-onset panic attacks.

Which of the following is the most appropriate treatment?

(A) Benzodiazepines plus an SSRI
(B) Benzodiazepines plus cognitive-behavioral therapy
(C) An SSRI plus cognitive-behavioral therapy
(D) Benzodiazepines plus nortriptyline
(E) Mirtazapine plus an SSRI

ANSWER: C

In at least one large-scale epidemiologic study, panic disorder was identified in about 1% of community-dwelling older adults. Classic panic disorder (ie, frequent, unexplained panic attacks with marked fear and autonomic symptoms) with first onset in late life appears to be rare. However, panic-like symptoms are common in late life, particularly in the context of cardiac or respiratory illness or Parkinson's disease. In addition, because panic disorder, like other anxiety disorders, tends to be chronic and relapsing, its recurrence or persistence in old age is unsurprising (SOE=B).

Benzodiazepines are among the most commonly prescribed medications in older adults. They are effective for anxiety symptoms, including panic attacks. The risk of dependence with these medications tends to be low in older adults, particularly if there is no history of alcohol or drug dependence. However, older adults are more likely to suffer falls, fall-related injury, delirium, and cognitive impairment when taking benzodiazepines, and chronic use can accelerate cognitive decline (SOE=B). Thus, benzodiazepines are not first-line treatment in anxiety disorders in older adults. Better options for this patient include a third-generation antidepressant (eg, SSRI or serotonin-norepinephrine–reuptake inhibitor) and cognitive-behavioral therapy. When beginning treatment with antidepressants, adjunctive treatment with benzodiazepines may be considered until therapeutic levels of the antidepressant are reached, as long as the trial is brief and the patient is aware of the risks (SOE=C).

References

1. Wetherell JL, Lenze EJ, Stanley MA. Evidence-based treatment of geriatric anxiety disorders. *Psychiatr Clin North Am.* 2005;28(4):871–896, ix.
2. Wu CS, Wang SC, Chang IS, et al. The association between dementia and long-term use of benzodiazepine in the elderly: nested case-control study using claims data. *Am J Geriatr Psychiatry.* 2009;17(7):614–620.

205. A 76-yr-old woman returns to the clinic for evaluation 1 mo after beginning treatment for stress incontinence. In accordance with the patient's preference, initial therapy comprised insertion of an estradiol vaginal ring and pelvic floor muscle exercises that were taught during pelvic examination and reinforced by an instruction booklet. Her symptoms are mostly unchanged, and she remains bothered by leakage with physical activity. History includes systolic hypertension, for which she is treated with hydrochlorothiazide.

Which of the following is the most appropriate next step?

(A) Remove the estradiol vaginal ring and begin oral estrogen therapy.
(B) Refer for biofeedback-assisted training of pelvic floor muscle.
(C) Refer for periurethral collagen injections.
(D) Begin pseudoephedrine 30 mg q8h.
(E) Begin oxybutynin 5 mg q8h.

ANSWER: B

The most appropriate next step in treating this patient would be biofeedback-assisted pelvic muscle training (SOE=C). Although some healthy, motivated older women can master pelvic muscle exercises taught during pelvic examination with reinforcement from educational materials, many benefit from biofeedback to assist in identifying the correct muscles and contracting them without simultaneously increasing abdominal pressure (SOE= C).

Oral estrogen replacement is associated with increased rates of urinary incontinence for previously continent women and worsening symptoms among women who are already incontinent (SOE=A). Referral to a surgeon is probably best reserved for older women who do not benefit from a trial of biofeedback-assisted training and who express a preference for surgical intervention (SOE=C). Pseudoephedrine can be helpful in some older women with stress incontinence, but hypertension is a relative contraindication to treatment (SOE=A). Duloxetine, a serotonin-norepinephrine–reuptake inhibitor, can improve quality of life in women with stress incontinence (SOE=A), but nausea and other adverse events are common. It is not currently approved for treatment of urinary incontinence in the United States. Oxybutynin is useful in urge urinary incontinence, not in stress incontinence; additionally, the oxybutynin option has too high a starting dosage (SOE=A).

References

1. Blackwell RE. Estrogen, progestin, and urinary incontinence. *JAMA*. 2005;294(21):2696–2697.
2. Burgio KL, Goode PS, Locher JL, et al. Behavioral training with and without biofeedback in the treatment of urge incontinence in older women: a randomized controlled trial. *JAMA*. 2002;288(18):2293–2299.
3. Rogers RG. Clinical practice: urinary stress incontinence in women. *N Engl J Med*. 2008;358(10):1029–1036.

206. What is the estimated lifetime prevalence of behavioral disturbance among adults with dementia?

(A) 20%–40%
(B) 40%–60%
(C) 60%–80%
(D) 80%–100%

ANSWER: D

Behavioral disturbances associated with dementia can be symptomatic of mood abnormalities, such as depression, anxiety, and apathy; agitation, as displayed by verbal and physical aggression; and psychoses, such as delusions and hallucinations. Other associated behaviors include wandering, pacing, rummaging, and disinhibition. The disturbances lead to greater functional impairment and cognitive decline, and increase caregiver burden and stress; they are a major reason for acute hospitalizations and long-term institutional placement. Early detection of behavioral disturbances and intervention can improve quality of life for patients and their caregivers.

Estimates of lifetime prevalence of behavioral disturbance among patients with dementia approach 100% (SOE=A). Most population-based epidemiologic studies agree that disturbances increase in frequency over the course of the illness. Although some appear to peak at different stages of dementia, for the most part they are especially prominent among patients with moderate or severe dementia. Over 50% of patients with dementia exhibit more than 2 types of behavioral disturbances. Nursing homes report up to a 75% prevalence of behavioral disturbances among their residents. Premorbid personality disorders may be related to a higher prevalence of later behavioral problems.

The reported population-based prevalence of behavioral disturbances in dementia patients varies widely, in part reflecting the type and location of the study (eg, longitudinal versus cross-sectional, community surveys versus data from clinics or nursing homes). Moreover, identification of symptoms and rating of severity in part depend on the reliability of the rating scale and the rater.

References
1. Cummings JL, Mackell J, Kaufer D. Behavioral effects of current Alzheimer's disease treatments: a descriptive review. *Alzheimers Dement.* 2008;4(1):49–60.
2. Lyketsos CG, Lopez O, Jones B, et al. Prevalence of neuropsychiatric symptoms in dementia and mild cognitive impairment: results from the cardiovascular health study. *JAMA.* 2002;288(12):1475–1483.
3. Sink KM, Holden KF, Yaffe K. Pharmacological treatment of neuropsychiatric symptoms of dementia: a review of the evidence. *JAMA.* 2005;293(5):596–608.
4. Steinberg M, Shao H, Zandi P, et al. Point and 5-year period prevalence of neuropsychiatric symptoms in dementia: the Cache County Study. *Int J Geriatr Psychiatry.* 2008;23(2):170–177.

207. An 80-yr-old woman who resides in a nursing facility is admitted to the hospital for fever. She is known to be colonized with methicillin-resistant *Staphyloccus aureus* (MRSA). The likely source of fever is a stage IV sacral decubitus ulcer (5 cm × 7 cm) with undermined tissue and erythema. The emergency room physicians obtained blood and urine cultures and swabbed the decubitus ulcer for culture, stating they could readily "probe to bone." She was treated empirically with vancomycin and piperacillin-tazobactam. Three days later she has defervesced, and her WBC count has dropped from 19,500 to 14,000/μL. The wound is less erythematous, and there is little drainage. Blood and urine cultures are negative. Culture of the ulcer is growing *Escherichia coli* susceptible to ceftriaxone and ciprofloxacin, and vancomycin-resistant enterococci susceptible to linezolid and daptomycin. CT of the back demonstrates erosion of the sacrum consistent with osteomyelitis.

What is the most appropriate next step in management?

(A) Continue the present antibiotics for 6 wk
(B) Request surgical consultation for bone biopsy and culture
(C) Change antibiotics to ceftriaxone plus linezolid for 6 wk
(D) Add ceftriaxone and linezolid to current regimen and continue for 6 wk
(E) Surgical consultation for bone debridement and flap closure.

ANSWER: B

Swab cultures have been shown to be of no value in determining the etiology of infection in the bone or even soft tissues underlying the ulcer (SOE=C). The appropriate course of therapy for osteomyelitis is 6 wk of antibiotics that are typically administered intravenously (although some data exist for oral ciprofloxacin). Any time such a prolonged antibiotic course is considered, particularly in older adults in whom complications are likely, therapy should be based on bone biopsy, which is well tolerated and can be obtained either surgically or via radiology-guided procedure through uninvolved skin (SOE=C). In this particular case, it is not at all certain that either the *E coli* or the vancomycin-resistant enterococci are even in the bone. Statistically, *S aureus*, including MRSA because this patient is known to be colonized, are most likely when swab cultures do not demonstrate the organism. Thus, surgical debridement and culture is the best choice in this patient (SOE=D). Primary closure is contraindicated in the presence of osteomyelitis.

References
1. Anderson DJ, Kaye KS. Skin and soft tissue infections in older adults. *Clin Geriatr Med.* 2007;23(3):595–613.
2. Wound, Ostomy, and Continence Nurses Society (WOCN). *Guideline for Prevention and Management of Pressure Ulcers.* Glenview, IL: Wound, Ostomy, and Continence Nurses Society (WOCN); 2003.

208. A 69-yr-old woman with a history of deep venous thrombosis of her right leg presents after diagnosis and surgical resection of estrogen and progesterone receptor-positive early stage breast cancer. She has been provided with a balanced discussion of the risks and benefits of adjuvant therapy in the setting of early stage breast cancer. Her most recent dual x-ray absorptiometry (DEXA) results revealed no evidence of osteopenia.

Which of the following therapies is the best option for adjuvant therapy to reduce risk of recurrence and increase survival?

(A) Chemotherapy
(B) Tamoxifen
(C) Raloxifene
(D) Aromatase inhibitor therapy

ANSWER: D

While the use of 5 yr of adjuvant tamoxifen is well known to significantly decrease tumor recurrence and mortality in women with hormone-receptor–positive breast cancer, both with or without chemotherapy, the prevalence of breast cancer recurrence at 15 yr remains high at 30% with tamoxifen. Furthermore, tamoxifen is associated with significant adverse events, including thromboembolism and cerebrovascular events. A randomized trial of letrozole versus placebo in a group of 5,187 postmenopausal women after 5 yr of tamoxifen therapy for early stage breast cancer revealed significantly improved disease-free survival with 5 yr of letrozole therapy after completion of standard tamoxifen regimen. These results led to further study comparing aromatase inhibitor alone, tamoxifen alone, and aromatase inhibitor plus tamoxifen.

Based on results of the Arimidex, Tamoxifen, Alone or in Combination (ATAC) trial, aromatase inhibitors are now recommended as adjuvant treatment for postmenopausal women with hormone-receptor–positive early stage breast cancer. This trial showed significant efficacy and tolerability advantages over tamoxifen during the treatment phase, including a significantly prolonged disease-free survival and time to recurrence, and fewer occurrences of thromboembolism, ischemic cerebrovascular events, and endometrial cancer. Based on the 100-mo follow-up analysis, lower recurrence rates are maintained with anastrazole, even after treatment has been completed. However, anastrazole was associated with an increase in fracture episodes as well as arthralgias.

Currently, most experts recommend that baseline bone mineral density examinations should be performed before aromatase inhibitor therapy is started in those suspected clinically to be at risk of osteopenia or osteoporosis.

Even though adjuvant chemotherapy is effective in treating breast cancer, by itself it is not as effective as either adjuvant tamoxifen or aromatase inhibitors in an older patient with estrogen- and progesterone-receptor–positive disease.

References

1. Clarke M, Coates AS, Darby SC, et al. Early Breast Cancer Trialists' Collaborative Group (EBCTCG). Adjuvant chemotherapy in oestrogen-receptor-poor breast cancer: patient-level meta-analysis of randomised trials. *Lancet*. 2008;371(9606):29-40.
2. Forbes JF, Cuzick J, Buzdar A, et al. Effect of anastrozole and tamoxifen as adjuvant treatment for early-stage breast cancer: 100-month analysis of the ATAC trial. *Lancet Oncol*. 2008;9(1):45–53.
3. Goss PE, Ingle JN, Martino S, et al. A randomized trial of letrozole in postmenopausal women after five years of tamoxifen therapy for early-stage breast cancer. *N Engl J Med*. 2003;349(19):1793–1802.
4. Howell A, Cuzick J, Baum M, et al. Results of the ATAC (Arimidex, Tamoxifen, Alone or in Combination) trial after completion of 5 years' adjuvant treatment for breast cancer. *Lancet*. 2005;365(9453):60–62.

209. An 82-yr-old man who lives in a nursing facility is evaluated because he has a facial rash. He has been taking ciprofloxacin therapy for 5 days for a urinary tract infection. History includes Parkinson's disease and dementia.

On examination, the rash comprises mild erythematous plaques with fine scales along the frontal hairline of the scalp as well as moderate erythema with increased scales along the nasolabial folds bilaterally.

Which of the following would be effective as an initial step in managing this patient's rash?

(A) Discontinue ciprofloxacin
(B) Open wet dressings
(C) 5% Fluorouracil ointment
(D) Ketoconazole cream and topical low-potency steroid
(E) Skin biopsy

ANSWER: D

This patient has an exacerbation of seborrheic dermatitis, which is common in men and in patients with Parkinson's disease. Exacerbations of dermatitis can be triggered by stress and illness (eg, urinary tract infection). Seborrheic dermatitis is diagnosed based on its appearance. The findings on examination in this case are typical: inflammatory changes with erythematous scaling, and pruritic plaques in the affected sites of the scalp and nasolabial folds. Treatment of seborrheic dermatitis includes an antifungal preparation, such as ketoconazole (SOE= A), to decrease colonization by yeast, and topical steroids to address the inflammatory and erythematous eruption. The need for combination therapy is based on the severity of symptoms and the degree of pruritus or erythema involved. A mild steroid (class IV-VI) should be used first, for a limited period of therapy. Although topical steroids are associated with several adverse events, including skin atrophy, discoloration, and telangiectasia, appropriate use of the least-potent steroid can minimize these outcomes. If response to the low-potency steroid is inadequate, a higher potency, class III steroid can be used. If response is still inadequate, a class II or I steroid may be considered, or a referral to a dermatologist.

The characteristics and location of the patient's lesions are not consistent with drug allergy reactions or actinic keratosis. Drug eruption can present with a fine erythematous maculopapular rash, hives, or scale, but the distribution should include the trunk and often the extremities. Open wet dressings can be useful for any inflammatory or pruritic eruption but would not specifically treat seborrheic dermatitis. Skin biopsy would be useful for diagnosing actinic keratosis or squamous cell carcinoma. Typically, actinic keratoses are slightly pink and rough to touch, but they may be skin colored or pigmented. Although lesions can be as large as several centimeters in diameter, more typically they average 5 mm. Actinic keratoses can be treated with 5% fluorouracil ointment.

References

1. Del Rosso J. Corticosteroids: options in the era of steroid-sparing therapy. *J Am Acad Dermatol.* 2005;53(1 Suppl 1):S50–58.
2. Elewski B. Efficacy and safety of a new once-daily topical ketoconazole 2% gel in the treatment of seborrheic dermatitis: a phase III trial. *J Drugs Dermatol.* 2006;5(7):646–650.
3. Gupta AK, Bluhm R. Seborrheic dermatitis. *J Eur Acad Dermatol Venereol.* 2004;18(1):13–26.
4. Swinyer LJ. Ketoconazole gel 2% in the treatment of moderate to severe seborrheic dermatitis. *Cutis.* 2007;79(6):475–482.

210. A 78-yr-old woman requires admission to a nursing facility after hospitalization for bilateral Colles' fractures sustained in a fall. Her daughter is concerned about the quality of care at the nursing home. She plans to look at the CMS Web site for the publicly reported nursing-home quality measures available on Nursing Home Compare.

Which of the following information is found on Nursing Home Compare?

(A) Information on any healthcare facility that is licensed at the state level
(B) Information about quality measures beyond the assessment data that nursing homes routinely collect
(C) Information about quality measures based on care provided to an individual resident
(D) Information that allows identification of nursing homes that provide above average or much above average care

ANSWER: D

Information on the CMS Web site should not be viewed as an endorsement or advertisement for any nursing home. Each nursing home that provides Medicare or Medicaid services is required to make results of its last full inspection available onsite for public review. The online report at www.medicare.gov/NHCompare gives information about quality measures, staffing patterns, and inspection results for all nursing homes that are certified by Medicare or Medicaid. The report also compares each nursing home's performance with national and regional average performances.

Nursing Home Compare provides information about nursing facilities. It does not cover other types of facilities that offer various levels of health care and assistance with ADLs; these are licensed only at the state level. State survey agencies may have information about any facility not found in the Nursing Home Compare database.

Publicly reported nursing-home quality measures are based on care provided to the population of residents in a facility, not to an individual resident. Most of the quality measures reflect a sample of residents' conditions for the 7 days before the facility was assessed. Therefore, the quality measures may not represent a resident's clinical condition during the time between assessments. Although quality measures are not intended to be used in litigation, plaintiffs have successfully introduced survey results to show a pattern of poor care in a nursing home. If a nursing home has no deficiencies, it has met the minimal standards at the time of survey by state inspectors. Surveys are mandated at least every 15 mo, and more frequently for cause.

The quality measures are generated from assessment data that nursing homes routinely collect on residents at specified intervals during their stay (referred to as the Minimum Data Set). The information collected pertains to the resident's physical and clinical condition, functional status, and care preferences. The set of current quality indicators based on Minimum Data Set items has been selected because it can be measured and does not require nursing homes to prepare additional reports. The quality of a nursing home can improve or deteriorate significantly in a relatively short time. Findings of inspections do not represent a complete picture of the quality of care provided by the nursing home.

The Five-Star Rating System was created to help consumers, their families, and providers compare the quality of care and services of nursing homes. The number of stars assigned to a facility, from 1 (much below average) to 5 (much above average), is determined by performance on quality measures, staffing ratios, and findings during regulatory inspections. However, deciding whether or not to choose a particular nursing home should not be based solely on the number of stars it earns. The Five-Star Rating System has limits; the best comparisons are made by looking at nursing homes within the same state while keeping in mind that information provided in the rating system is a "snap shot" of the care in an individual nursing home.

Patients or family should visit nursing homes to meet the staff and care teams and to observe living conditions and the general environment. For the most current information about a nursing home, the U.S. Department of Health and Human Services recommends contacting a local ombudsman's office or the state survey agency.

References

1. Centers for Medicare and Medicaid Services. *Nursing Home Quality Initiatives: Quality Measures.* http://www.cms.hhs.gov/NursingHomeQualityInits/10_NHQIQualityMeasures.asp (accessed Nov 2009).
2. *Nursing Home Compare.* http://www.medicare.gov/NHCompare/ (accessed Nov 2009).

211. When should the rapid plasma reagin test be included in the evaluation for dementia?

(A) Routinely in patients undergoing initial assessment for dementia
(B) When symptoms of dementia appear in a patient <65 yr old
(C) If there is a specific risk factor for syphilis
(D) When symptoms of dementia progress rapidly
(E) Rapid plasma reagin test is not part of the initial evaluation for dementia.

ANSWER: C

The diagnostic evaluation for dementia has changed over time, with additional changes likely as neuroimaging and biochemical techniques become more sophisticated.

At present, there is no single, universally accepted, evidence-based guideline for the initial assessment of dementia. The American Academy of Neurology guidelines recommend that the routine diagnostic evaluation for dementia include structural neuroimaging (noncontrast CT or MRI) and screening for major depressive disorder, vitamin B_{12} deficiency, and hypothyroidism (SOE=C). The guidelines no longer include syphilis serology among laboratory tests to be obtained in the initial evaluation of dementia unless the patient has "a specific risk factor or evidence of prior syphilitic infection, or resides in one of the few areas in the United States with high numbers of syphilis cases," mostly concentrated in the midwestern and southeastern regions of the country. The guidelines note further that "except in these high-incidence regions, screening for the disorder in patients with dementia without an increased pretest probability would appear to be ill-supported because positive serum Venereal Disease Research Laboratory, rapid plasma reagin, and fluorescent treponemal antibody tests are non-specific" (SOE=B). Except in these high-incidence regions, screening for the disorder in patients with dementia without an increased pretest probability would appear to be ill-supported because positive serum Venereal Disease Research Laboratory, rapid plasma reagin, and fluorescent treponemal antibody tests are nonspecific.

Early onset (before age 65) and rapid progression are not typical of most dementias, except for frontotemporal dementia, in which onset can occur in patients in their 50s, and in prion disease, which often progresses rapidly.

In assessing a dementia with an atypical presentation, history and physical signs consistent with possible neurosyphilis should guide decision making.

In addition to screening for vitamin B_{12} deficiency and hypothyroidism to exclude potentially reversible causes of dementia, most practitioners obtain a CBC, serum chemistries, liver function tests, and possibly other tests (eg, for HIV or Lyme disease), depending on the specific history and physical examination. In the past decade, studies have found that reversible dementia is exceedingly rare, on the order of 1% (SOE=A).

References

1. Brayne C, Fox C, Boustani M. Dementia screening in primary care: is it time? *JAMA.* 2007;298(20):2409–2411.
2. Clarfield AM. The decreasing prevalence of reversible dementias: an updated meta-analysis. *Arch Int Med.* 2003;163(18):2219–2229.
3. Feil DG, MacLean C, Sultzer D. Quality indicators for the care of dementia in vulnerable elders. *J Am Geriatr Soc.* 2007;55(Suppl 2):S293–S301.
4. Knopman DS, DeKosky ST, Cummings JL, et al. Practice parameter: diagnosis of dementia (an evidence-based review): Report of the Quality Standards Subcommittee of the American Academy of Neurology. *Neurology.* 2001;56(9):1143–1153.

212. A 76-yr-old woman with end-stage heart failure (New York Heart Association class IV) has worsening dyspnea at rest and has become dependent in all ADLs except feeding. She sometimes feels as though she is suffocating and becomes very anxious. She began home hospice care 4 mo ago. She had been feeling relatively well since an increase in her furosemide dosage and the addition of supplemental oxygen last month. The cardiologist believes that she would not benefit from increasing her current dosages of carvedilol, enalapril, and spironolactone, and she has been compliant with her medication regimen and diet.

On a home visit by the hospice nurse, the patient is alert, oriented, and in mild distress. Temperature is 36.5°C (97.7°F), blood pressure is 126/64 mmHg, heart rate is 105 beats per minute, respiratory rate is 24 breaths per minute, and O_2 saturation is 97% on 4 L/min oxygen by nasal cannula. She has decreased breath sounds at the right base with dullness on percussion approximately one-fourth of the way up; a few crackles are heard at the left

base. Jugular venous pressure is 12 mmHg. Hepatojugular reflex is positive, and leg edema is minimal.

The hospice nurse calls to discuss the care plan and recommends increasing the dosage of furosemide.

Which of the following is the most appropriate next step for this patient?

(A) Admit to the hospital for inpatient diuresis.
(B) Increase dosage of furosemide and arrange for outpatient, ultrasound-guided pleurocentesis.
(C) Increase dosage of furosemide and increase oxygen to 6 L/min by nasal cannula.
(D) Increase dosage of furosemide and add nebulized albuterol 2.5 mL q4h as needed for dyspnea.
(E) Increase dosage of furosemide and start morphine 5 mg po q3h as needed for dyspnea.

ANSWER: E

Dyspnea is common in many patients with advanced heart failure, even in those who are not in overt fluid overload. This patient shows evidence of mild fluid overload, and her furosemide dosage should be adjusted as recommended by the home hospice nurse. Because the cardiologist does not think her symptoms would improve by adjusting her other current medications, the addition of opioids should be considered (SOE=C). In patients who are not already taking an opioid, morphine, 5 mg po q3–6h as needed, can offer significant relief. Given this patient's persistent and distressing dyspnea, the morphine should be started at a low dosage as needed and adjusted for symptom relief.

Admission for inpatient diuresis is not indicated. If this patient's dyspnea was moderate or severe, and the hospice nurse and physician did not believe that her symptoms could be managed effectively at home, then admission to the hospital for general inpatient care under the Medicare Hospice Benefit would be recommended. Although she likely has a right-sided pleural effusion, pleurocentesis is not likely to relieve her dyspnea and may cause significant complications, eg, pneumothorax. In addition, the effusion may improve with an increase in the furosemide dosage.

Supplemental oxygen can improve dyspnea in patients with heart failure, including those who are not hypoxemic. However, this patient is already on a moderate amount of supplemental oxygen, with normal O_2 saturation. Increasing supplemental oxygen to 6 L/min is unlikely to provide additional benefit. Nonpharmacologic methods that may be effective in the treatment of dyspnea include breathing training, walking aids, neuroelectrical muscle stimulation, and chest wall vibration (SOE=B). The use of fans and fresh air can also provide relief in patients with dyspnea (SOE=D).

There is no evidence to suggest that addition of nebulized albuterol relieves dyspnea in patients with heart failure without bronchospasm. This patient does not have evidence of reactive airway disease, she has no history of asthma or COPD, and she has no wheezing or other signs of obstruction. The addition of nebulized albuterol could exacerbate her tachycardia and dyspnea.

References

1. Bausewein C, Booth S, Gysels M, et al. Non-pharmacological interventions for breathlessness in advanced stages of malignant and non-malignant diseases. *Cochrane Database Syst Rev*. 2008;(2):CD005623.
2. Johnson MJ, McDonagh TA, Harkness A, et al. Morphine for the relief of breathlessness in patients with chronic heart failure—a pilot study. *Eur J Heart Fail*. 2002; 4(6):753–756.
3. Pantilat SZ, Steimle AE. Palliative care for patients with heart failure. *JAMA*. 2004;291(20):2476–2482.

213. A 75-yr-old man comes to the office for a routine physical examination. He feels well. He is on hemodialysis for chronic kidney disease; history also includes long-term type 2 diabetes mellitus, peripheral vascular disease, and coronary artery disease. Medications include insulin, metoprolol, sevelamer, and calcitriol. Examination is unremarkable.

Laboratory results (blood sample drawn at dialysis):

BUN	20 mg/dL
Creatinine	6.5 mg/dL
Sodium	140 mEq/L
Potassium	4.4 mEq/L
Hemoglobin	10 g/dL

Which of the following is the most appropriate next step?

(A) Begin epoetin-α with a target hemoglobin concentration of 13–14 mg/dL.
(B) Begin epoetin-α with a target hemoglobin concentration of 11–12 mg/dL.
(C) Begin epoetin-α if hemoglobin concentration falls to <9 mg/dL.
(D) Begin epoetin-α if symptoms develop.

ANSWER: B

Erythropoietin has become a standard part of therapy for patients with chronic or end-stage renal disease, because it improves both physiologic and clinical parameters and quality of life (SOE=A). Recommendations are to treat patients with anemia of chronic renal disease when the hemoglobin concentration falls to <11 g/dL (SOE=C), better outcomes have been with a target hemoglobin concentration of 11–12 g/dL (hematocrit 33%–36%) (SOE=B). Evidence is increasing for worse clinical outcomes when hemoglobin concentration ≥13 g/dL (hematocrit ≥39%) is targeted and maintained in dialysis and predialysis patients (SOE=B). The U.S. Normal Hematocrit Study was terminated prematurely because patients in the group targeted to normal hematocrit values had a higher mortality that approached statistical significance. Other possible adverse consequences associated with normal or near-normal hemoglobin concentrations include stroke, arteriovenous access thrombosis, and hypertension. The updated 2007 guidelines from the National Kidney Foundation Dialysis Outcomes Quality Initiative (DOQI) recommend target hemoglobin concentrations of 11–12 g/dL, not to exceed 13 g/dL (SOE=B). Similar target levels are recommended in Canadian, European, and Japanese guidelines.

References

1. K/DOQI. K/DOQI Clinical Practice Guidelines and Clinical Practice Recommendations for anemia in chronic kidney disease: 2007 update of hemoglobin target. *Am J Kidney Dis*. 2007;50:471–530.
2. Phrommintikul A, Haas SJ, Elsik M, et al. Mortality and target haemoglobin concentrations in anaemic patients with chronic kidney disease treated with erythropoietin: a meta-analysis. *Lancet*. 2007;369(9559):381–388.
3. Singh AK, Szczech L, Tang KL, et al. Correction of anemia with epoetin alfa in chronic kidney disease. *N Engl J Med*. 2006;355(20):2085–2098.

214. A 70-yr-old woman comes to the office for a routine examination. She is cognitively intact and has a history of hypertension, macular degeneration, and osteoarthritis, mainly in her knees. She takes a multivitamin, lisinopril, and extra-strength acetaminophen as needed for pain.

Physical examination is normal, except that she wears pads. She reluctantly admits to having "accidents." She is embarrassed and worried, and has given up weekly bridge sessions. Lately she has been rushing to the bathroom frequently to prevent accidents. Which of the following is the most appropriate next step?

(A) Start an oxybutynin trial and schedule follow-up in 2 wk.
(B) Ask patient to keep a voiding diary and schedule follow-up in 2 wk.
(C) Start bladder retraining program and schedule follow-up in 2 wk.
(D) Obtain urology consultation.
(E) No further intervention is necessary.

ANSWER: B

This patient has involuntary loss of urine severe enough to affect her quality of life. From the history, it is not clear what type of incontinence she has. A voiding diary can help identify her exact symptoms and the severity of the problem. In addition, a medication review is indicated. Urinary incontinence is not a part of normal aging, although prevalence of the syndrome increases with age. Prevalence is higher in women than in men up to age 80, after which the prevalence is equal.

Conservative measures are highly effective for urinary incontinence in women. Kegel exercises significantly reduce symptoms of stress incontinence, although the cure rate is low (SOE=A). Bladder training should be first-line treatment for overactive bladder, because it is as effective as medication (SOE=A). Because the type of incontinence and its possible precipitants are unknown at this point, a trial of oxybutynin is premature and could be harmful. Clinical practice guide-lines for urinary incontinence in adults recommend referral to specialists when there is no clear diagnosis, poor correlation between symptoms and clinical findings, inadequate response to therapy, hematuria without infection, comorbid conditions, or when surgery is a consideration (SOE=C).

References

1. Rogers RG. Urinary stress incontinence in women. *N Engl J Med.* 2008;358(10):1029–1036.
2. Shamliyan TA, Kane RL, Wyman J, et al. Systematic review: randomized, controlled trials of nonsurgical treatments for urinary incontinence in women. *Ann Intern Med.* 2008;148(6):459–473.

215. A 69-yr-old woman comes to the office for a follow-up visit. She has had type 2 diabetes mellitus, dyslipidemia, and hypertension for 5 yr. In addition to lisinopril, pravastatin, and aspirin, she takes metformin 1000 mg q12h, glipizide 10 mg q12h, and rosiglitazone 4 mg/d. Hemoglobin A_{1c} has ranged from 7.5% to 8.5% since diagnosis, and she is frustrated that she has never "achieved target."

On physical examination, weight is 95 kg (210 lb), up 4 kg (9 lb) from 6 mo ago. Blood pressure is 128/82 mmHg and pulse is 76 beats per minute. She has a III/VI systolic ejection murmur and 1+ bilateral leg edema. The remainder of the examination, including sensation to monofilament, is normal. Her most recent hemoglobin A_{1c} was 8.5%. A recent ophthalmology examination showed no retinopathy or macular edema. Rosiglitazone is discontinued because of her leg edema.

Which of the following should be initiated to improve her glycemic control?

(A) Sitagliptin
(B) Increased glipizide dose
(C) Long-acting insulin
(D) Exenatide

ANSWER: C

Adding a long-acting insulin is likely to achieve the target hemoglobin A_{1c} goal of <7%. Unlike the dosage limitations of oral medications, the dosage of basal insulin can be increased by several units every few days until fasting glucose concentrations reach target. Although insulin is associated with modest weight gain, this is more pronounced with prandial insulin, and the benefits of improved glycemic control would likely outweigh the possible modest increase in weight (SOE=B).

Adding a glucagon-like peptide-1 receptor agonist (exenatide) or dipeptidyl peptidase-4 inhibitor (sitagliptin) may also achieve the hemoglobin A_{1c} target, but there are no data on long-term safety for these newer classes of medications (SOE=C). The patient is already on the maximal dosage of glipizide of 20 mg/d.

References

1. Drazen JM, Morrissey S, Curfman GD. Rosiglitazone—continued uncertainty about safety. *N Engl J Med.* 2007;357(1):63–64.
2. Drucker DJ, Nauck MA. The incretin system: glucagon-like peptide-1 receptor agonists and dipeptidyl peptidase-4 inhibitors in type 2 diabetes. *Lancet.* 2006;368(9548):1696–1705.
3. Nathan DM. Rosiglitazone and cardiotoxicity—weighing the evidence. *N Engl J Med.* 2007;357(1):64–66.
4. Nissen SE, Wolski K. Effect of rosiglitazone on the risk of myocardial infarction and death from cardio-vascular causes. *N Engl J Med.* 2007;356(24):2457–2471.
5. Richter B, Bandiera-Echtler E, Bergerhoff K, et al. Rosiglitazone for type 2 diabetes mellitus. *Cochrane Database Syst Rev.* 2007;(3):CD006063.

216. A 67-yr-old woman comes to the office to request hormone therapy for her vaginal atrophy symptoms that have not responded to topical estrogen.

Which of the following is an additional indication for starting therapy?

(A) Stress incontinence
(B) Moderate to severe hot flushes
(C) Coronary heart disease
(D) Dementia

ANSWER: B

Vasomotor symptoms are seen most often in late menopausal transition and soon after menopause. Although there are alternative treatments for vasomotor symptoms, none are as effective as estrogen (SOE=A). Estrogen is a reasonable short-term (2- to 3-yr) option for most symptomatic postmenopausal women unless they have a history of, or are at high risk of, breast cancer, coronary heart disease, or venous thromboembolism.

Data from the Women's Health Initiative (WHI) and the Heart and Estrogen/Progestin Replacement Study (HERS) have led to changes in recommendations for postmenopausal hormone therapy. If estrogen is prescribed, even if it is used short-term, routine mammography and breast examinations are essential. A progestin should be added for women who have not had a hysterectomy (SOE=A). Both the WHI and HERS trials provided data on combined continuous conjugated estrogens (0.625 mg) and medroxyprogesterone acetate (2.5 mg).

Long-term hormone therapy is no longer recommended for primary or secondary prevention of coronary heart disease. Estrogen as first-line therapy for osteoporosis has been replaced by bisphosphonates or raloxifene, but estrogen can be considered for women with no contraindications who cannot take bisphosphonates or raloxifene.

Hormone therapy should not be started in women ≥65 yr old to prevent dementia. Insufficient evidence exists at this time about estrogen use in perimenopausal women to prevent later dementia. Evidence is also lacking to recommend systemic estrogen to treat stress incontinence and is insufficient to recommend topical estrogen for urge or stress incontinence.

References

1. Col NF, Weber G, Stiggelbout A, et al. Short-term menopausal hormone therapy for symptom relief: an updated decision model. *Arch Intern Med.* 2004;164(15):1634–1640.
2. North American Menopause Society. Estrogen and progestogen use in peri- and postmenopausal women: March 2007 position statement of The North American Menopause Society. *Menopause.* 2007;14(2):168–182.
3. Rossouw JE, Prentice RL, Manson JE, et al. Postmenopausal hormone therapy and risk of cardio-vascular disease by age and years since menopause. *JAMA.* 2007;297(13):1465–1477.
4. Utian WH, Archer DF, Bachmann GA, et al. Estrogen and progestogen use in postmenopausal women: July 2008 position statement of The North American Menopause Society. *Menopause.* 2008;15(4 Pt 1):584–602.

217. A 90-yr-old woman comes to the office to establish care. She has difficulty breathing with exertion and awakens several times each night to urinate. These symptoms began a year ago. She has a history of chronic poorly controlled hypertension, diabetes mellitus controlled by diet, and rheumatoid arthritis. On examination, jugular venous pressure is 9 cm H_2O. Lungs are clear. The abdomen is mildly distended with no tenderness, and there is 1+ edema in her legs. Brain natriuretic peptide (BNP) concentration is 76 pg/mL.

Which of the following is the most likely diagnosis?

(A) Deconditioning
(B) Heart failure with diastolic dysfunction
(C) Interstitial lung disease
(D) Pulmonary embolism
(E) Cirrhosis of the liver

ANSWER: B

Heart failure with diastolic dysfunction is common in patients with chronic hypertension, particularly women. Findings include dyspnea, edema, and increased jugular venous pressure. However, it is difficult on physical examination to differentiate systolic from diastolic heart failure. Lung examination is often normal in patients with chronic heart failure, despite evidence on physical examination of volume overload such as increased jugular venous pressure and edema. BNP is secreted by the myocardium as a result of increased stretch of the ventricular myocytes. BNP levels can be normal in patients with heart failure. Diagnosis of heart failure should therefore be based on physical signs and symptoms of heart failure, not on serum testing of BNP alone.

Deconditioning does not lead to increased jugular venous pressure. Interstitial lung disease due to rheumatoid arthritis is usually associated with an abnormal respiratory examination. While chronic pulmonary embolism could cause this patient's symptoms, diastolic dysfunction is more likely, given her chronic hypertension. Cirrhosis of the liver is unlikely to cause shortness of breath in the absence of significant ascites.

References

1. Devereux RB, Roman MJ, Liu JE. Congestive heart failure despite normal left ventricular systolic function in a population-based sample: the Strong Heart Study. *Am J Cardiol.* 2000;86(10):1090–1096.
2. Kitzman DW, Gardin JM, Gottdiener JS. Cardiovascular Health Study Research Group. Importance of heart failure with preserved systolic function in patients > or = 65 years of age. CHS Research Group. Cardiovascular Health Study. *Am J Cardiol.* 2001;87(4):413–419.
3. Maurer MS, Burkhoff D, Fried LP. Ventricular structure and function in hypertensive participants with heart failure and a normal ejection fraction: the Cardiovascular Health Study. *J Am Coll Cardiol.* 2007;49(9):972–981.

218. Which of the following experimental observations pertaining to specific theories of aging is true?

(A) Alterations in local microenvironments and systemic physiologic changes at the level of an entire organism can both contribute to decreased tissue homeostasis and repair.
(B) Aging is associated with evidence of chronic inflammation, increased levels of circulating autoantibodies, and increased production of antibodies targeted to novel antigenic stimuli.
(C) Low-impact exercise and physical activity contribute to accelerated aging on a cellular level by inducing oxidative stress, DNA damage, and the development of tissue inflammation.
(D) Dietary changes are unlikely to affect development of tissue inflammation and fibrosis.

ANSWER: A

Individual tissues vary in terms of their regenerative potential and cellular turnover. Adult stem cells are present in most mammalian tissues. Tissue-specific decline in stem-cell function, alterations in the local microenvironment, as well as systemic changes associated with aging or disease can all contribute to decreased tissue plasticity with aging.

Aging, frailty, and chronic diseases common to aging are all associated with increases in peripheral levels of pro-inflammatory cytokines and other inflammatory markers, as well as in increased levels of circulating autoantibodies. At the same time, older adults exhibit a decreased ability to respond to specific infections and vaccines.

Increased oxidative stress can accelerate aging (free radical theory of aging), while also contributing to a number of disease processes. Advanced glycation end products represent a class of modified proteins that accumulate with both aging (protein modification theory of aging) and with specific disease processes (eg, glycosylated hemoglobin in diabetes). Dietary advanced glycation end products can contribute to oxidative stress and renal injury in animal models, thus offering the potential for modifying this type of tissue injury via nutritional manipulation.

While acute intense physical exercise has the ability to induce muscle damage and oxidative stress, habitual participation in low-impact exercise or increased physical activity appears to allow for an upregulation in endogenous antioxidant defenses.

References

1. Bloomer RJ. Effect of exercise on oxidative stress biomarkers. *Adv Clin Chem.* 2008;46:1–50.
2. Pawelec G, Larbi A. Immunity and ageing in man: Annual Review 2006/2007. *Exp Gerontol.* 2008;43(1):34–38.
3. Rando TA. Stem cells, ageing and the quest for immortality. *Nature* 2006;441(7097):1080–1086.
4. Vlassara H, Uribarri J, Cai W, et al. Advanced glycation end product homeostasis: exogenous oxidants and innate defenses. *Ann N Y Acad Sci.* 2008;1126:46–52.

219. A 72-yr-old woman comes to the office because her shoulders and thighs ache. She believes the aches are related to a new exercise program. For the past few days, she has not been able to exercise because of fatigue. She has no fever, chills, sweats, or weight loss.

On examination, the pain is reproduced on passive motion of her shoulders and on internal rotation of her hips. She has no other joint abnormalities. Westergren sedimentation rate is 52 mm/h and hematocrit is 36%; muscle and liver enzymes and thyroid profile are normal.

Polymyalgia rheumatica is diagnosed, and prednisone 20 mg/d is started. On follow-up, she is symptom free after 8 days of therapy, and prednisone is reduced to 10 mg/d. Two weeks later, she again reports that her shoulders and thighs ache.

Which of the following is the most appropriate next step?

(A) Add naproxen 500 mg q12h.
(B) Increase prednisone to 20 mg/d.
(C) Increase prednisone to 50 mg/d and obtain surgical consultation.
(D) Initiate oral methotrexate 5 mg weekly.
(E) Initiate amitriptyline 10 mg nightly.

ANSWER: B

Polymyalgia rheumatica is an inflammatory condition that causes pain or stiffness of the upper arms, shoulders, hips, or thighs, and constitutional symptoms of fatigue, low-grade fever, and weight loss. Symptoms abate quickly in response to a regimen of prednisone 10–20 mg/d. The regimen must be maintained for 4–6 wk before gradual tapering (by 1 mg each month) is attempted. The total duration of treatment required varies considerably, from 3 mo to several years. The most appropriate intervention for this patient is to resume prednisone 20 mg/d and verify laboratory and symptom response (SOE=C).

Had symptoms returned despite correct tapering of the prednisone, consideration of overlapping giant cell arteritis or an alternative diagnosis of rheumatoid arthritis would be appropriate. Increasing the prednisone beyond 20 mg and obtaining a surgical consultation are inappropriate because there is no mention of claudicatory symptoms or vascular abnormalities at the time of symptom recurrence. Methotrexate has marginal benefit as a steroid-sparing agent in management of temporal arteritis and has not shown benefit in management of polymyalgia rheumatica. A short-acting NSAID may be useful for symptom control during prednisone taper but is inappropriate at this time given the premature and overly aggressive taper. Amitriptyline has numerous adverse events in older adults; in addition, this medication will not treat the underlying problem.

References

1. Dasgupta B, Matteson EL, Maradit-Kremers H, et al. Management guidelines and outcome measures in polymyalgia rheumatica (PMR). *Clin Exp Rheumatol.* 2007;25(6 Suppl 47):130–136.
2. Hennell S, Busteed S, George E, et al. Evidence-based management for polymyalgia rheumatica for rheumatology practitioners, nurses and physiotherapists. *Musculoskeletal Care.* 2007;5(2):65–71.
3. Sengupta R, Kyle V. Recognising polymyalgia rheumatica. *Practitioner.* 2006;250(1688):40–44, 47.

220. An 86-yr-old woman with asthma comes to the office during a community outbreak of influenza. She had previously deferred receiving the influenza vaccine but now wants to do everything possible to prevent getting influenza.

Which of the following is true regarding prevention of influenza during a community outbreak?

(A) Adamantanes are not as effective as neuraminidase inhibitors (oseltamivir and zanamivir) for chemoprophylaxis.
(B) Vaccination is of little benefit once an outbreak has begun.
(C) Chemoprophylactic agents should be used for 5 days.
(D) Chemoprophylactic agents have few significant adverse events.
(E) The influenza vaccine has not been shown to prevent pneumonia or death.

ANSWER: A

Influenza is typically seen during late fall and winter. The influenza strain changes each year and involves both influenza A and B viruses. Prevention is mainly through vaccination. Although vaccination clearly decreases the incidence of pneumonia and death, many older adults in the community do not receive the vaccine.

Morbidity and mortality are highest for adults ≥65 yr old, for children <2 yr old, and for anyone with a comorbidity. People at high risk should be vaccinated even if an outbreak has already begun. Because antibodies do not develop for approximately 2 wk, chemoprophylaxis can be used to provide protection until immunity is likely. In the case presented here, the patient should be vaccinated and, after discussing adverse events, offered chemoprophylaxis for 2 wk.

In the United States, adamantanes are no longer recommended for prophylaxis because influenza strains have shown increased resistance to them. In community studies, oseltamivir and zanamivir appear similarly effective in preventing influenza in adults. Only oseltamivir has been studied in institutional settings. Recently, increased resistance to oseltamivir has been seen.

Adverse events of oseltamivir include nausea and vomiting. Postmarket surveillance suggests that it can also cause transient neuropsychiatric events (delirium or self-harm). The FDA recommends monitoring for unusual behavior. Zanamivir is not recommended for those with underlying airway disease.

References
1. Fiore AE, Shay DK, Haber P, et al. Prevention and control of influenza. Recommendations of the Advisory Committee on Immunization Practices. *MMWR Recomm Rep.* 2007;56(RR-6):1–54.
2. Nichol KL, Nordin JD, Nelson DB, et al. Effectiveness of the influenza vaccine in the community dwelling elderly. *N Engl J Med.* 2007;357(14):1373–1381.

221. A 77-yr-old woman with a 40-yr history of depression is evaluated in an outpatient clinic for change in behavior. Her marriage was stable up until 10 yr ago, when her relationship with her husband became stormy. The clinic staff perceives her as manipulative, noting increasingly needy, frustration-intolerant, and rejection-sensitive behavior. For example, she moans at regular intervals, requests help with simple tasks, becomes enraged by perceived rejection, and is suspicious that others are lying to her. Records include findings of "focal atrophy in the right frontal region of unclear etiology" on MRI, and her family reports that she had a "blood clot in her brain" about 10 yr ago.

On examination, she has no focal neurologic signs. Score on Mini–Mental State Examination is 26/30. Neuropsychologic evaluation reveals intact verbal memory but impaired initiation and executive functioning consistent with mild cognitive impairment. She admits to feeling depressed, worthless, and unable to experience pleasure, and she reports chronic passive suicidal ideation, insomnia, and fatigue. She exhibits no gross perceptual abnormalities or delusions.

Which of the following is the most likely cause of the patient's behavior?

(A) Recurrent major depressive disorder and dependent personality disorder
(B) Recurrent major depressive disorder and borderline personality disorder
(C) Recurrent major depressive disorder and personality change due to a medical disorder
(D) Recurrent major depressive disorder

ANSWER: C

This patient exhibits personality change due to a medical disorder, but her behavior may be mistaken for personality disorder. Mild cognitive impairment, or a static or slowly progressing neurocognitive disorder, may go undetected, overshadowed by prominent, persisting behaviors. Symptoms that seem to represent an amplification of premorbid personality traits can particularly confuse family members. Dysfunction in four neuroanatomic areas can result in behavioral syndromes that amplify underlying personality traits: 1) orbital frontal lobe dysfunction, resulting in reduced empathy and disinhibition; 2) dorsolateral frontal lobe dysfunction, resulting in impaired initiation, planning, and social awareness; 3) parietal and temporal lobe dysfunction, resulting in misperception of sensory stimuli and of the emotional content of speech; and 4) anterior cingulate syndrome, resulting in apathy.

Although some features of this patient's behavior suggest borderline or dependent personality disorder superimposed on symptoms of major depressive disorder, the features must be present since young adulthood to meet criteria for personality disorder. The late onset of this patient's personality changes, the neuroimaging and neuropsychologic findings suggestive of frontal lobe impairment, and the temporal relationship between cognitive findings and personality changes argue against a diagnosis of personality disorder. Major depressive disorder alone is also insufficient to explain this constellation of symptoms.

References

1. Lyketsos CG, Lopez O, Jones B, et al. Prevalence of neuropsychiatric symptoms in dementia and mild cognitive impairment: results from the cardiovascular health study. *JAMA*. 2002;288(12):1475–1483.
2. Oxman TE. Personality disorders. In: Blazer DG, Steffens DC, eds. *The American Psychiatric Publishing Textbook of Geriatric Psychiatry*. 4th ed. Washington, DC: American Psychiatric Publishing Inc; 2009.
3. Zweig RA, Agronin ME. Personality disorders in late life. In: Agronin M, Maletta G, eds. *Principles and Practice of Geriatric Psychiatry*. Philadelphia, PA: Lippincott, Williams & Wilkins; 2006:449–469.

222. A 65-yr-old man has problems parking his van too close to the garage wall; recently, while backing out his car, he hit the door and damaged the car and garage. He has driven a truck for the past 50 yr with no incident. His wife schedules an appointment with his ophthalmologist, whom he has not seen for 4 yr. He sees his internist regularly.

Which of the following is the most likely diagnosis?

(A) Cataracts
(B) Diabetic retinopathy
(C) Glaucoma
(D) Macular degeneration

ANSWER: C

Primary open-angle glaucoma slowly causes restriction of the visual field without other symptoms. The optic nerve atrophies, with loss of retinal ganglion cells and axons. Chronic optic neuropathy causes the loss and is often associated with increased intraocular pressure, although the increased pressure need not be present for the damage to occur. In this patient, progressive glaucoma has restricted the visual field such that he is unable to see the garage wall (SOE=A).

Macular degeneration causes loss of central vision. A person with macular degeneration can have difficulty reading signs, but peripheral vision is not impaired. Rather than hitting the garage wall, a patient with macular degeneration might have difficulty reading a road sign in front of the car.

Cataracts cause blurring of vision and possibly light sensitivity and glare. Visual impairment from cataracts usually progresses slowly. Loss of peripheral vision is unlikely to be an early symptom.

Diabetic retinopathy severe enough to cause visual field loss is usually associated with systemic findings of diabetes. Field loss from diabetes can be associated with vitreous hemorrhage, which would most likely affect central vision as well. Field loss is also found in diabetic individuals who have had extensive pan-retinal photocoagulation for retinopathy. This treatment can result in a field loss in dimly illuminated areas, such as a poorly lit tunnel.

References

1. American Academy of Ophthalmology. *Preferred Practice Patterns*. San Francisco, CA: American Academy of Ophthalmology; 2006. Available at: http://one.aao.org/CE/PracticeGuidelines/PPP.aspx (accessed Nov 2009).
2. Caprioli J, Coleman AL. Intraocular pressure fluctuation: a risk factor for visual field progression at low intraocular pressures in the Advanced Glaucoma Intervention Study. *Ophthalmology.* 2008;115(7):1123–1129.
3. Much JW, Liu C, Piltz-Seymour JR. Long-term survival of central visual field in end-stage glaucoma. *Ophthalmology.* 2008;115(7):1162–1166.

223. A 68-yr-old man is brought to the office by his wife for evaluation. His wife reports a 9-mo history of increasing problems with "saying what he wants to say." The patient agrees that he often knows what he wants to say but has difficulty "getting the words out." The patient is a college graduate and recently retired from an accounting firm. He has no trouble driving, maintains his investment portfolio, and enjoys cooking in his new kitchen, for which he oversaw the remodeling 6 mo earlier. History includes dyslipidemia controlled by diet, and mild hypertension, for which he takes hydrochlorothiazide daily.

On examination, the patient is fully oriented and demonstrates normal memory on a screening test. He names 8 items beginning with the letter S in 60 seconds, and he struggles to copy intersecting pentagons. The remainder of the neurologic examination is nonfocal. Neuropsychologic assessment shows moderate impairment on the Boston Naming and Clock Drawing tests, confirming the initial clinical impression of impairment in the language and visuospatial domains of cognition. Laboratory evaluation is within normal limits. Noncontrast CT of the head reveals mild periventricular white matter disease and a lacunar infarct in the left basal ganglia.

Which of the following is the most likely diagnosis?

(A) Vascular dementia
(B) Mild cognitive impairment
(C) Lewy body dementia
(D) Frontotemporal dementia
(E) Alzheimer's disease

ANSWER: B

This patient displays a deficit in language (evident on tests of verbal fluency and confrontational naming) and a deficit in visuospatial abilities (evident in poor figure-copying and clock drawing). The neurologic and subsequent neuropsychologic evaluations did not reveal a memory deficit, and his function appears to be maintained. Despite the 9-mo history of progressive symptoms, the patient does not meet the diagnostic criteria for dementia because he does not have memory impairment or significant decline in ADLs. The clinical examination and neuropsychologic testing indicate that he has impairment in two nonmemory domains of cognition (language ability and visuospatial skills). The most appropriate diagnosis at this time is multiple-domain, nonamnestic mild cognitive impairment.

The diagnostic construct of mild cognitive impairment (MCI) has been in use since the late 1990s. In its original form, MCI was meant to characterize incipient dementia, most often Alzheimer's disease. The initial criteria for MCI therefore focused on memory impairment. More recently, through epidemiologic research on MCI and through better characterization of the non-Alzheimer's dementias, the definition of MCI has been broadened to include cognitive domains in addition to memory. The original criteria, which included subjective and objective memory dysfunction in the setting of preserved general cognition and intact ADLs, now represent a possible variant of MCI. Currently, diagnosis of MCI requires objective evidence of cognitive decline in at least one domain, with preservation of baseline function. If memory is the affected domain, then the MCI is designated amnestic; if memory is preserved, the MCI is nonamnestic. Cognitive dysfunction can be limited to a single domain or involve multiple domains. Therefore, "amnestic MCI" can be designated either single or multiple domain, depending on whether any cognitive domain in addition to memory is impaired. Similarly, "nonamnestic MCI" can be either single or multiple domain, depending on whether cognition is impaired in only one or in more than one nonmemory cognitive domain.

MCI may progress to a variety of dementing disorders. However, MCI does not progress to dementia in most cases. Many patients remain stable, and some revert to normal cognition. In a recent validation study of the revised MCI criteria, MCI reverted to normal in approximately 20% of participants ≥75 yr old (SOE=B). In a typical clinical practice, about 10%–15% of patients diagnosed with MCI progress to dementia each year. The best predictors of progression from MCI to dementia have not been identified. Currently, candidate predictors include clinical severity, *APOE* carrier status, MRI volumetric studies, positron emission tomography, amyloid imaging, and biomarkers for colony-stimulating factor.

The patient has some evidence of cerebrovascular disease on structural neuroimaging. The mild degree of white matter disease is common with multiple vascular risk factors such as hypertension and dyslipidemia. Without memory impairment and functional loss, dementia cannot be diagnosed.

Visuospatial cognitive deficits can develop early and prominently in Lewy body dementia, while memory is often preserved in the early stages. This patient does not meet other essential criteria for Lewy body dementia, which require presence of dementia plus at least one core feature of the disease (ie, fluctuating cognition, recurrent visual hallucinations, or spontaneous features of parkinsonism).

Frontotemporal dementia is unlikely in a patient who demonstrates good insight into his cognitive problems, has a stable personality, and has no signs of emotional blunting. However, early language dysfunction can be a feature of the nonfluent aphasia variant of frontotemporal dementia (previously called primary progressive aphasia), which is characterized by effortful speech and articulatory deficits without the changes in behavior and personality common in the behavioral variant of frontotemporal dementia.

In the absence of memory impairment, Alzheimer's disease is highly unlikely.

References

1. Busse A, Hensel A, Gühne U, et al. Mild cognitive impairment: long-term course of four clinical subtypes. *Neurology*. 2006;67(12):2176–2185.
2. Ellison JM. A 60-year-old woman with mild memory impairment. Review of mild cognitive impairment as a diagnostic entity. *JAMA*. 2008;300(13):1566–1574.
3. Gauthier S, Reisberg B, Zaudig M, et al. Mild cognitive impairment. *Lancet*. 2006;367(9518):1262–1279.
4. Jack CR, Weigand SD, Shiung MM, et al. Atrophy rates accelerate in amnestic mild cognitive impairment. *Neurology*. 2008;70(19 Pt 2):1740–1752.
5. McKeith IG, Dickson DW, Lowe J, et al. Diagnosis and management of dementia with Lewy bodies: third report of the DLB consortium. *Neurology*. 2005;65(12):1863–1872.

224. Which of the following is meant by culturally competent care?

(A) Allocation of resources in proportion to the cultural composition of the community.
(B) Delivery of health services according to the cultural practices of the caregiver.
(C) Delivery of health services that acknowledge cultural diversity in the clinical setting.
(D) Characterizing patients based on their cultural backgrounds rather than their individual preferences.

ANSWER: C

Over the last few decades, globalization and changing geopolitics have caused major changes in immigration trends in the United States. In contrast to the predominantly European immigration during the earlier part of the 20th century, large numbers of people are migrating from other regions, especially Asia and Africa, thereby increasing the ethnic and cultural diversity of older Americans. Cultural diversity of older Americans poses significant challenges for optimal delivery of health care: clinical encounters should be characterized by a patient-centered approach to and respect for cultural, social, and ethnic differences—ie, cultural competency.

Culturally competent care involves delivery of health services in a manner consonant with customs, beliefs, values, behaviors, and norms of an individual patient. It involves aspects that directly or indirectly affect delivery of health care, including language, communication style, attire, food, reaction to pain, and participation in decision making. All of these components influence patients' decisions regarding acceptance of and adherence to treatment plans.

Allocation of resources according to the cultural composition of the community is not consistent with equitable, nondiscriminatory, need-based distribution that would ensure health care for all segments of the community.

The beliefs and cultural practices of the patient, not of the care provider, should influence care. Attempts should be made to identify and incorporate a patient's health beliefs, social values, family dynamics, dietary practices, and privacy issues, and to overcome language barriers.

Beliefs and attitudes vary greatly even among specific cultural groups. Hence, to provide culturally competent care, it is essential to treat each patient as an individual rather than as a cultural, religious, socioeconomic, or ethnic stereotype.

References

1. American Geriatrics Society. *Doorway Thoughts. Volume III: Cross-Cultural Healthcare for Older Adults.* Sudbury, MA: Jones & Bartlett; 2008.
2. Brach C, Fraser I. Can cultural competency reduce racial and ethnic disparities? A review and conceptual model. *Med Care Res Rev.* 2000;57(Suppl 1):181–217.
3. https://cia.gov/cia/publications/factbook/geos/xx.html (accessed Nov 2009).

225. A 70-yr-old man comes to the office because he has diarrhea with associated crampy abdominal pain and low-grade fever. The diarrhea began 3 days earlier; he is passing up to 5 watery, nonbloody bowel movements daily. History includes venous insufficiency, and he was recently treated with a 7-day course of cephalexin for lower-extremity cellulitis.

On examination, he does not look ill, and vital signs are normal. Abdominal examination demonstrates mild, nonspecific diffuse tenderness without guarding or rebound. Bowel sounds are present. Laboratory results are normal except for a WBC count of 11,000/μL. Abdominal radiography demonstrates a nonspecific gas pattern. Enzyme immunoassay detects the presence of *Clostridium difficile* toxin A. His symptoms improve with a 10-day course of oral metronidazole, but diarrhea recurs within 1 week, and enzyme immunoassay again detects *C difficile* toxin A.

Which of the following should be prescribed next?

(A) Rifampin and metronidazole
(B) Metronidazole
(C) Vancomycin
(D) Cholestyramine
(E) *Saccharomyces boulardii*

ANSWER: B

Clostridium difficile, the most common enteric pathogen, can colonize the large intestine of patients taking antibiotics. Infection can be asymptomatic, or symptoms can range from mild diarrhea to fulminant pseudomembranous colitis. Recent outbreaks of *C difficile* infection in North America have been due to a more virulent and possibly more resistant strain (BI/NAP1) that causes more severe disease.

The offending antibiotic must be stopped immediately, and medications with antiperistaltic activity avoided unless absolutely necessary. The CDC recommends that oral metronidazole be used as first-line therapy rather than vancomycin for all but seriously ill patients and those with complicated or fulminant infections or multiple recurrences. Most sources suggest stopping treatment after 10 days if symptoms have resolved (SOE=C); complicated cases may require longer or individualized treatment regimens (SOE=D). Metronidazole is less expensive than vancomycin, and its use avoids the risk of colonization with vancomycin-resistant organisms. Metronidazole and vancomycin are equally effective for treatment of mild *C difficile*–associated disease; vancomycin is superior for treating severe *C difficile*–associated disease (SOE=A). A trial of combination rifampin and metronidazole therapy for first-episode cases found the combination to be no better than therapy with metronidazole alone.

Despite successful initial therapy, *C difficile* infection recurs in >20% of patients. Typically, relapse does not result in progression of disease or symptom severity. First relapses should be treated with the original medical regimen: up to 90% of cases can be treated successfully on first recurrence with the agent that was initially used (SOE=C).

Different regimens are used for patients with multiple relapses. These include continuous or pulsed dosing of oral vancomycin, anion exchange resins such as cholestyramine or colestipol that bind to *C difficile* toxins in the colon, probiotics (ie, *Saccharomyces boulardii, Lactobacillus rhamnosus* strain GG, and *Lactobacillus acidophilus*), intravenous immunoglobulin, and feces transplant. All of these measures are successful some of the time, but none is successful all of the time.

References

1. Bartlett JG. Historical perspectives on studies of *Clostridium difficile* and *C. difficile* infection. *Clin Infect Dis*. 2008;46(Suppl 1):S4–11.
2. Gerding DN, Muto CA, Owens RC Jr. Treatment of *Clostridium difficile* infection. *Clin Infect Dis*. 2008;46(Suppl 1):S32–42.
3. Kelly CP, LaMont, JT. *Clostridium difficile*—more difficult than ever. *N Engl J Med*. 2008;359(18):1932–1940.
4. Surowiec D, Kuyumjian AG, Wynd MA, et al. Past, present, and future therapies for *Clostridium difficile*-associated disease. *Ann Pharmacother*. 2006;40(12):2155–2163.
5. Zar FA, Bakkanagari SR, Moorthi KM, et al. A comparison of vancomycin and metronidazole for the treatment of *Clostridium difficile*-associated diarrhea, stratified by disease severity. *Clin Infect Dis*. 2007;45(3):302–307.
6. http://www.cdc.gov/ncidod/dhqp/id_Cdiff.html (accessed Nov 2009).

226. Which of the following is the mostly likely cause of new onset vaginal bleeding in a 70-yr-old woman?

(A) Pyometra
(B) Endometrial cancer
(C) Endometrial hyperplasia
(D) Vaginal atrophy
(E) Hormonal effect

ANSWER: D

Vaginal atrophy is the most common cause of postmenopausal bleeding (SOE=A). In a series of 1,138 postmenopausal women (49–91 yr old) who had bleeding, atrophy was the histopathologic diagnosis in 59% of cases. Polyp was the next most frequent cause (12% of cases). Endometrial cancer and hyperplasia caused about 10% of cases, and hormonal effect caused 7%. Cervical cancer accounted for <1% of postmenopausal bleeding. Other causes (eg, hydrometra, pyometra, and hematometra) combined accounted for 2%. Even though 95% of postmenopausal bleeding is due to benign causes, all postmenopausal women with unexpected vaginal bleeding should be evaluated for endometrial cancer, because it is highly treatable.

Vaginal and endometrial atrophy is caused by hypoestrogenism. Classic findings include a pale, dry vaginal epithelium that is smooth and shiny, is easily friable, and has decreased rugae. Atrophic endometrial surfaces in the uterus contain little or no fluid to prevent intracavitary friction. This results in microerosions of the surface epithelium and subsequent chronic inflammatory reaction. The inflammatory reaction produces a chronic endometritis, which is prone to light bleeding or spotting.

The main objective in evaluating postmenopausal bleeding is to exclude cancer. Endometrial biopsy is the initial diagnostic test. If the patient cannot tolerate biopsy in the office, then transvaginal ultrasonography is an alternative. A biopsy is not required if the endometrial lining is <4–5 mm thick and appears homogeneous, without increased echogenicity (SOE=A).

Unless contraindicated, systemic or local estrogen is the most effective treatment for vaginal atrophy. Vaginal administration minimizes systemic absorption, although it can increase plasma levels of estrogen. Local estrogen applications include low-dose creams, rings, and tablets. One strategy is low-dose vaginal estrogen cream 0.5 g/d for 3 wk, with twice-weekly administration thereafter. The estradiol ring (Estring) delivers 6–9 mcg of estradiol to the vagina daily for 3 mo. The vaginal estrogen tablet (Vagifem) is usually recommended every day for 2 wk, then twice weekly. Progestins are not prescribed routinely for women treated with low-dose vaginal estrogen. In women with breast cancer, vaginal estrogen is not used for symptoms of urogenital atrophy unless recommended by the woman's oncologist.

References

1. Ferenczy A. Pathophysiology of endometrial bleeding. *Maturitas*. 2003;45(1):1–14.
2. Moodley M, Roberts C. Clinical pathway for the evaluation of postmenopausal bleeding with an emphasis on endometrial cancer detection. *J Obstet Gynaecol*. 2008;24(7):736–741.

227. A 69-yr-old woman is brought to the emergency department because she has uncontrolled pain. Yesterday, she woke up with excruciating pain in her left hip and lower spine, leaving her unable to walk. She has breast cancer with known metastases in the spine and liver. Until now she had been comfortable with a standing dose of hydrocodone 5 mg and acetaminophen 500 mg q8h. Examination in the emergency department reveals new metastatic lesions in her left femur and in her L1 and L2 vertebrae.

She is admitted to the hospital and started on patient-controlled analgesia with intravenous hydromorphone. Her pain is well controlled within 1 hour and she is able to rest. Several hours later, nausea develops, and she has 2 episodes of vomiting. The next morning, she is pain free, but nausea is still present. Repeat physical examination and laboratory studies disclose no new findings.

Which of the following is most appropriate for this patient?

(A) Discontinue patient-controlled hydromorphone.
(B) Halve the dosage of hydromorphone.
(C) Start metoclopramide 5 mg po q6h around the clock for 2 days.
(D) Start metoclopramide 5 mg po q6h as needed for nausea and vomiting.
(E) Start ondansetron 8 mg po q12h as needed for nausea and vomiting.

ANSWER: C

Short-term, around-the-clock metoclopramide is the best treatment choice for this patient's nausea and vomiting (SOE=C). Nausea and vomiting develop in up to 40% of patients receiving opioids. Typically, opioid-induced nausea and vomiting occur with initiation or dose escalation of the opioid. Usually symptoms resolve within 3–5 days of continued opioid use. Opioid-related nausea and vomiting can be caused by constipation, stimulation of the chemoreceptor trigger zone (CTZ), and gastroparesis. The effects in the CTZ are primarily mediated by central dopamine type 2 (D_2) receptors, and gastroparesis is mostly mediated by peripheral D_2 receptors. Metoclopramide is a central and peripheral D_2-receptor antagonist. It has central antiemetic effects by blocking D_2 receptors in the CTZ, and peripheral antiemetic effects by blocking peripheral D_2 receptors and improving motility. Metoclopramide should be prescribed around-the-clock for the first several days and then tapered off. Because the patient's nausea is persistent and is expected to last only a few days, the metoclopramide should not be offered only as needed.

Because the patient's pain is under excellent control, discontinuation of hydromorphone is not appropriate, nor should the dosage be halved, which would likely result in inadequate analgesia. If nausea persists after 3–5 days of treatment with hydromorphone despite a trial of around-the-clock metoclopramide, then reducing the hydromorphone dosage by 10%–20% may be reasonable. If her nausea does not resolve or analgesia is ineffective, then discontinuation of hydromorphone and a trial of a different opioid are appropriate.

Ondansetron is a serotonin 5-HT$_3$ receptor antagonist that reduces the activity of the vagus nerve, which activates the vomiting center in the medulla oblongata and blocks central serotonin receptors in the CTZ and peripheral serotonin receptors in the gut. It does not have any effect on dopamine receptors or muscarinic receptors. It typically is used to treat nausea and vomiting caused by chemotherapy. Ondansetron is costly and should not be used as first-line therapy in opioid-induced nausea.

References

1. Naeim A, Dy SM, Lorenz KA, et al. Evidence-based recommendations for cancer nausea and vomiting. *J Clin Oncol.* 2008;26(23):3903–3910.
2. Wood GJ, Shega JW, Lynch B, et al. Management of intractable nausea and vomiting in patients at the end of life "I was feeling nauseous all of the time . . . nothing was working." *JAMA.* 2007;298(10):1196–1207.

228. A 75-yr-old man comes to the office for his annual visit. He has a family history of heart disease and wonders whether he would benefit from taking aspirin. He exercises frequently. History includes borderline dyslipidemia. On examination, blood pressure is 130/70 mmHg.

Which of the following is true about the role of aspirin in primary prevention?

(A) Enteric coating decreases the risk of aspirin-related GI bleeding.
(B) The recommended dosage for primary prevention is 325 mg/d.
(C) Aspirin reduces the number of cardiovascular events in men.
(D) Aspirin reduces the risk of ischemic stroke in men.

ANSWER: C

The role of aspirin in primary prevention of ischemic stroke and cardiovascular events has been studied with varying results for years. Several randomized, controlled trials demonstrate that aspirin reduces the risk of myocardial infarction in men (SOE=A). Depending on the study and the risk factors of the cohort, the number needed to treat to prevent one myocardial infarction over 5 yr ranges from 65 to 667. The randomized trials did not show a reduction in death or ischemic stroke, but they were underpowered to assess these outcomes.

Study results have been mixed regarding the role of aspirin in primary prevention of heart disease in women. In the Nurses' Health Study, fewer cardiovascular events were observed in women ≥55 yr old who used aspirin, but aspirin did not prevent stroke or death from any cause. In contrast, the Women's Health Study showed a decrease in stroke but not in cardiovascular events for women taking aspirin 100 mg every other day.

The current consensus is to consider the individual patient's risk of coronary artery disease, including sex, age, diabetes, cholesterol level, blood pressure, and smoking and family history. Organizations such as the U.S. Preventive Services Task Force recommend aspirin for patients in whom the risk of coronary artery disease in 5 yr is ≥3%.

The optimal dose of aspirin for men appears to be between 75 mg and 160 mg daily or every other day. Enteric-coated preparations do not decrease the risk of GI bleeding. Over a 5-yr period, aspirin causes GI bleeding in 4 to 12 per 1,000 older adults, and hemorrhagic stroke in 0 to 2 per 1,000 adults. These risks are likely higher in patients who have uncontrolled hypertension, use NSAIDs, or are >75 yr old, and in patients taking higher dosages of aspirin.

References

1. Berger JS, Roncaglioni MC, Avanzini F, et al. Aspirin for the primary prevention of cardiovascular events in women and men: a sex-specific meta-analysis of randomized controlled trials. *JAMA*. 2006;295(17):306–313.
2. U.S. Preventive Services Task Force. Aspirin for the primary prevention of cardiovascular events: recommendations and rationale. *Ann Intern Med*. 2002;136(2):157–160.

229. A 75-yr-old man comes to the office because he has increased pain related to osteoarthritis. At his last office visit 2 wk earlier, pain level was 3 of 10; it is now 5 of 10. In addition to osteoarthritis, he has type 2 diabetes mellitus, chronic kidney disease, and major depressive disorder, which was diagnosed at his last office visit. His current medications include codeine 30 mg/acetaminophen 300 mg, 2 tablets q6h; glipizide 10 mg q12h; NPH insulin 20 U at bedtime; aspirin 81 mg/d; and most recently, paroxetine 20 mg/d.

Which of the following is the best option for managing his pain?

(A) Increase codeine/acetaminophen dosage.
(B) Change codeine/acetaminophen to oxycodone/acetaminophen.
(C) Change codeine/acetaminophen to propoxyphene/acetaminophen.
(D) Add ibuprofen 200 mg q6h.
(E) Discontinue paroxetine.

ANSWER: B

This patient may have less pain relief with codeine because of an interaction between paroxetine and codeine. Codeine, a prodrug, essentially has no analgesic activity. In the liver, it is metabolized by CYP2D6 to the active metabolite (ie, morphine), thereby providing pain relief. Paroxetine is a potent inhibitor of CYP2D6 enzyme in the liver; concomitant administration of paroxetine and codeine can result in less of the active metabolite. Although pain relief can be achieved by increasing the dosage of codeine/acetaminophen, changing the narcotic (eg, oxycodone/acetaminophen) is a better choice because the chance of inappropriate acetaminophen dosage is lessened.

Because this patient has chronic kidney disease, ibuprofen should be avoided because it may cause renal function to deteriorate (SOE=A). Propoxyphene should be avoided in older adults because it is not more effective than acetaminophen or ibuprofen (SOE=A), and it has narcotic-related adverse events, including an increased risk of hip fracture (SOE=A). Stopping paroxetine without initiating another treatment for major depressive disorder is not appropriate.

References

1. Hersh EV, Pinto A, Moore PA. Adverse drug interactions involving common prescription and over-the-counter analgesic agents. *Clin Ther*. 2007;29(Suppl):2477–2497.

2. MacLean CH, Pencharz JN, Saag KG. Quality indicators for the care of osteoarthritis in vulnerable elders. *J Am Geriatr Soc.* 2007;55(Suppl 2):S383–391.

3. Shrank WH, Polinski JM, Avorn J. Quality indicators for medication use in vulnerable elders. *J Am Geriatr Soc.* 2007;55(Suppl 2):S373–382.

230. An 85-yr-old woman is brought to the emergency department after she is found on the bathroom floor at home. She has retrograde amnesia for the circumstances surrounding the episode, and denies any confusion after the episode. There were no witnesses. History includes hypertension, for which she takes atenolol 25 mg/d and hydrochlorothiazide 25 mg/d.

On physical examination, she has a right periorbital ecchymosis. Blood pressure is 152/84 mmHg while supine and 146/86 mmHg while upright, and heart rate is 76 beats per minute while supine and 86 beats per minute while upright. There is no jugular venous distension or carotid bruit. Lungs are clear. Carotid upstroke is delayed, with a II/VI midpeaking systolic murmur at the base; the second heart sound is not audible.

CT of the head and facial bones shows a large, right periorbital contusion and no fractures.

Which of the following is the most appropriate next step in the evaluation of this patient?

(A) Blood tests
(B) Echocardiography
(C) Holter monitoring
(D) Event monitor
(E) Tilt-table test

ANSWER: B

This patient's clinical history suggests syncope, although in the absence of a definitive history, an unexplained fall is also possible. In older adults, syncope and unexplained falls can be indistinguishable clinical manifestations of the same pathophysiologic process, and for this reason many physicians treat them as the same. This patient's physical examination suggests significant aortic stenosis. While the murmur is not loud and is midpeaking, the absence of a second heart sound indicates potentially severe aortic stenosis. Echocardiography can characterize the degree of aortic stenosis noninvasively. Because structural heart disease is the most important risk factor in unexplained syncope, echocardiography should be the next test ordered.

Echocardiographic findings of severe valvular abnormalities, ventricular hypertrophy with outflow obstruction, severe pulmonary hypertension, and atrial myxoma or thrombus are rare in the absence of a suggestive initial evaluation. In a study of 650 consecutive patients with syncope (average age 60 yr, with 44% of patients ≥75 yr old), echocardiography was useful mainly in confirming suspected severe aortic stenosis and for using ejection fraction to stratify patients with known cardiac disease. Echocardiography was normal or irrelevant in all patients who had no history, physical examination, or electrocardiography suggesting cardiac disease (SOE=A).

Blood tests have an extremely low diagnostic yield for patients with unexplained syncope. For example, hypoglycemia does not result in a transient loss of consciousness but rather requires intervention to reverse the metabolic derangement that could be contributing to symptoms. Unless it uncovers frequent ventricular ectopy or nonsustained ventricular tachycardia, short-term continuous electrocardiographic monitoring, such as telemetry, Holter monitor, or an event monitor, is not useful for identifying the cause of syncope because weeks, months, or even years can pass before the next arrhythmia-related event. Also, most arrhythmias detected in patients with syncope are brief and result in no symptoms.

Triage decisions and management should be based on preexisting cardiac disease or echocardiographic abnormalities, which are important predictors of arrhythmic syncope and mortality, rather than on symptoms. A tilt-table test would be appropriate only after structural heart disease has been excluded.

References
1. Otto CM. Valvular aortic stenosis: disease severity and timing of intervention. *J Am Coll Cardiol.* 2006;47(11):2141–2151.

2. Pires LA, Ganji JR, Jarandila R, et al. Diagnostic patterns and temporal trends in the evaluation of adult patients hospitalized with syncope. *Arch Intern Med.* 2001;161(15):1889–1895.

3. Sarasin FP, Junod AF, Carballo D, et al. Role of echocardiography in the evaluation of syncope: a prospective study. *Heart.* 2002;88(4):363–367.

231. A 69-yr-old black man comes to the office for evaluation because routine laboratory tests showed an increased total calcium concentration (10.8 mg/dL). Three years ago, the concentration was 10.6 mg/dL. He has no symptoms of hypercalcemia, such as nausea, constipation, personality changes, or renal stones. There is a family history of hypertension; he is unaware of any family history of calcium disorders. The patient has an enlarged prostate and hypertension. Medications include amlodipine, hydrochlorothiazide, and saw palmetto. He does not take any vitamin supplements.

On physical examination, blood pressure is 140/80 mmHg, and he has mild prostatic hyperplasia. The remainder of the physical examination is normal. Levels of creatinine and $1,25(OH)_2D$ are normal. Parathyroid hormone concentration is 78 pg/mL and thyrotropin concentration is 2.1 mU/L.

Which of the following tests should be ordered next?

(A) Genetic testing for familial benign hypercalcemia hypocalciuria mutation
(B) 25(OH)D
(C) Parathyroid sestamibi (nuclear scan)
(D) A 24-hour urine collection for calcium and creatinine
(E) Dual x-ray absorptiometry (DEXA) scan of the spine, hip, and forearm

ANSWER: B

Although this patient's increased calcium and parathyroid hormone levels suggest primary hyperparathyroidism, it is also possible that the hypercalcemia is due to the thiazide he takes, and that the increased parathyroid hormone is secondary to vitamin D deficiency. An appropriate approach would be to switch to a different class of antihypertensive medications and to check the level of 25(OH)D, which is the best measure of the body's vitamin D stores. The $1,25(OH)_2D$ level is often not helpful in diagnosing vitamin D deficiency because its production is tightly regulated by the kidney, and the serum concentration is often normal (SOE=C).

Vitamin D deficiency is found in up to 50% of older adults. Darker-skinned people have reduced synthesis of vitamin D because of decreased absorption of ultraviolet B radiation. Epidemiologic studies have shown that low levels of vitamin D are linked not only to decreased calcium absorption and bone mineralization, but also to poorer physical performance (SOE=B), frailty, falls (SOE=A), risk of cardiovascular disease (SOE=B), and increased incidence of cancers (SOE=B).

Genetic testing for familial benign hypercalcemia hypocalciuria is not indicated until the previous steps are taken, and then only if hypocalciuria is confirmed on a 24-hour urine collection for calcium and creatinine. Familial benign hypercalcemia hypocalciuria is usually asymptomatic. Previously increased calcium concentrations are an important diagnostic clue (SOE=C).

Parathyroid sestamibi (nuclear scan) and DEXA scans of the forearm would be appropriate if primary hyperparathyroidism turns out to be the diagnosis. Localization of an adenoma via nuclear scan would allow a surgeon to remove a gland through minimally invasive surgery. The DEXA scan, together with other laboratory findings and patient symptoms, would help in determining whether the primary hyperparathyroidism should be managed medically or surgically (SOE=C). No randomized trials demonstrate a reduction in fractures in patients undergoing surgery rather than medical treatment.

References

1. Broe KE, Chen TC, Weinberg J, et al. A higher dose of vitamin D reduces the risk of falls in nursing home residents. *J Am Geriatr Soc.* 2007;55(2):234–239.
2. Holick MF. Vitamin D deficiency. *N Engl J Med.* 2007;357(3):266–281.
3. Lappe JM, Travers-Gustafson D, Davies KM, et al. Vitamin D and calcium supplementation reduces cancer risk. *Am J Clin Nutr.* 2007;85(6):1586–1591.
4. Wang TJ, Pencina MJ, Booth SL, et al. Vitamin D deficiency and risk of cardiovascular disease. *Circulation.* 2008;117(4):503–511.
5. Wicherts IS, van Schoor NM, Boeke JP, et al. Vitamin D status predicts physical performance and its decline in older persons. *J Clin Endocrinol Metab.* 2007;92(6):2058–2065.

232. Which of the following is most likely to facilitate recovery of gait after a stroke?

(A) Neurophysiologic approaches (Bobath approach)
(B) Neuromuscular facilitation
(C) Transcutaneous electrical stimulation
(D) Electromechanics-assisted gait training with physical therapy

ANSWER: D

Recovery of gait is one of the most desired functions after a stroke, because it reduces caregiver burden and promotes independence. Several interventions have been developed to facilitate recovery of gait, but there is little evidence from randomized, controlled trials in regard to their effectiveness.

A Cochrane Collaboration review of trials showed that electromechanics-assisted gait training combined with physical therapy increased the likelihood of independence in walking and increased walking capacity, but did not increase walking speed significantly (SOE=A). However, another Cochrane review found no evidence that the outcomes vary according to different traditional physical therapy approaches (SOE=A). While it is clear that a multidisciplinary, stroke-specific rehabilitation program leads to better outcomes, it is difficult to show that one specific therapy technique is better than another.

References

1. Mehrholz J, Werner C, Kugler J, et al. Electromechanical-assisted training for walking after stroke. *Cochrane Database Syst Rev.* 2007;(4):CD006185.
2. Pollock A, Baer G, Pomeroy V, et al. Physiotherapy treatment approaches for the recovery of postural control and lower limb function following stroke. *Cochrane Database Syst Rev.* 2007;(1):CD001920.

233. A 68-yr-old woman comes to the office for follow-up related to asthma. She has had asthma for 50 yr. For the past 4 mo, she has had intermittent wheezing, cough, and dyspnea approximately 3 days per week, relieved by 2 puffs of albuterol. In the last month she has awakened 3 times coughing and wheezing. Asthma does not impair her ability to do normal activities. Her last exacerbation requiring oral corticosteroids was 2 yr ago. Her asthma control test (ACT) score is 18. She uses low-dose inhaled corticosteroid every day and albuterol as needed. Vital signs and lung and cardiac examination are normal. Peak flow is normal.

Which of the following is the most appropriate next step?

(A) Add a leukotriene-modifying agent.
(B) Add a long-acting β_2-agonist.
(C) Add a long-acting anticholinergic agent.
(D) Discontinue the inhaled corticosteroid.
(E) Continue the present regimen.

ANSWER: B

The first step is to determine whether the patient's asthma is adequately controlled. Guidelines from the National Asthma Education and Prevention Program, which are not age specific, divide asthma status into well controlled, not well controlled, and very poorly controlled. The components of control are differentiated by impairment and risk. Determinants of *impairment* include symptom frequency, frequency of need for short-acting β_2-agonist (does not include use for prevention of exercise-induced bronchospasm), interference with normal activity, answers to validated questionnaires such as the ACT, and objective measures of lung function (FEV$_1$ or peak expiratory flow [PEF]). Determinants of *risk* include frequency of exacerbations, progressive loss of lung function, and treatment-related adverse events.

A patient's asthma is considered well controlled if *all* of the following criteria are met: Symptoms occur ≤2 days per week; short-acting β_2-agonist is used for symptom control ≤2 days per week; nocturnal awakenings are ≤2 per month; there is no interference with normal activity; ACT score is ≥20; FEV$_1$ or PEF is >80% of predicted or personal best (preferred); and there is ≤1 exacerbation per year.

Asthma is not well controlled if *any* of the following criteria are met: Symptoms occur >2 days per week but not throughout the day; short-acting β_2-agonist is used for symptom control >2 days per week but not several times per day; there are ≥3 nocturnal awakenings per month; there is some (limited) interference with normal activity; ACT score is between 16 and 19; FEV$_1$ or PEF is between 60% and 80% of predicted or personal best; and there are 2 or 3 exacerbations per year.

Asthma is considered very poorly controlled if it exceeds *any* of the criteria for not well controlled. A patient is placed in the highest category for which he or she has even a single criterion.

If asthma has been well controlled for ≥3 mo, therapy can be decreased (step-down). Asthma that is not well controlled or that is very poorly controlled requires an increase (step-up) in therapy; for asthma that is very poorly controlled, increasing therapy by 2 steps plus a short course of oral corticosteroids may be appropriate.

This patient's asthma meets criteria for not well controlled, and she requires a step-up in treatment. The best step-up treatment for a patient on low-dose inhaled corticosteroid is the addition of a long-acting β_2-agonist such as formoterol or salmeterol (SOE=A). A long-acting β_2-agonist plus low-dose inhaled corticosteroid results in superior asthma control compared with increasing the dosage of inhaled corticosteroid and adding a leukotriene-modifying agent such as montelukast or zafirlukast (SOE=A). If there is concern about the potential adverse events of long-acting β_2-agonists, increasing the dosage of inhaled corticosteroids is a reasonable option (SOE=A).

References

1. Ind PW, Dal Negro R, Colman NC, et al. Addition of salmeterol to fluticasone propionate treatment in moderate-to-severe asthma. *Respir Med.* 2003;97(5):555–562.
2. Masoli M, Weatherall M, Holt S, et al. Moderate dose inhaled corticosteroids plus salmeterol versus higher doses of inhaled corticosteroids in symptomatic asthma. *Thorax.* 2005;60(9):730–734.
3. Nelson HS, Weiss ST, Bleecker ER, et al. The Salmeterol Multicenter Asthma Research Trial: a comparison of usual pharmacotherapy for asthma or usual pharmacotherapy plus salmeterol. *Chest.* 2006;129(1):15–26. Erratum in: *Chest* 2006;129(5):1393.
4. National Heart, Lung and Blood Institute. Expert panel report (EPR) 3: Guidelines for the diagnosis and management of asthma; 2007. http://www.nhlbi.nih.gov/guidelines/asthma/asthgdln.htm (accessed Nov 2009).

234. An 82-yr-old man living in a nursing facility is evaluated because of gradual functional decline. He has lost 4.5 kg (7% of body weight) since he entered the nursing facility 6 mo ago after hospitalization for acute myocardial infarction. During that hospitalization, type 2 diabetes was diagnosed. In the nursing home he has remained hyperglycemic, with periodic blood glucose concentrations spiking to 300 mg/dL and a recent hemoglobin A_{1c} level of 7.9 g/dL. He is on an American Diabetic Association low-fat diet. He takes several medications, including glipizide, pravastatin, hydrochlorothiazide, metoprolol, lisinopril, and aspirin.

Laboratory results:

Creatinine	1.4 mg/dL
Low-density lipoprotein	100 mg/dL
High-density lipoprotein	34 mg/dL
Triglycerides	170 mg/dL

Which of the following is the most appropriate next step in management of this patient?

(A) Increase glipizide dosage.
(B) Add metformin.
(C) Add acarbose.
(D) Add niacin.
(E) Liberalize his diet.

ANSWER: E

Older adults with recently diagnosed diabetes, other chronic disease, and functional impairment are at high risk of micro- and especially macrovascular complications of diabetes. This patient is at especially grave risk of medical complications and death because of his weight loss and functional decline. Moreover, changes in his medication regimen carry added risk for him. The most rational approach in this exceptionally vulnerable patient is also the most conservative: make no change in his (already complex) regimen of multiple medications and increase his caloric intake (SOE=D).

Increasing the dose of glipizide to lower this patient's hemoglobin A_{1c} level (to below <7 g/dL) might increase his risk of hypoglycemia and death (SOE=A). Marginal renal function is likely, given his creatinine level of 1.4 mg/dL and probable low muscle mass. Adding metformin to glipizide might increase anorexia and the risk of lactic acidosis. When this approach was tried in the United Kingdom Prospective Diabetes Study (albeit in individuals who were overweight and diabetic), the death rate was unexpectedly increased (SOE=A).

Adding acarbose to his current dose of glipizide might reduce his hyperglycemia and possibly moderate postprandial glycemic excursions. However, acarbose has common and predictable GI adverse events (eg, flatulence, diarrhea) that often limit compliance in patients with diabetes. In this patient with progressive weight loss and functional decline, acarbose is inappropriate and perhaps unsafe (SOE =D). Also, addition of acarbose would complicate an already complex regimen. The first priority is to stop his weight loss.

Niacin is associated with increased levels of high-density lipoprotein and reduced triglyceride levels. It would be unlikely to lower this patient's low-density lipoprotein level (the additional benefit of which would be controversial in any event); moreover, his high-density lipoprotein and triglyceride levels are as likely attributable to his frailty and marginal nutritional status as to his diabetes (SOE=D). Niacin also might exacerbate his hyperglycemia.

References

1. Abraira C, Colwell J, Nuttall F, et al. Cardiovascular events and correlates in the Veterans Affairs Diabetes Feasibility Trial. Veterans Affairs Cooperative Study on Glycemic Control and Complications in Type II Diabetes. *Arch Intern Med*. 1997;157(2):181–188.
2. American Diabetes Association. Standards of medical care in diabetes—2008. *Diabetes Care*. 2008;31(Suppl 1):S1–11.
3. California Healthcare Foundation/American Geriatrics Society Panel on Improving Care for Elders with Diabetes. Guidelines for Improving the Care of the Older Person with Diabetes Mellitus. *J Am Geriatr Soc*. 2003;51(5 Suppl Guidelines):S265–280. http://www.americangeriatrics.org/products/positionpapers/JAGSfinal05.pdf (accessed Nov 2009).
4. Chang AM, Halter JB. Diabetes mellitus. In: Halter JB, Hazzard WR, Ouslander JG, et al. *Hazzard's Geriatric Medicine and Gerontology*, 6th ed. NY: McGraw-Hill; 2009:1305–1324.

235. A 65-yr-old woman comes to the office because she has a deep, burning pain and drainage of clear fluid in the left ear. In addition, 4 days after onset of ear pain, spontaneous vertigo developed, and she noted a high-pitched tinnitus in the left ear.

On examination, she has a right-beating, horizontal-torsional nystagmus that increases when she looks to the right and decreases when she looks to the left. She has hearing loss in the left ear, and Weber test lateralizes to the right. She also has upper and lower left facial paralysis.

Which of the following is the most appropriate treatment?

(A) Positioning maneuver
(B) Antibiotics and intravenous fluids
(C) Steroids and antiviral agents
(D) Intravenous tissue plasminogen activator
(E) Surgical correction with prosthesis

ANSWER: C

The most likely diagnosis is herpes zoster oticus, a varicella zoster viral infection of the eighth cranial nerve (Ramsay Hunt syndrome). This usually begins with a deep, burning pain in the ear, followed by a vesicular eruption in the external auditory canal and concha. There may be associated hearing loss, vertigo, and peripheral facial weakness (upper and lower). MRI with gadolinium may be indicated to exclude other infectious causes, eg, suppu-

rative bacterial labyrinthitis. Treatment of Ramsay Hunt syndrome with combination high-dose steroids and acyclovir appears to be superior to treatment with steroids alone (SOE=A).

A positioning maneuver, used for benign paroxysmal positional vertigo, is not indicated for Ramsay Hunt syndrome. Antibiotics would be indicated for suppurative labyrinthitis with purulent exudate. Surgical correction with a prosthesis can be used in otosclerosis for correction of air-bone gap hearing loss.

References

1. Kinishi M, Amatsu M, Mohri M, et al. Acyclovir improves recovery rate of facial nerve palsy in Ramsay Hunt Syndrome. *Auris Nasus Larynx*. 2001;28(3):223–226.
2. Uscategui T, Dorée C, Chamberlain IJ, et al. Antiviral therapy for Ramsay Hunt syndrome (herpes zoster oticus with facial palsy) in adults. *Cochrane Database System Rev*. 2008;(4):CD006851.
3. Van Den Bossche P, Van Den Bossche K, Vanpoucke H. Laryngeal zoster with multiple cranial nerve palsies. *Eur Arch Otorhinolaryngol*. 2008;265(3):365–367.

236. Which of the following is the most accurate office screening tool for physiologic hearing loss in older adults?

(A) Whisper test
(B) Hearing Handicap Inventory for the Elderly–Screening Version
(C) Handheld audioscope
(D) Rubbing fingers next to the patient's ears
(E) Holding vibrating tuning fork next to the patient's ears

ANSWER: C

Hearing loss affects 25%–40% of adults ≥65 yr old in the United States. Age-associated hearing loss is insidious and is often not reported by patients until it is moderate or severe. Hearing loss can be a major handicap and cause functional decline, depression, and delirium in susceptible people (SOE=B). The U.S. Preventive Services Task Force recommends routine screening of hearing for all adults ≥65 yr old (SOE=C). The AudioScope is an otoscope that emits 20-, 25-, and 40-dB hearing level tones at 500 Hz, 1000 Hz, 2000 Hz, and 4000 Hz. The device is recommended by the Canadian Task Force on the Periodic Health Examination (SOE=C). It is a physiologic test and most accurate with the 40-dB tone at 2000 Hz (94% sensitivity and 69%–80% specificity for hearing loss). Further evaluation is recommended for patients who cannot hear this tone in either ear.

The Hearing Handicap Inventory for the Elderly–Screening Version comprises 10 questions and has acceptable sensitivity and specificity, but it tests for functional hearing loss and often misses mild hearing loss.

The whisper test is not a standardized reproducible test. Its results can vary from one examiner to the next, because hearing is affected by distance, content of speech, and background noise. Rubbing fingers and holding a vibrating tuning fork next to the patient's ears are also not accurate or reproducible tests.

References

1. Medwetsky L. Hearing loss. In: Duthie EH, Katz PR, Malone ML, eds. *Practice of Geriatrics*. 4th ed. Philadelphia: Saunders; 2007:41–53.
2. Yueh B, Collins MP, Souza PE, et al. Screening for Auditory Impairment–Which Hearing Assessment Test (SAI–WHAT): RCT design and baseline characteristics. *Contemp Clin Trials*. 2007;28(3):303–315.
3. Yueh B, Shapiro N, MacLean CH, et al. Screening and management of adult hearing loss in primary care: scientific review. *JAMA*. 2003;289(15):1976–1985.

237. A 77-yr-old woman comes to the office because she has frequent falls. She has difficulty walking unassisted and frequently feels that her feet get tangled together. She is also urinating more frequently. She has no burning on urination, fever, chills, or flank pain.

On examination, there are no significant abnormalities of joints in the limbs. There is good mobility of the lumbar spine and mild immobility of the cervical spine, with 45-degree rotation to the right and left and limited extension. Arm reflexes are 2+, with occasional fasciculations in the biceps and triceps muscles. Hoffmann's sign is present in both hands. There is increased tone in the lower extremities. Reflexes are 3+ at the knees and ankles. Both toes are upgoing.

Which of the following is the most appropriate next step?

(A) Bone scan
(B) MRI of the lumbar spine
(C) MRI of the cervical spine
(D) Radiography of the cervical spine
(E) Radiography of the thoracic spine

ANSWER: C

This patient has symptoms and signs of cervical spinal stenosis (ie, cervical myelopathy). The most significant physical findings are upper motor neuron signs in the legs (increased muscle tone, increased reflexes, and upgoing toes) with both lower (fasciculations) and upper motor neuron signs (Hoffmann's signs) in the hands. Hoffmann's test involves flicking the terminal phalanx of the third finger; if the terminal phalanx of the thumb flexes into the palm, the test is positive. (This is analogous to the Babinski sign for the lower extremities.) The presence of Hoffmann's sign indicates interruption of the corticospinal tract, usually in the cervical spine.

Any patient with gait disorders and increased frequency of urination should be evaluated for cervical myelopathy. MRI of the cervical spine is the most appropriate study (SOE=D).

MRI of the lumbar spine would not be helpful, because this patient has upper motor neuron signs indicating disease above L1 (SOE=D). Tumor of the cervical spine rarely causes cervical myelopathy. A much more common cause is cervical spinal stenosis. Plain radiography of the cervical spine is not likely to be helpful, because 80% of radiographs are abnormal in adults ≥55 yr old (SOE=D).

Radiography of the thoracic spine would not be helpful, because the presence of Hoffmann's sign in both hands indicates stenosis of the cervical spine, not the thoracic spine (SOE=D). A bone scan cannot demonstrate compression of the spinal cord and is not indicated in this patient.

References

1. Baron EM, Young W. Cervical spondylitic myelopathy: a brief review of its pathophysiology, clinical course, and diagnosis. *Neurosurgery*. 2007;60(Suppl 1):35–41.
2. Rao R. Neck pain, cervical radiculopathy, and cervical myelopathy. *J Bone Joint Surg*. 2002;84A:1872–1881.
3. Salvi FJ, Jones JC, Weigert BJ. The assessment of cervical myelopathy. *Spine J*. 2006;6(6 Suppl):182S–189S.

238. Which of the following statements describing response to common homeostatic challenges is true?

(A) Aging is associated with increased complexity of responses to auditory frequencies.
(B) Aging is associated with a decreased ability to respond to glucose challenges.
(C) Hypothermia in older adults exposed to cold temperatures is caused primarily by decreased thermogenesis.
(D) When exposed to stress, older adults have a shorter period of activation of the sympathetic nervous system than younger adults.

ANSWER: B

Aging is associated with a variety of well-described deficits in the ability of cells, tissues, and organisms to respond to common homeostatic challenges. For example, older adults are less able to maintain normal glucose levels in response to oral or intravenous glucose challenges. While both insulin secretion and tissue sensitivity to insulin decline in old age, tissue insulin responsiveness is heavily influenced by changes in body composition and physical activity.

Although many physiologic parameters remain relatively unchanged with age when measured at a single point in time, the complexity of their behavior often declines with aging when more extensive measurements and analyses are conducted. Examples of physiologic variables that decline in terms of complexity with age include narrowing of auditory frequency responsiveness, decreased long-range correlations in time-series data such as blood pressure measurements, and increased randomness or stochastic activity in terms of cardiac intervals. Together with declines in structural complexity of bone microarchitecture and brain connectivity, these changes increase the vulnerability of older adults when confronting common homeostatic challenges.

Older adults are less able to maintain a normal body temperature when exposed to low environmental temperatures. Multiple relevant mechanisms include decreased sensation of cold, declines in shivering intensity, inadequate thermogenesis, and poor vasoconstriction; inadequate thermogenesis is not the primary cause.

When exposed to physical or emotional stress, older adults demonstrate greater and more prolonged activation of both sympathetic (eg, norepinephrine levels) and hypothalamic-pituitary-adrenal (eg, cortisol levels) systems than younger adults.

A key impact of aging on homeostatic mechanisms is also reflected in the observation that older adults are often able to respond adequately to individual homeostatic challenges, yet become vulnerable when exposed to more than one concurrent challenge. For example, many healthy older adults who maintain normal blood pressure in response to orthostasis or mild diuretic-induced sodium depletion are unable to do so in the face of both challenges.

References

1. Kuchel GA. Aging and Homeostatic Regulation. In: Halter JB, Hazzard WR, Ouslander JG, et al, eds. *Hazzard's Principles of Geriatric Medicine and Gerontology*, 6th ed. New York: McGraw Hill; 2009.
2. Lipsitz LA. Dynamics of stability: the physiologic basis of functional health and frailty. *J Gerontol A Biol Sci Med Sci*. 2002;57(3):B115–B125.
3. Szoke E, Shrayyef MZ, Messing S, et al. Effect of aging on glucose homeostasis: accelerated deterioration of beta-cell function in individuals with impaired glucose tolerance. *Diabetes Care*. 2008;31(3):539–543.

239. A 74-yr-old woman comes to the clinic because she has urinary incontinence. She loses urine when she coughs, laughs, sneezes, and lifts objects, but not on her way to the bathroom or when she washes her hands. She has no urinary urgency. She uses estrogen cream vaginally.

On pelvic examination, a cough produces a dribble and a slight anterior-to-posterior bulge of the bladder and vagina. The vaginal mucosa is pink and not friable. There is no fecal impaction. Prevoid ultrasonography of the bladder shows 200 mL of urine. A cough test when the patient stands upright demonstrates urine leakage, with spots covering one-third of a washcloth that she held against her perineum. After normal emptying of the bladder, ultrasonography shows postvoid residual volume of 15 mL.

Which of the following is the most appropriate next step?

(A) Discuss the different benefits and risks of behavioral management and surgery.
(B) Assess cognitive status before beginning oxybutynin.
(C) Review breast cancer history before beginning oral estrogen therapy.
(D) Administer antibiotic prophylaxis before urodynamic testing.
(E) Measure orthostatic blood pressure and pulse before beginning an α-blocker.

ANSWER: A

Patients' preferences for treatment of urinary incontinence should be elicited before starting therapy (SOE=C). In this patient, the demonstration of urine leakage with a standing cough test is highly predictive of stress urinary incontinence (SOE=A). There are far fewer pharmacologic treatments for stress incontinence than for urge incontinence. Behavioral therapy (including exercises of the pelvic floor muscle) and surgery are more effective than pharmacologic agents for stress incontinence in women (SOE=A). Oxybutynin is not effective for stress incontinence (SOE=A).

Oral estrogen therapy worsens symptoms of urinary incontinence; indeed, its use increases the likelihood that incontinence will develop (SOE=A). α-Adrenergic antagonists (α-blockers) are not effective for stress incontinence in women (SOE=B).

Urodynamic testing can help determine whether uninhibited detrusor contractions are present during the filling phase of a diagnostic study (SOE=A). Uninhibited detrusor contractions are associated with persistence of urge incontinence after surgery. It is premature to begin urodynamic testing until treatment preferences are determined.

References

1. Hendrix SL, Cochrane BB, Nygaard IE, et al. Effects of estrogen with and without progestin on urinary incontinence. *JAMA*. 2005;293(8):935–948.
2. Holroyd-Leduc JM, Tannenbaum C, Thorpe KE, et al. What type of urinary incontinence does this woman have? *JAMA*. 2008;299(12):1446–1456.
3. Rogers RG. Clinical practice. Urinary stress incontinence in women. *N Engl J Med*. 2008;358(10):1029–1036.
4. Shamliyan TA, Kane RL, Wyman J, et al. Systemic review: randomized, controlled trials of nonsurgical treatments for urinary incontinence in women. *Ann Intern Med*. 2008;148(6):459–473.

240. A 72-yr-old woman comes to the office because of persistent pain in her left hip. History includes osteoarthritis, as well as a life-threatening episode of GI bleeding related to use of NSAIDs. Oral acetaminophen 1000 mg q6h decreases the pain for a short time. She follows her physical therapy regimen routinely.

Which of the following is the most appropriate intervention?

(A) Increase acetaminophen to 1,000 mg q4h.
(B) Start ibuprofen 600 mg q6h.
(C) Start oxycodone 2.5 mg q4h as needed.
(D) Start long-acting morphine 15 mg q12h.

ANSWER: C

Following the dosage dictum to "start low and go slow" for older adults, the most appropriate next step is to prescribe oral oxycodone 2.5 mg q4h as needed (SOE=B). If the pain relief remains inadequate, then the dosage can be increased to 5 mg q4h. If the pain relief is adequate and adverse events are tolerable, a long-acting regimen can be introduced. All patients beginning opioid therapy should also be started on a scheduled bowel regimen of an osmotic laxative (eg, lactulose) and a stimulant laxative (eg, senna), with a rescue regimen (eg, bisacodyl suppository or enema).

Increasing the acetaminophen dosage to q4h would be incorrect because the total daily dose would be above the limit for liver toxicity of 4,000 mg/d. Starting ibuprofen is inappropriate given this patient's history of life-threatening GI bleeding with NSAIDs. In an opioid-naive patient, starting long-acting morphine is unsafe before completing a dose-finding trial with a short-acting opioid. If long-acting morphine is started, the patient may have excessive drowsiness or respiratory depression. Once an effective opioid dose is found, changing the patient to a long-acting opioid would be appropriate.

References

1. Lorenz KA, Lynn J, Dy SM, et al. Evidence for improving palliative care at the end of life: a systematic review. *Ann Intern Med*. 2008;148(2):147–159.
2. Stevenson KM, Dahl JL, Berry PH, et al. Institutionalizing effective pain management practices: practice change programs to improve the quality of pain management in small health care organizations. *J Pain Symptom Manage*. 2006;31(3):248–261.

241. A 72-yr-old woman comes to the office to discuss her husband's treatment for recently diagnosed major depressive disorder compounded by anxiety. He is 79, wheelchair-bound, and somewhat less demanding after 4 wk of antidepressant medication at the recommended dosage. She acknowledges he is somewhat better, but she feels nearly "burnt out." You want to reassure her by providing an evidence-based prognosis.

Which of the following is the best advice?

(A) Be patient; depression with anxiety responds as well to antidepressant treatment as does depression alone.
(B) A benzodiazepine can always be added if his symptoms become intolerable.
(C) His partial response predicts a great likelihood of full remission.
(D) Supportive therapy for her will accelerate his response.
(E) It is time to add a second antidepressant (augmentation) to the treatment regimen.

ANSWER: C

The patient's partial response at 4 wk increases the likelihood of full remission (SOE=B). Comorbidity of anxiety and major depressive disorder in later life presents a more severe and treatment-resistant illness than either disorder alone. Functional MRI has demonstrated that the condition is associated with excessive amygdala activity in response to affective stimuli. This is demonstrated clinically by excessive or prolonged rumination about adverse events (SOE=A). Anticipating the adverse events serves to reduce the efficacy of the target medications. The husband may also have mild cognitive decline associated with the prolonged stress of anxiety.

Often, older adults may not achieve full remission with initial antidepressant treatment. In this respect, the Sequenced Treatment Alternatives to Relieve Depression (STAR-D) can provide guidance. Several medications have shown promise in anxious major depressive disorder in older adults, including third-generation antidepressant agents (eg, SSRIs, dual-reuptake inhibitors), first-generation agents (eg, secondary amine tricyclic antidepressants), and second-generation antipsychotics (SOE=A). However, it is too soon to add a second medication.

Psychotherapy may be useful to manage residual anxiety after partial remission and to reduce likelihood of recurrence. Data do not support the use of benzodiazepines or supportive therapy for the spouse.

References

1. Ayers CR, Sorrell JT, Thorp SR, et al. Evidence-based psychological treatments for late-life anxiety. *Psychol Aging.* 2007;22(1):8–17.
2. Gildengers AG, Houck PR, Mulsant BH, et al. Trajectories of treatment response in late-life depression: psychosocial and clinical correlates. *J Clin Psychopharmacol.* 2005;25(4):S8–S13.
3. Jeste ND, Hays JC, Steffens DC. Clinical correlates of anxious depression among elderly patients with depression. *J Affect Disord.* 2006;90(1):37–41.
4. Kennedy GJ. The Sequenced Treatment Alternatives to Relieve Depression (STAR*D) studies: How applicable are the results for older adults? *Prim Psychiatry.* 2006:13(11):33–36.
5. Lenze E. Anxious depression in the elderly. *Perspectives in Psychiatry: A Clinical Update.* 2007;2(4):3–6.
6. Siegle GJ, Steinhauer SR, Thase ME, et al. Can't shake that feeling: event-related fMRI assessment of sustained amygdala activity in response to emotional information in depressed individuals. *Biol Psychiatry.* 2002;51(9):693–707.

242. An 84-yr-old woman had a total thyroidectomy 3 mo ago because of gradually worsening compression symptoms. The symptoms were due to a benign multinodular goiter. Since thyroidectomy, the patient has taken levothyroxine 88 mcg/d. She also takes calcium and vitamin D for osteopenia.

After thyroidectomy, the patient's thyrotropin and free T_4 levels increased and total T_3 level decreased.

Laboratory results:	Before thyroidectomy	After thyroidectomy
Thyrotropin	1.2 mIU/L	1.6 mIU/L
Free T_4	1.1 ng/dL	1.4 ng/dL
Total T_3	140 ng/dL	119 ng/dL

Which of the following is the best management option?

(A) Continue levothyroxine 88 mcg/d.
(B) Increase levothyroxine to 100 mcg/d.
(C) Add liothyronine 25 mcg/d.
(D) Switch to Armour desiccated thyroid 60 mg/d.

ANSWER: A

The thyrotropin concentration is the best monitor during treatment for hypothyroidism. Because this patient's thyrotropin concentration remains normal, no changes to therapy are needed. The thyroid gland makes T_4 and to a lesser extent T_3, most of which is derived through peripheral conversion of T_4. After thyroidectomy, the peripheral conversion of levothyroxine to T_3 maintains the concentration of total T_3 similar to that before thyroidectomy (SOE=C). Often, however, the free T_4 concentration on levothyroxine therapy is significantly higher than the free T_4 concentration before thyroidectomy.

Increasing the levothyroxine dosage can lower the thyrotropin concentration below the lower limit of normal, and can increase bone turnover and the incidence of atrial fibrillation (SOE=B).

There is no proven benefit to combination therapy of levothyroxine and T_3 (liothyronine) versus levothyroxine alone (SOE=B). Many studies of combination therapy are limited by small sample size, iatrogenic hyperthyroidism, and different thyrotropin levels between treatment groups. The serum concentration of T_3 can fluctuate widely depending on the time of ingestion of T_3.

Most endocrinologists do not recommend therapy with Armour thyroid because the amount of desiccated animal T_4 and T_3 is not consistent (SOE=D).

Many substances, such as calcium, iron, and multivitamins, interfere with absorption of thyroid medications. Because this patient takes medication for both hypothyroidism and osteopenia, the schedule for medication administration should be structured and followed carefully.

References

1. Escobar-Morreale HF, Botella-Carretero JI, Gomez-Bueno M, et al. Thyroid hormone replacement therapy in primary hypothyroidism: a randomized trial comparing L-thyroxine plus liothyronine with L-thyroxine alone. *Ann Intern Med.* 2005;142:412–424.
2. Jonklaas J, Davidson B, Bhagat S, et al. Triiodothyronine levels in athyreotic individuals during levothyroxine therapy. *JAMA.* 2008;299:769–777.
3. Saravanan P, Simmons DJ, Greenwood R, et al. Partial substitution of thyroxine (T_4) with triiodothyronine in patients on T_4 replacement therapy. *J Clin Endocrinol Metab.* 2005;90:805–812.

243. Which of the following is true regarding how the nursing-home population has changed since 1985?

(A) The number of residents has increased.
(B) Among adults ≥85 yr old, men now outnumber women.
(C) The level of disability has declined.
(D) The number of admissions has increased.

ANSWER: D

The number of nursing home admissions has increased since 1994, because more facilities now offer short-term medical services and rehabilitation care after a hospitalization. The number of nursing-home residents has remained approximately constant since 1985; overall, the percentage of older people living in nursing homes has actually declined. In the United States, about 2% of adults 65–84 yr old, and about 14% of adults ≥85 yr old, live in nursing homes. Nationally, the occupancy rates in nursing homes have declined from about 92% to about 88% in the last 20 yr.

The level of disability among nursing-home residents has increased over the past decade. Dementia remains the most prevalent condition, affecting an estimated 50%–70% of residents. Between 48% and 65% of residents have urinary or fecal incontinence, and more than half are confined to a wheelchair or bed. About 25% require assistance with 1 or 2 ADLs, and about 75% require assistance with 3 or more.

According to the National Nursing Home Survey, 674,000 adults ≥85 yr old lived in nursing homes in 2004; of those, 18% were men and 82% were women.

References

1. AARP Public Policy Institute analysis of the 2004 National Nursing Home Survey (NNHS) and US Census Bureau population estimates, http://www.aarp.org/ppi (accessed Nov 2009).
2. The AGS Foundation for Health and Aging. *Nursing home care.* http://www.healthinaging.org (accessed Nov 2009).
3. Centers for Disease Control and Prevention, Trends in Health and Aging, http://www.CDC.gov/NCHS/NNAS2004.htm (accessed Nov 2009).
4. Elon RD, Katz PR. Nursing facility care. In: Duthie EH, Katz PR, Malone M, eds. *Practice of Geriatrics.* 4th ed. Philadelphia, PA: Saunders Elsevier; 2007:93–101.

244. A 73-yr-old man in a rehabilitation facility is evaluated for irritable mood, poor motivation for rehabilitation, and demanding and verbally abusive behavior toward staff. He entered rehabilitation after an above-knee amputation. He acknowledges having felt depressed and anxious for a long time, and he has taken a low dose of an antidepressant for several years. Family members report that he previously was extroverted and tended to be provocative and hot-tempered. In recent years, he has had increasing difficulty tolerating disability and reliance on others, prompting arguments that have frayed already estranged relations with his children. He admits to frequent verbal outbursts toward staff because "I need help and they just walk by!" Staff members believe he is just seeking attention. He has pervasive irritable mood, anhedonia, feelings of worthlessness, reduced appetite, poor sleep, and low energy. He inconsistently attends physical therapy sessions.

Cognitive examination and thyroid function are normal, and his symptoms are not due to medication or substance abuse.

Which of the following is most likely to improve this patient's behavior?

(A) Increase dosage of antidepressant and refer for psychotherapy.
(B) Maintain and monitor on current dosage of antidepressant.
(C) Discontinue antidepressant treatment and screen for mania.
(D) Advise staff to ignore attention-seeking behavior.

ANSWER: A

Some older adults have chronic, unremitting major depressive disorder. If the behavior is of long duration and characterized by irritable mood and an abrasive interpersonal style, a mood disorder may be mistaken for an Axis II personality disorder. Although major depression and personality disorders can coexist, features of personality disorder can overshadow depressive symptoms. Distinguishing a personality disorder from persisting mood disorder is challenging and may be possible only after adequate treatment for depressive disorder (SOE=C).

This patient may have major depression superimposed on medical illness and an underlying personality disorder. The continuation of his symptoms despite long-term, low-dose treatment with an antidepressant suggests that

the dosage is inadequate and should be reevaluated. In contrast to that for major depressive disorder, the goal of treating personality disorders in older adults is not remission but reduction in frequency and intensity of symptoms.

It is unlikely that this patient's behavior would disappear if ignored by staff. Although irritability can be a symptom of mania, it is also common in older depressed adults. In patients with depressive symptoms, irritability does not suggest mania if symptoms of mania (eg, inflated self-esteem, decreased need for sleep, increased involvement in pleasurable activity) are absent.

References

1. Lynch TR, Cheavens JS, Cukrowicz KC, et al. Treatment of older adults with co-morbid personality disorder and depression: a dialectical behavior therapy approach. *Int J Geriatric Psychiatry.* 2007;22(2):131–143.
2. Reynolds CJ 3rd, Dew MA, Pollack BG, et al. Maintenance treatment of major depression in old age. *N Engl J Med.* 2006;354(11):1130–1138.
3. Thompson DJ, Borson S. Major depression and related disorders in late life. In: Agronin ME, Maletta GJ, eds. *Principles and Practice of Geriatric Psychiatry.* Philadelphia, PA: Lippincott Williams & Wilkins; 2006:349–368.

245. Which of the following improves functional communication with hearing aids?

(A) Patient purchase of hearing aid on the Internet
(B) Instructional brochures that explain how the hearing aids work
(C) Group instruction about hearing aids and effective communication
(D) Waiving physical examination of the ear to shorten time between determination of hearing loss and use of hearing aids

ANSWER: C

Hearing aids can be purchased from state-licensed audiologists or hearing-instrument specialists. When hearing aids are delivered in the context of a client-centered comprehensive rehabilitation program, their functionality is enhanced (SOE=A). Such a program can be offered in a group setting or with the patient and his or her partner or caregiver alone, and may require 3 to 6 counseling sessions that cover personal adjustment, operation and use of the device, communication strategies, and hearing-assistive technologies that supplement hearing aids. In addition, realistic expectations must be established early, because patient satisfaction is maximized when their expectations match the performance capabilities of the hearing aid.

Consumers can purchase hearing-assistive devices without assistance from a hearing specialist via the Internet, through mail order, or OTC; some of these devices are not considered hearing aids in accordance with FDA specifications. (The FDA classifies medical devices into three categories, ranging from Class I devices, the simplest and subject to the least regulatory control, to Class III devices, which are subject to regulatory control.) Devices that are available OTC are limited in their frequency range and may provide amplification that can damage residual hearing. The devices are less expensive than custom hearing aids: in 2007, the average price of state-of-the-art hearing aids was approximately $1,986.

The FDA and licensure laws in some states mandate that manufacturers' instructional brochures accompany hearing aids. The brochures illustrate and describe the operation, use, and care of the particular hearing aid and list sources for repair and maintenance. The brochures should include a statement that the use of a hearing aid may be only part of a rehabilitative program. There is no evidence that the instructional brochure enhances benefit from hearing aids.

Before the advent of antibiotics and surgical treatment for conductive hearing loss due to middle ear disease, hearing aids were the treatment of choice. However, most diseases of the middle ear that result in conductive hearing loss can be treated medically (eg, stapedectomy for otosclerosis, removal of impacted cerumen, antibiotics for chronic middle ear infection). The FDA requires that hearing specialists obtain a written statement from the patient confirming that his or her ears have been medically evaluated and that the patient is approved for fitting of a hearing aid. The statement must be signed by a licensed physician and dated within the previous 6 mo. Patients ≥18 yr old can sign a waiver for a medical examination, but dispensers must avoid encouraging the patient to waive the medical evaluation requirement.

References

1. Callaway S, Punch J. An electroacoustic analysis of over-the counter hearing aids. *Am J Audiol.* 2008;17(1):14–24.

2. Hawkins D. Effectiveness of counseling-based adult group aural rehabilitation programs: A systematic review of the evidence. *J Am Acad Audiol.* 2005;16(7):485–493.

246. An 84-yr-old woman is admitted to the hospital with chest pains. Myocardial infarction is diagnosed, and supportive treatment initiated. Three days into hospitalization, she becomes extremely anxious and nervous, and has anxiety attacks. She denies alcohol use, which is substantiated by family. A review of her current medications reveals that no anxiogenic medications were recently started or increased. She is taking a β-blocker. She has no history of panic disorder, but she is vague about the medications she was taking before admission. She is cognitively intact. Vital signs and laboratory tests are normal. A mild hand tremor is noted.

What is the most likely cause of this patient's anxiety?

(A) New-onset panic disorder
(B) Discontinuation of a benzodiazepine on admission
(C) Discontinuation of an SSRI on admission
(D) Adjustment reaction to myocardial infarction and hospitalization
(E) Alcohol withdrawal

ANSWER: B

Inadvertent discontinuation of a medication is a common cause of new-onset anxiety in a hospitalized patient. Many older adults are unaware of all the medications they are taking or why, and discontinuation of psychiatric medications during hospitalization is common. Serotonin withdrawal sometimes occurs when short-acting SSRIs are discontinued without taper, but withdrawal is more commonly marked by flu-like symptoms, including headache, dizziness, and nausea.

Benzodiazepine withdrawal is marked by increased anxiety and other emotional distress, together with tremor and tachycardia. However, peripheral manifestations might be masked or blocked by medications such as β-blockers (SOE=C). Benzodiazepine withdrawal is a potentially serious problem, similar to alcohol withdrawal.

Although signs and symptoms of benzodiazepine withdrawal are virtually indistinguishable from those of alcohol withdrawal, the history provided by family and the patient's vagueness about medications suggest the former rather than the latter. The timing and precipitous onset of this patient's anxiety attacks are more consistent with withdrawal than new-onset panic disorder.

Reference

1. Wu CS, Wang SC, Chang IS, et al. The association between dementia and long-term use of benzodiazepine in the elderly: nested case-control study using claims data. *Am J Geriatr Psychiatry.* 2009;17(7):614–620.

247. An 83-yr-old woman is brought to the local emergency department because she is unresponsive to efforts to awaken her from a 3-hour nap. She had complained of fatigue before the nap. She has a history of hypertension and hyperlipidemia. Medications include a thiazide diuretic, a calcium channel blocker, and a statin.

On examination, she can be aroused but is extremely lethargic and unable to answer questions. Blood pressure is 100 mmHg systolic, and pulse is 90 beats per minute. Neck veins are mildly distended, and scattered rales are audible. There are no murmurs, gallops, or edema, and no focal neurologic deficits.

Initial ECG shows ST elevations in leads II, III, aVF, and V5-V6 and depressions in a VL and V1-V2. The emergency room physicians initiated the acute myocardial infarction protocol and administered aspirin, oxygen, and a β-blocker. The local hospital does not have a catheterization laboratory, and the emergency room physician contacts you because he wants to transfer the patient to the nearest large hospital, which is 20 min away. The patient's husband is unsure about the recommendations and contacts her primary care physician for advice.

Which of the following is the most appropriate advice?

(A) Continue with conservative management (no fibrinolysis or percutaneous intervention [PCI] because of her age and indeterminate presentation.
(B) Begin fibrinolysis as soon as possible.
(C) Transfer to the outside hospital for PCI.
(D) Transfer to the outside hospital for urgent coronary artery bypass grafting.

ANSWER: C

Presentation of myocardial infarction is commonly atypical in older adults and can include symptoms of shortness of breath, indigestion, fatigue, or altered mental status. A 12-lead ECG should be ordered promptly in any older adult presenting with symptoms that are consistent with myocardial infarction or that are vague and not otherwise explainable. The 12-lead ECG is at the center of the therapeutic decision pathway. The ECG in this patient demonstrates ST-segment elevation in the inferior and lateral leads. For patients with ST-segment elevation, the diagnosis of ST-elevation myocardial infarction (STEMI) is secure.

The decision regarding reperfusion therapy should be made in the emergency department based on a predetermined, institution-specific, written protocol (SOE=A). Starting reperfusion therapy should not be delayed for results of a cardiac biomarker assay (such as CPK-MB or cardiac troponin). Flow in the infarct artery can be promptly and completely restored by pharmacologic means (fibrinolysis), PCI (balloon angioplasty with or without deployment of an intracoronary stent under the support of pharmacologic measures to prevent thrombosis), or surgical measures. It is not usually possible to provide surgical reperfusion in a timely fashion; therefore, patients with STEMI who are candidates for reperfusion routinely receive either fibrinolysis or a catheter-based treatment. However, in multiple randomized trials, survival with high-quality PCI was better than that with fibrinolysis, with a lower rate of intracranial hemorrhage and recurrent myocardial infarction (SOE=A). The 2007 update of the ACC/AHA Guidelines for the Management of Patients with STEMI recommends the use of primary PCI for any patient with an acute STEMI who can undergo the procedure within 90 min of first medical contact by persons skilled in the procedure.

If the expected "door-to-balloon" time exceeds the expected "door-to-needle" time by >60 min, fibrinolysis should be considered unless contraindicated. Controlled clinical trials have demonstrated the potential for functional, clinical, and mortality benefits only if fibrinolysis is done within 12 hours. Thus, older adults with indeterminate presentations often do not present within the window of possible therapeutic benefit of reperfusion.

In adults >75 yr old, the overall risk of mortality from myocardial infarction is high with and without therapy, and the data on adults >80–85 yr old are difficult to interpret. Fibrinolytic trials showed absolute mortality reductions of about 30 per 1,000 for those presenting within 0–6 hours and of about 20 per 1,000 for those presenting 7–12 hours from onset, with statistically uncertain benefit of about 10 per 1,000 for those presenting at 13–18 hours. However, the relative benefit appears to vary by age, with a smaller relative reduction in risk for the oldest patients. In some observational trials, patients >80–85 yr old showed no mortality benefit, and possible harm, with fibrinolysis (SOE=B).

The major risk of pharmacologic reperfusion therapy is life-threatening hemorrhage. Older age, female sex, black race, prior stroke, systolic blood pressure ≥160 mmHg, lower weight (≤65 kg for women, ≤80 kg for men), excessive anticoagulation (INR ≥4), and choice of fibrinolytic therapy (tissue plasminogen activator associated with greater risk than streptokinase) are risk factors for intracranial bleeding. Many absolute and relative contraindications to fibrinolysis exist; these should be reviewed for each patient by emergency department personnel involved in STEMI protocol implementation.

Although this woman's presentation was somewhat indeterminate and atypical, her symptoms apparently began about 3 hours before presentation, well within the potential window of benefit from reperfusion therapy. In this case, the delay associated with transfer (<60 min) is not sufficient to outweigh the benefits of PCI over fibrinolysis. If PCI had not been available, fibrinolytic therapy should have been initiated because she has no known contraindications.

References

1. Alexander KP, Newby LK, Armstrong PW, et al. Acute coronary care in the elderly, part II: ST-segment-elevation myocardial infarction: a scientific statement for healthcare professionals from the American Heart Association Council on Clinical Cardiology: in collaboration with the Society of Geriatric Cardiology. *Circulation*. 2007;115(19):2570–2589.

2. Antman EM, Anbe DT, Armstrong PW, et al. ACC/AHA guidelines for the management of patients with ST-elevation myocardial infarction: a report of the American College of Cardiology/American Heart Association Task Force on Practice Guidelines (Committee to Revise the 1999 Guidelines for the Management of Patients With Acute Myocardial Infarction). *J Am Coll Cardiol*. 2004;44(3):E1–211.

248. An 82-yr-old woman who lives in a nursing home has a follow-up evaluation for a symptomatic urinary tract infection that was diagnosed 3 wk ago. Although the patient's fever responded rapidly to a course of amoxicillin, she is somewhat lethargic and has not recovered to her baseline level of alertness and physical activity. No other specific problems are evident. Chart documentation indicates that she is eating 75%–100% of food served at most meals but is no longer going to the residents' dining room for meals. History includes Alzheimer's disease. On her last Minimum Data Set evaluation, she was independent in eating.

On examination, the resident weighs 69.4 kg (153 lb; body mass index, 26 kg/m^2), which is unchanged from previous monthly records over the last year. Temperature is 37°C (98.6°F). Lungs are clear, and jugular venous pressure is <5 cm. She has 2+ to 3+ pretibial and presacral edema that was not evident on previous examinations. Otherwise, the examination is unchanged from baseline.

In laboratory results from 2 days ago, her WBC count, electrolytes, and renal function tests are in the normal range and unchanged from baseline. Urinalysis is normal. Given the resident's slow recovery, recent development of dependent edema, and unchanged weight, her nutritional status is checked.

Which of the following should be undertaken to assess the patient's nutritional risk?

(A) Obtain serum albumin level.
(B) Obtain serum prealbumin level.
(C) Order calorie counts for 3 days.
(D) Measure biceps and triceps skinfold thickness and arm muscle circumference.
(E) Screen for depression.

ANSWER: C

At this point, it is important to know how well the resident is eating. The combination of bed rest, acute disease-induced inflammation, and anorexia can result in rapid loss of both lean tissue mass and fat stores in older adults. This resident seems to be at particular risk of nutritional deterioration given her slow recovery from the recent urinary tract infection. Her level of alertness and physical activity is noticeably different than at baseline, her weight is unchanged, and she has significant amounts of edema. This would suggest that her nonfluid weight has declined. Given her clinical course, it is likely that she is not eating as well as in the past. The nursing home diet records may not accurately reflect her nutrient intake. Several studies indicate that nursing home personnel often overestimate how much residents are eating. Residents who are assessed to be independent in eating are often the ones at greatest risk of having unrecognized poor nutrient intake. Consequently, formal calorie counts must be obtained for high-risk patients. Although it is advisable to order calorie counts for 3 days, the data should be assessed as it is collected. A very low nutrient intake would be apparent in the calorie count data collected within the first 24 hours. Calorie counts for 3 days are helpful in assessing residents with fluctuating or borderline nutrient intake.

The serum secretory proteins albumin and prealbumin would not be of much value in assessing the resident's nutritional risk at this time. Both lack sensitivity and specificity as markers of nutritional status in older adults. Prealbumin has a shorter half-life and is considered to be more responsive to nutrient intake than albumin. However, recent studies suggest it is not an adequate substitute for calorie counts in assessing the nutrient intake in older adults recovering from an acute illness (SOE=A).

Measurements of skinfold and arm muscle circumference provide an indirect assessment of a resident's nutritional reserves. However, the usefulness of serial measurements is limited by poor retest reliability and inadequate sensitivity to change in nutritional status, especially over 1–2 mo. Although it is reasonable to assess the patient for depressive symptoms, this will not provide specific infor

mation regarding her nutrient intake. The most important information currently needed to assess this resident's nutritional risk is an accurate assessment of her nutrient intake.

References

1. Dennis RA, Johnson LE, Roberson PK, et al. Changes in prealbumin, nutrient intake, and systemic inflammation in elderly recuperative care patients. *J Am Geriatr Soc.* 2008;56(7):1270–1275.
2. Seres DS. Surrogate nutrition markers, malnutrition, and adequacy of nutrition support. *Nutr Clin Prac.* 2005;20(3):308–313.
3. Simmons SF. Quality improvement for feeding assistance care in nursing homes. *J Am Med Dir Assoc.* 2007;(3 Suppl):S12–S17.
4. Simmons SF, Reuben D. Nutritional intake monitoring for nursing home residents: a comparison of staff documentation, direct observation, and photography methods. *J Am Geriatr Soc.* 2000;48(2):209–213.

249. An 80-yr-old obese man comes to the office because he has excessive daytime sleepiness. His wife notes that he is more irritable and is snoring more than in the past. The patient has hypertension poorly controlled by several medications.

Which of the following is most likely to establish this patient's diagnosis?

(A) Electrocardiography
(B) Chest radiography
(C) Polysomnography
(D) CT of the head
(E) CBC

ANSWER: C

This patient has classic signs and symptoms of obstructive sleep apnea, which is a failure of breathing during sleep brought about by obstruction of the upper airway, in the presence of continued efforts to breathe. Polysomnography is used to evaluate patients during sleep for episodes of apnea (cessation of breathing or airflow for ≥10 sec) and hypopnea (decreased airflow with arterial oxygen saturation decreased by >4%). Polysomnography yields an apnea-hypopnea index or respiratory disturbance index; both indices refer to the total number of apnea and hypopnea events per hour of sleep. The respiratory disturbance index also incorporates respiratory events less severe than apnea or hypopnea but that nonetheless disrupt sleep. It can be used to determine the severity of obstructive sleep apnea (SOE=B).

Obstructive sleep apnea is more common in men (4:1), increases with age, and is associated with obesity, sedative agents such as alcohol and benzodiazepines, and hypothyroidism. Large tonsils; anatomic abnormalities of the soft palate, uvula, and tongue; and retrognathic mandible may be contributing factors.

Electrocardiography and chest radiography are unlikely to identify obstructive sleep apnea. These tests are part of the subsequent evaluation, because the disorder is associated with cardiovascular disease. Neither CT of the head nor a CBC has a role in diagnosis of sleep apnea.

References

1. Benjamin JA, Lewis KE. Sleep-disordered breathing and cardiovascular disease. *Postgrad Med J.* 2008;84(987):15–22.
2. Launois SH, Pepin JL, Levy P. Sleep apnea in the elderly: a specific entity? *Sleep Med Rev.* 2007;11(2):87–97.

250. A 70-yr-old woman comes to the office because her vision seems less clear and she has trouble reading, especially with her right eye, and she misses letters in the middle of words. History includes chronic type 2 diabetes mellitus and, beginning 6 mo ago, severe respiratory problems that necessitated oral steroids. Since then, she has been hospitalized repeatedly for respiratory infections, with resulting difficulty in controlling the diabetes. She sees her ophthalmologist annually to check for diabetic retinopathy and has received a good report at each visit.

Which of the following is the most likely cause of her visual symptoms?

(A) Cataracts
(B) Diabetic macular edema
(C) Open-angle glaucoma
(D) Vitreous hemorrhage

ANSWER: B

Diabetic macular edema causes a loss of clear vision centrally. Often the vision is distorted, and individuals will describe letters missing in the middle of a word. The symptoms are similar to those experienced by those with age-related macular degeneration. Macular edema is a leading cause of vision loss in people with diabetic retinopathy. This patient's hospitalizations for infections necessitating steroid treatment are likely to have been

associated with poor glucose control and worsening of retinopathy (SOE=A).

Developing cataracts are more likely to cause glare and generalized blurring. Posterior subcapsular cataracts can affect reading, but blurriness in the center of a word is more likely to indicate a macular change.

Open-angle glaucoma does not cause central distortion and blur; visual field constriction is more likely (SOE=A).

The symptoms of vitreous hemorrhage are generalized blur or loss of more vision than just a distortion in the center of words. There can be a sudden drop in vision involving a large portion of the visual field.

References

1. American Academy of Ophthalmology. *Cataract in the Adult Eye, Preferred Practice Pattern.* San Francisco, CA: American Academy of Ophthalmology; 2006. Available at: http://one.aao.org/CE/PracticeGuidelines/PPP.aspx (accessed Nov 2009).
2. Mohamed Q, Gillies MC, Wong TY. Management of diabetic retinopathy: a systematic review. *JAMA.* 2007;298(8):902–916.
3. Tranos PG, Wickremasinghe SS, Stangos NT, et al. Macular edema. *Surv Ophthalm.* 2004;49(5):470–490.

251. A 65-yr-old woman comes to the office because over the past week she has had an episode of vertigo every time she laid down or rolled over in bed. Each episode lasted about 30 sec and left her feeling queasy and unsteady. The vertigo was also triggered in the morning when she tilted her head back to reach a cup on a high kitchen shelf. She has no other symptoms, including no other problems with gait or balance. She feels fine between episodes and has not had any spontaneous spells. History includes hypertension well controlled by hydrochlorothiazides.

Her general physical examination is normal. Her vertigo is recreated by a Dix-Hallpike test when she hangs her head to the left.

Which of the following is most likely to benefit this patient?

(A) Gait and balance therapy
(B) Surgical ablation of the vestibular nerve
(C) Low-salt diet and diuretics
(D) Positioning maneuver
(E) White-noise generator

ANSWER: D

This patient has the characteristic clinical features of benign paroxysmal positional vertigo (BPPV). It is the most common cause of dizziness seen in neurotology clinics. In an epidemiologic study in Germany, the 1-y prevalence of BPPV in adults ≥60 yr old was 3.4%, nearly 7-fold higher than the prevalence in adults 18–39 yr old. Detachment of the otoconium presumably occurs more readily with age: the cumulative incidence of BPPV reaches almost 10% at age 80. BPPV, which is commonly worse in the early morning, occurs when otolithic calcium-carbonate crystals fall into and are loose in the posterior semicircular canal. When the patient is placed in position for the Dix-Hallpike test, with head hanging to the side of the BPPV, there is a characteristic upbeat-torsional geotropic (beating toward the ground) nystagmus that lasts <1 min and fatigues with repeated positioning. The canalith repositioning procedure (modified Epley's maneuver) is an effective and safe therapy for this condition (SOE=A).

Gait and balance therapy is often useful after both acute vestibulopathy and cerebellar strokes. Surgical ablation is not indicated because the canalith repositioning maneuver is effective and noninvasive. Low-salt diet and diuretics may be used in Meniere disease, and a white-noise generator may be useful in some cases of tinnitus.

References

1. Fife TD, Iverson DJ, Lempert T, et al. Quality Standards Subcommittee of the American Academy of Neurology. Practice parameter: therapies for benign paroxysmal positional vertigo (an evidence-based review): report of the Quality Standards Subcommittee of the American Academy of Neurology. *Neurology.* 2008;70(22):2067–2074.
2. von Brevern M, Radtke A, Lezius F, et al. Epidemiology of benign paroxysmal positional vertigo. A population-based study. *J Neurol Neurosurg Psychiatry.* 2007;78(7):710–715.

252. A 74-yr-old man has a chief complaint of chronic diabetes and difficulty finding shoes. History reveals fairly well controlled type 2 diabetes; the right fifth digit was amputated 3 yr ago. Physical examination reveals absent pulses bilaterally, loss of sensation to the 5.07 Semmes-Weinstein monofilament, moderate hallux valgus deformity with hammertoe digits bilaterally, and a well healed surgical site at the right fifth digit. His last hemoglobin A_{1c} was 7.4%.

Which of this patient's features places him at highest risk of future ulceration?

(A) Hammertoes
(B) Previous amputation
(C) Hemoglobin A_{1c}
(D) Loss of protective sensation
(E) Absent pedal pulses

ANSWER: B

Amputation prevention for diabetic patients has been well studied and has led to the development of a risk stratification based on risk factors for ulceration. Ulceration risk factors include loss of protective sensation due to peripheral neuropathy, peripheral vascular disease, foot deformities, and previous ulcerations and/or amputations. Hemoglobin A_{1c}, unless consistently increased, does not place a patient at high risk of ulceration. A history of amputation places this patient at greatest risk of recurrent ulceration (SOE=B).

Reference

1. Frykberg RG, Zgonis T, Armstrong DG, et al. Diabetic foot disorders: a clinical practice guideline (2006 Revision). *J Foot Ankle Surg.* 2006;45(5 Suppl):S1–S66.

253. An 80-yr-old man comes to the office for a routine visit. He is enrolled in traditional fee-for-service Medicare Parts A and B and has a Part D policy. He has seen advertisements for an insurance plan called SeniorGold, which is described as a Medicare Advantage organization with a Medicare contract. He wishes to discuss advantages and disadvantages of switching his insurance coverage to this plan.

Which of the following is most likely to occur if he switches insurance coverage to SeniorGold?

(A) He would lose some Part A benefits.
(B) He would lose some Part B benefits.
(C) He would have to drop Part D prescription drug coverage.
(D) He would not get coverage for vision examination and eyeglasses.
(E) He would not get to choose his physicians.

ANSWER: E

A potential disadvantage of a Medicare Advantage plan is that the provider network may be restricted, because this is a key strategy for controlling costs in managed-care systems. Medicare Advantage plans are required by law to provide all services covered in traditional Medicare Parts A and B. Participants may enroll in a Medicare Advantage plan and have a separate, stand-alone Part D policy, or attach a Part D policy to the Medicare Advantage plan. Traditional Medicare does not cover vision examination and eyeglasses; many Medicare Advantage plans cover such services as an enticement to get patients to enroll.

References

1. Centers for Medicare & Medicaid Services. *Medicare & You 2008.* http://www.medicare.gov/Publications/Pubs/pdf/10050.pdf, p. 38 (accessed Nov 2009).
2. Kaiser Family Foundation. Medicare Advantage Plans. In: *Talking About Medicare: Your Guide to Understanding the Program, 2009.* http://www.kff.org/medicare/7067/med_advantage.cfm (accessed Nov 2009).

254. A 79-yr-old woman was discharged from the hospital yesterday after a 2-wk stay for diverticular bleeding. She underwent transfusion with 8 units of RBCs and declined surgery. She has diabetes and osteoarthritis and was in bed for most of the past 2 wk. Her husband calls to report that she is very weak. She needs follow-up laboratory tests in 2 days in compliance with hospital discharge instructions, but he does not think he can transport her to the office. He wants to know if she can receive home health care to address her needs.

Which of the following is an allowable indication for home health care in this patient?

(A) Follow-up laboratory testing
(B) Physical therapy
(C) Home aide services
(D) Monitoring of glycemic control
(E) Durable medical equipment

ANSWER: B

This patient qualifies for Medicare Part A home health agency care, both for nursing assessment and teaching, and for rehabilitative physical and occupational therapy. Physical therapy to help a homebound patient recover functionally from deconditioning that resulted from a recent illness is a qualifying service;

the patient does not need to have nursing care to begin Part A home health services.

Drawing blood for laboratory testing was removed as an independent qualifying service need, effective February 1998 as part of the Balanced Budget Act of 1997. Drawing blood as part of a care plan to actively manage a recently unstable medical condition is permitted.

Although home health agencies must provide home health aide care as part of their service portfolio, agencies are not required to provide home health aide services to each patient, and the amount of service to be provided is under the agency's control. Requiring only a home health aide is not sufficient to qualify for home health services under Medicare Part A.

Teaching related to diabetes care can be the primary indication for home health care in a homebound patient if the diabetes has been newly diagnosed or is newly unstable, or if the patient lacks knowledge and ability in self-care of this condition. However, overseeing glycemic control is not an indication for home health care, and there is no suggestion that this patient's diabetes has recently been uncontrolled.

Unlike hospice, in which some home medical equipment is arranged or paid for by the hospice, in Medicare Part A home health care, the agency's responsibility is limited to providing services (eg, nursing, physical therapy) plus some related supplies (eg, wound care). In general, durable medical equipment is covered by Medicare Part B, and medications are covered by Medicare Part D (for those who are enrolled in Part D). Home health services are not required to provide durable medical equipment covered by Part B.

Reference

1. Home Health Agency Center. Centers for Medicare and Medicaid Services. United States Department of Health and Human Services. http://www.cms.hhs.gov/center/hha.asp (accessed Nov 2009).

255. An 80-yr-old man has been evaluated, after an uncomplicated myocardial infarction, with an exercise stress test. He was able to maintain maximal heart rate for 15 min without angina or electrocardiographic changes. Although somewhat anxious, the patient would like to proceed with therapy for erectile dysfunction, which developed after his myocardial infarction. Medications include aspirin, atorvastatin, and atenolol.

Which of the following treatments is most appropriate for him?

(A) Psychotherapy
(B) Yohimbine
(C) Testosterone patches
(D) Sildenafil

ANSWER: D

Phosphodiesterase inhibitors have become the standard of care for erectile dysfunction (SOE=A), but they are contraindicated in patients taking nitrates. This patient's stress test indicates that he can achieve a maximal heart rate during exercise (and, by extension, during intercourse) without having angina. He should be cautioned not to take sildenafil or any other phosphodiesterase inhibitor within 24 hours of using nitroglycerin. Typical adverse events of phosphodiesterase inhibitors include headache, flushing, and loss of vision or hearing.

Yohimbine is not approved for treatment of erectile dysfunction and may be associated with increases in blood pressure. The patient's situational anxiety is normal. Thus, psycho-therapy is not indicated unless his anxiety increases due to a poor response to medical therapy, or if he becomes afraid to attempt intercourse.

This patient's erectile dysfunction, occurring after an myocardial infarction, is mostly likely due to vascular causes, which are the most common causes of erectile dysfunction in older men (SOE=B). Testosterone is not first-line treatment for erectile dysfunction in men.

References

1. Feifer A, Carrier S. Pharmacotherapy for erectile dysfunction. *Expert Opinion Invest Drugs.* 2008;17(5):679–690.
2. Hatzimouratidis K, Hatzichristou DG. Looking to the future for erectile dysfunction therapies. *Drugs.* 2008;68(2):231–250.
3. Seidman SN. Exploring the relationship between depression and erectile dysfunction in aging men. *J Clin Psychiatry.* 2002;63 Suppl 5:5–12.

256. A 75-yr-old man is brought to the office because he has recently had visual hallucina-tions. History includes moderate dementia and repeated falls. Therapy is initiated with a low-dose second-generation antipsychotic agent. Shortly thereafter, the family calls because the patient is walking with great difficulty and has muscle stiffness and occasional tremors.

Which of the following is the most likely diagnosis?

(A) Alzheimer's disease
(B) Lewy body dementia
(C) Vascular dementia
(D) Mixed Alzheimer's disease and vascular dementia

ANSWER: B

First- and second-generation antipsychotic agents have high rates of adverse events yet some efficacy for behavioral disturbances associated with dementia. Among the most prominent adverse events associated with use of antipsychotics are extrapyramidal symptoms and tardive dyskinesia. Second-generation antipsychotic agents (eg, clozapine, risperidone, quetiapine, olanzapine, aripiprazole) are less likely than first-generation agents to cause extrapyramidal symptoms.

Lewy body dementia has an especially strong association with hallucinations. Patients with Lewy body dementia are uniquely sensitive to antipsychotic adverse events (SOE=A). This sensitivity to neuroleptics is characterized by rigidity, immobility, sedation, and confusion, and is singular enough to be included in consensus criteria for the diagnosis of Lewy body dementia. Reduction of dopaminergic innervation in the basal ganglia may account for this phenomenon. Because the risk of extrapyramidal symptoms is smaller with second- than with first-generation antipsychotics, second-generation agents have been used to control behavioral disturbances in patients with Lewy body dementia. However, even these agents can induce rigidity and immobility in patients with Lewy body dementia (SOE=B).

References

1. Baskys A. Lewy body dementia: the litmus test for neuroleptic sensitivity and extrapyramidal symptoms. *J Clin Psychiatry.* 2004;65(Suppl 11):16–22.
2. Jacobson SA, Pies RW, Katz IR. Medications to treat dementias and other cognitive disorders. In: *Clinical Manual of Geriatric Psychopharmacology.* Washington, DC: American Psychiatric Publishing, Inc; 2007:543–606.
3. Kobayashi A, Kawanishi C, Matsumura T, et al. Quetiapine-induced neuroleptic malignant syndrome in dementia with Lewy bodies: a case report. *Prog Neuropsychopharmacol Biol Psychiatry.* 2006;30(6):1170–1172.
4. McKeith IG, Dickson DW, Lowe J, et al. Diagnosis and management of dementia with Lewy bodies: third report of the DLB Consortium. *Neurology.* 2005;65(12):1863–1872.

257. A 70-yr-old woman comes to the office to establish care. She has been on estrogen and progesterone therapy for 15 yr, since menopause. She would like to discontinue therapy, despite tolerating it well, because she has heard that estrogen therapy is dangerous.

Which of the following is true about this patient's projected risks 3 yr after stopping estrogen therapy compared with the risks of other women of a similar age who did not use estrogen therapy?

(A) She has a higher risk of invasive breast cancer.
(B) She has a lower risk of fracture.
(C) She has the same risk of death.
(D) She has a higher risk of coronary heart disease.
(E) She has a higher risk of deep venous thrombosis.

ANSWER: C

After stopping estrogen therapy, this patient would have the same all-cause mortality as women who had not taken hormone replacements for the previous 5 yr (SOE=A). In the Women's Health Initiative, the higher risks of all cardiovascular events and of invasive breast cancer seen in women taking combination estrogen and progesterone were not sustained after therapy was discontinued (SOE=A). Likewise, the reduction in fractures was not sustained after estrogen therapy was discontinued (SOE=A). There was no statistically significant difference in any outcome between women who had been on placebo and those who had taken the estrogen and progesterone combination. Whereas the global index suggested a higher risk-to-benefit ratio during hormone replacement, the index was neutral in the 2.4-yr follow-up of the Women's Health Initiative.

There is much confusion regarding the conclusions of the Women's Health Initiative. Many patients believe that replacement therapy, including estrogen alone, is harmful. Although women randomly assigned to the estrogen plus progesterone group had a statistically significant greater incidence of invasive breast cancer and cardiovascular disease (SOE=A), this was not the case for women in the estrogen-only arm.

References
1. Anderson GL, Limacher M, Assaf AR, et al. Effects of conjugated equine estrogen in postmenopausal women with hysterectomy: the Women's Health Initiative Randomized Controlled Trial. *JAMA.* 2004;291(14):1701–1712.
2. Heiss G, Wallace R, Anderson GL, et al. Health risks and benefits 3 years after stopping randomized treatment with estrogen and progestin. *JAMA.* 2008;299(9):1036–1045.
3. Roussouw JE, Anderson GL, Prentice RL, et al. Risks and benefits of estrogen plus progestin in healthy postmenopausal women: principal results from the Women's Health Initiative randomized controlled trial. *JAMA.* 2002;288(3):321–333.

258. An 82-yr-old man comes to the office because he has had excessive daytime sleepiness for about 6 mo. He falls asleep during the day, particularly in the late morning. He falls asleep easily around 8 PM, but wakes up every 2–3 hours throughout the night. His wife's sleep is often disturbed by his awakenings, and they have not been able to participate in social activities because of his intermittent daytime napping. History includes stroke (with residual mild leg weakness), hypertension, and mild cognitive impairment.

The patient is referred for actigraphy, a 24-hour graphing of sleep and wake intervals that uses a unit (actigraph) worn on the nondominant wrist. Results show 3 sleep intervals during the 24-hour test, with no single, clearly defined major nocturnal sleep period.

Which of the following is the most likely diagnosis?

(A) Idiopathic hypersomnia
(B) Advanced sleep phase disorder
(C) Irregular sleep/wake rhythm disorder
(D) Sundowning
(E) REM sleep behavior disorder

ANSWER: C

The patient's sleep pattern is consistent with circadian rhythm sleep disorder, irregular sleep/wake rhythm type. This condition is characterized by fragmented nocturnal sleep and daytime napping (SOE=B): there are at least 3 sleep periods throughout the 24-hour cycle, with no clearly defined, single, major nocturnal sleep period. The disorder is common in older adults with dementia; lack of structured exposure to light and to social and physical activities can precipitate or perpetuate the problem. A combination of increased light exposure and increased social and physical activity during the day is often recommended (SOE=B).

Although the patient complains of daytime sleepiness, the history indicates daytime napping and lack of consolidation of nocturnal sleep. The frequent daytime napping is most likely due to a decrease in the amplitude of the circadian rhythm, rather than to idiopathic hypersomnia. Advanced sleep phase disorder is characterized by one major nocturnal sleep period that is advanced relative to conventional sleep-wake times. This patient does not have one major sleep period, but rather several irregular periods of sleep and wake during the 24-hour cycle. The history does not indicate abnormal behavior during sleep (REM sleep behavior disorder) or agitation in the evening (sundowning).

References

1. Barion A, Zee PC. A clinical approach to circadian rhythm sleep disorders. *Sleep Med*. 2007;8(6):566–577.
2. Morgenthaler TI, Lee-Chiong T, Alessi C, et al. Practice parameters for the clinical evaluation and treatment of circadian rhythm sleep disorders. An American Academy of Sleep Medicine report. *Sleep*. 2007;30:1445–1459.
3. Sack RL, Auckley D, Auger RR, et al; American Academy of Sleep Medicine. Circadian rhythm sleep disorders: part II, advanced sleep phase disorder, delayed sleep phase disorder, free-running disorder, and irregular sleep-wake rhythm. An American Academy of Sleep Medicine review. *Sleep*. 2007;30(11):1484–1501.

259. An active 75-yr-old man with no significant medical history has a chief complaint of dry scaling feet and thickened nails. The patient indicates that, for >20 yr, he has had thick nails starting in the great toes. Over the last few years, this has spread to his lesser digits. His main complaint is chronic itching and scaling feet. Self-care has included nail trimming and OTC hand cream, which he applies a few times a week. Physical examination shows dry erythematous scaling in a moccasin distribution bilaterally, web-space scaling, and thickened yellow nails. Neurovascular examination is within normal limits.

What is the most likely causative organism?

(A) *Candida albicans*
(B) *Microsporum canis*
(C) *Trichophyton rubrum*
(D) *Corneum bacterium*

ANSWER: C

The incidence of onychomycosis rises with age and often leads to chronic athlete's feet. It is usually caused by a dermatophyte infection. *Trichophyton rubrum* has been reported to be the infecting organism in up to 90% of cases (SOE=A). *Microsporum canis*, another dermatophyte, has been demonstrated to cause onychomycosis, although this type of infection is rare. Yeast infections do not usually involve the toenails, and more commonly cause fingernail infections in patients chronically exposed to water. Bacterial infections do affect the feet but do not present with chronic scaling. *Corneum bacterium* is associated with pitted keratolysis and presents with moisture and odor limited to web spaces and weight-bearing plantar skin.

References

1. Hainer BL Dermatophyte infections. *Am Fam Physician*. 2003;67(1):101–108.
2. Eckhard M, Lengler A, Liersch J, et al. Fungal foot infections in patients with diabetes mellitus—results of two independent investigations. *Mycoses*. 2007;50 Suppl 2:14–19.
3. Seebacher C, Bouchara JP, Mignon B. Updates on the epidemiology of dermatophyte infections. *Mycopathologia*. 2008;166(5-6):335–352.

260. A 67-yr-old woman comes to the office for a routine examination. She wants to quit smoking, but having failed in 6 previous attempts, has no confidence in her ability to do so. She has smoked 2 packs of cigarettes daily for 40 yr; her husband also smokes. In prior efforts to quit, she used either the nicotine patch or nicotine gum, but never both together. She has had no difficulty with withdrawal symptoms. She resumed smoking each time largely because of weight gain. History is notable for a depressive disorder for 5 yr. She takes no medications. Physical examination is normal.

Which of the following is the most appropriate pharmacotherapy for this patient?

(A) Nicotine gum
(B) Nicotine patch
(C) Nortriptyline
(D) Sustained-release bupropion
(E) Clonidine

ANSWER: D

First-line pharmacotherapy for smoking cessation includes sustained-release bupropion, varenicline, and the various forms of nicotine replacement therapy (eg, transdermal patch, gum, tablet/lozenge, inhaler, nasal spray) (SOE=A).

This patient's gender, history of depression, concern about weight gain, and prior attempts to quit are factors to consider when determining the most appropriate pharmacotherapy. Sustained-release bupropion appears to be effective in patients with depression (SOE=B) and may be preferred in this situation. Nicotine replacement therapy may be less effective in women (SOE=B) and had not worked for this patient in the past.

Sustained-release bupropion and nicotine replacement therapy, in particular, higher-dosage gum and lozenges (4 mg dosage for either), appear to be effective in delaying weight gain after quitting (SOE=B). Moreover, there appears to be a dose-response relationship between the total amount of gum use and weight suppression (ie, the greater the gum use, the less weight gain) (SOE=B). However, once either nicotine gum or sustained-release bupropion is stopped, weight gain begins, and the gain is approximately the same as if the individual had not used these medications. Prior successful experience (sustained abstinence with the medication) suggests that the medication may be helpful in a subsequent attempt to quit, especially if the patient found the medication tolerable and easy to use. However, it is difficult to draw firm conclusions from prior failure with a medication. Pragmatic factors can also influence selection of pharmacotherapy, such as insurance coverage, out-of-pocket costs, likelihood of adherence, use of dentures (when considering gum therapy), or dermatitis (when considering transdermal therapy).

Although they are effective in achieving abstinence, clonidine and nortriptyline are second-line agents (SOE=A) because of their associated warnings, adverse events, and lack of FDA approval for smoking cessation. Second-line agents should be used only if there are contraindications to first-line agents or if first-line agents have been ineffective.

References

1. Eisenberg MJ, Filion KB, Yavin D, et al. Pharmacotherapies for smoking cessation: a meta-analysis of randomized trials. *CMAJ*. 2008;179(2):135–144.
2. Fiore MC, Jaen CR, Baker TB, et al. *Treating Tobacco Use and Dependence: 2008 Update*. Clinical Practice Guideline. Rockville, MD: U.S. Department of Health and Human Services. Public Health Service; May 2008.
3. Ranney L, Melvin C, Lux L, et al. *Tobacco Use: Prevention, Cessation, and Control*. Evidence Report/Technology Assessment No. 140. (Prepared by the RTI International–University of North Carolina Evidence-Based Practice Center under Contract No. 290-02-0016). AHRQ Publication No. 06-E015. Rockville, MD: Agency for Healthcare Research and Quality. June 2006.

261. An 81-yr-old woman is brought to the office by her family because she has increasing abdominal distension, nausea, and vomiting. She recently immigrated to the United States from India after the death of her husband. Thorough evaluation confirms a diagnosis of pancreatic cancer with liver metastases. The family believes that she will not be able to tolerate this news because she has just lost her husband, and requests that the diagnosis be withheld from her. The patient is anxious and wants to know what is wrong with her.

Which of the following is the most appropriate course of action?

(A) Inform the patient of the diagnosis.
(B) Tell the patient that she has a minor illness that will soon resolve.
(C) Meet with the patient and the family together to explore their concerns.
(D) Seek advice from the legal department of the local hospital.

ANSWER: C

The most appropriate course of action is to set up a meeting with the patient and her family as soon as possible to discuss their concerns and expectations. One goal of the meeting should be to assess how much the patient knows about her condition and the extent to which she wants to participate in decisions about her care. The physician cannot ethically, legally, or morally withhold her healthcare information from her. Physicians are ethically responsible to provide, with compassion, as much information as the patient requests.

Although the fiduciary patient-physician relationship requires that the patient be informed of the diagnosis, the family's request to withhold the diagnosis from the patient cannot be ignored, for ethical, moral, and legal reasons. Involving both the patient and family in decision-making reduces emotional distress, increases patient satisfaction, improves compliance, and reduces the risk of a malpractice claim.

Lying to the patient is unethical. It is the physician's responsibility to truthfully divulge as much information as the patient requests in a culturally sensitive manner. It is up to the patient to determine her involvement in making decisions.

If the physician is uncomfortable with the situation, the matter should be referred to the local ethics committee rather than to the legal department of the local hospital.

References

1. Arnold SJ, Koczwara B. Breaking bad news: learning through experience. *J Clin Oncol.* 2006;24(31):5098–5100.
2. Lapine A, Wang-Cheng R, Goldstein M, et al. When cultures clash: physician, patient, and family wishes in truth disclosure for dying patients. *J Pall Med.* 2001;4(4):475–480.
3. Matthew DB. Race, religion, and informed consent—lessons from social science. *J Law Med Ethics.* 2008;36(1):150–173.

262. A 74-yr-old woman comes to the office because she has a rash on her neck. It has been present for a few months and is getting thicker and redder. The area is itchy, and sometimes she finds herself scratching without realizing she is doing so; it is difficult for her to stop scratching, especially when she is worried and tired. She has been under stress recently because she is in the process of selling her house, to move in with her daughter. She does not use make-up or jewelry and has not changed detergent. Her usual emollient cream has not helped the rash.

On examination, she is afebrile and appears well. She has a 9-cm lichenified plaque on her neck that is erythematous, with areas of more intense erythema where it was recently scratched. The plaque feels thick and leathery to touch and is not warmer than the surrounding skin.

Which of the following is the most likely diagnosis?

(A) Nodular prurigo
(B) Xerosis
(C) Lichen simplex chronicus
(D) Asteatotic dermatitis
(E) Dyshidrotic eczematous dermatitis

ANSWER: C

The location of this patient's lesion is consistent with psoriasis, but the clinical description is more consistent with lichen simplex chronicus (neurodermatitis). Lichen simplex chronicus is a localized area of lichenification caused by repetitive rubbing and scratching. It involves areas that are easily reached by the dominant hand: legs, ankles, arms, scrotal skin, neck, and upper trunk. Many patients have a history of atopic dermatitis and have anxiety disorders or emotional stresses. It is difficult to treat unless the patient stops scratching. Treatment includes education on the importance of breaking the itch-scratch-itch cycle, addressing psychologic factors, and application of topical steroids with occlusive dressing.

Psychogenic factors also play a role in nodular prurigo, in which emotional tensions induce a self-perpetuating pruritic sensation, but patients scratch in multiple locations and develop dome-shaped nodules rather than plaques. The nodules can be several millimeters to 2 cm in diameter; they can be excoriated and ulcerated when the patient picks at them with fingernails.

Dyshidrotic eczematous dermatitis is a vesicular dermatitis that involves palms, fingers, and soles. It starts with pruritic vesicles that can progress to scaling fissures and lichenification.

Xerosis, or dry skin, is a common cause of generalized itching in older adults. It gets worse in winter with low humidity and frequent bathing. Clinically, the skin is dry and scaly; in more severe cases, the skin becomes inflamed, with fissuring or cracking of the stratum corneum that resembles "cracked porcelain" (erythema craquelé or asteatotic dermatitis). Xerosis usually involves legs, arms, and hands, rather than the neck.

References

1. Chuh A, Wong W. The skin and the mind. *Aust Fam Physician.* 2006;35(9):723–725.
2. Eczema/Dermatitis. In: Fitzpatrick TB, ed. *Fitzpatrick's Color Atlas and Synopsis of Clinical Dermatology.* 5th ed. NY: The McGraw-Hill Companies; 2005.
3. Lotti T, Buggiani G, Prignano F. Prurigo nodularis and lichen simplex chronicus. *Dermatol Ther.* 2008;21(1):42–26.

263. A 75-yr-old man comes to the office with several vague complaints and concerns. He is retired and has been married for 50 yr. Over the past 6 mo, he has come to the office repeatedly and has become increasingly homebound. He describes leg weakness, fatigue, and overall malaise that prevent him from engaging in once-pleasurable activities, such as playing cards at the senior center. He has become fearful of driving and of being alone, and his sleep and appetite are poor. He has lost approximately 4.5 kg (10 lb). History includes hypertension and spinal stenosis. Major depressive disorder is diagnosed, and a trial of an antidepressant is begun.

Which of the following is characteristic of late-life major depressive disorder?

(A) Strong family history of mood disorder
(B) Sudden onset of symptoms
(C) Preferential response to treatment with first-generation antidepressants
(D) Higher prevalence of somatic symptoms

ANSWER: D

In general, major depressive disorder presents with sad mood and a variety of symptoms affecting energy level, sleep, appetite, cognitive skills, and overall ability to derive enjoyment from activities. It can be complicated by psychotic symptoms (eg, delusions or hallucinations) and suicidal ideation. It is a recurring illness, and it is more prevalent in family members of patients.

When major depressive disorder is first seen after age 65, the presentation is distinctive. Dementia is described in up to one-third of patients within 5 yr of the depression. The family history of mood disorder is weaker than in younger patients. The onset of symptoms is slow, subtle, and insidious. Psychotic symptoms and somatic complaints are more prevalent. Nonetheless, recommendations for treatment are similar in those for major depressive disorder with onset before age 65: because of their more favorable adverse event profile and low rates of death in overdose, second-generation antidepressants are first-line treatment for major depressive disorder in adults, regardless of age at onset. There is no evidence that any class of antidepressants is superior to another for treatment of late-life depressive disorder. Tolerability and potential drug-drug interactions in patients on several medications should guide the choice of treatment.

References
1. American Psychiatric Association. *Diagnostic and Statistical Manual of Mental Disorders, Fourth Edition, Text Revision.* Washington, DC, American Psychiatric Association; 2000.
2. Kennedy GJ. Reducing the risk of late-life suicide through improved depression care. *Primary Psychiatry.* 2007;14(1):26–28, 31–34.
3. Taylor WD, Doraiswamy PM. A systematic review of antidepressant placebo-controlled trials for geriatric depression: limitation of current data and directions for the future. *Neuropsychopharmacology.* 2004;29(12):2285–2299.
4. Wilson RS, Barnes LL, Mendes de Leon CF, et al. Depressive symptoms, cognitive decline, and risk of AD in older persons. *Neurology.* 2002;59(3):364–370.

264. Two residents of a for-profit nursing home want to share a bed but can do so only with the cooperation of the staff. One is a 90-yr-old man who is blind and a double-amputee with well-controlled heart failure. The other is an 86-yr-old woman with severe rheumatoid arthritis and a colostomy. Both have outlived spouses after long marriages and have been residents in the facility for some time; both have a normal mental status. The residents have had two falls when in her single room alone, and they have asked for staff assistance to undress and share a bed. Some staff members are uncomfortable and want the medical director to call the families to stop this behavior. Both residents say that they do not want their families informed. There is no relevant statement regarding the facility's protocols or limitations in the materials provided at admission.

Which of the following is the best course of action?

(A) Have a private conversation with the lead family member in each family.
(B) Research civil rights laws to determine the legality of the couple's request.
(C) Pursue a compromise, such as working only with volunteer staff or getting married, with the couple and the staff.
(D) Advise the couple that sexual activity is hazardous to their health and cannot be allowed.

ANSWER: C

Sexual activity among residents in nursing homes usually raises questions of competence, exploitation, harassment of staff, or other adverse behaviors that can justify efforts to eliminate the behavior. However, disabled adults generally have the right to create and follow relationships on the same grounds as nondisabled adults. They do not have to notify children or justify their choices. Yet the facility has to respect the sentiments of staff members and cannot dictate that staff members cooperate, especially if there is strong support in the community for limiting sexual activity to marriage. A reasonable compromise may be possible. Very likely, some staff members are not personally troubled and are willing to assist the couple. Senior leaders (the nursing director, medical director, and social work director) will need to take a strong stand of being willing to be among those helping out. Local advocates for people living with disabilities could be of help, or some volunteers at the nursing home may be supportive.

Informing the families over the explicit objections of competent adults is contrary to medical ethical principles and probably illegal. Legal advice from responsible public agencies is unlikely to help the situation or to be authoritative. Advising the couple that sexual activity would be hazardous to their health is generally not true, because people with well-controlled heart failure, stable arthritis, and colostomies can enjoy sex without harm. Furthermore, even if there is some risk, the nursing home cannot require that the couple make their decisions in accordance with the nursing home's view of risk.

References

1. Hajjar RR, Kamel HK. Sexuality in the nursing home, part 1: attitudes and barriers to sexual expression. *J Am Med Dir Assoc.* 2004;5(2 Suppl):S42–47.
2. Medicare. Resident Rights. http://www.medicare.gov/Nursing/ResidentRights.asp (accessed Nov 2009).
3. *The Merck Manual of Geriatrics.* Section 14. Men's and women's health issues: Chapter 114. Sexuality. At http://www.merck.com/mkgr/mmg/sec14/ch114/ch114a.jsp (accessed Nov 2009).
4. National Citizens Coalition for Nursing Home Reform. *Resident Rights.* http://www.nccnhr.org/public/50_156_449.cfm (accessed Nov 2009).

265. A 75-yr-old man comes to the office for a routine evaluation. He states that recently he has had considerable difficulty understanding speech, even when the speaker's face is within 6 ft of his own. He wears hearing aids because he has had sensorineural hearing loss for many years, previously described by his audiologist as severe, high-frequency, bilateral symmetric loss. The patient reports that he has cut back on social engagements because the hearing aids no longer help.

On examination, his score on the Mini–Mental State Examination is 5 points lower than it was last year. His score on the Hearing Handicap Inventory for the Elderly (HHIE) is now 28, increased from 20 last year. He is referred to his audiologist, who finds that the patient's hearing has declined to the level of profound hearing loss and that speech comprehension is consistent with the severity of hearing loss.

Which of the following is the most appropriate recommendation for this patient?

(A) Cochlear implant
(B) Inteo hearing aid
(C) Bone-anchored hearing aid
(D) Auditory brain-stem implant

ANSWER: A

This patient's hearing has deteriorated to the profound level, and his hearing aids are no longer adequate. Of the choices, a cochlear implant is most likely to improve his profound hearing loss. Cochlear implants are small, commercially available electronic devices that are effective in older adults with long-term severe to profound hearing loss. This type of hearing loss is typically unrelated to aging. The device is surgically implanted into the inner ear such that the arrays of electrodes bypass the damaged hair cells and are inserted into the auditory nerve, directly stimulating the nerve. Cochlear implants are a viable option for approximately 300,000 older adults with profound hearing loss. The implants improve the ability to hear verbal communication and environmental sounds, and they can enhance telephone communication and enjoyment of music. In studies including older adults, a cochlear implant in one ear reduced the emotional consequences of hearing loss, as measured using the HHIE. Bilateral implantation further reduced the social and situational consequences of severe hearing loss (SOE=B). Age at implantation had a minimal effect on postoperative outcome for older recipients. The variables most predictive of success were the percentage of life spent with a severe to profound sensorineural hearing loss and residual speech-recognition ability (SOE=B). In older adults with a good auditory foundation, late-onset hearing loss mitigates the potentially negative physiologic effects of age. Medicare covers cochlear implants and surgery. The procedure requires anesthesia and can be completed in about 3 hours.

Only 23% of the 31 million people with hearing loss use hearing aids. Because Medicare does not cover hearing aids, these devices may be a value-added benefit for commercial health plans. Data continue to demonstrate the quality-of-life benefits of hearing aids, especially among older adults. Use of hearing aids is associated with decreased depression and delayed declines in functional status. The Inteo hearing aid can be useful for hearing loss that is not at the profound level. It uses integrated signal processing with adaptive directional microphones, feedback cancellation, multiple channels, and advanced noise-reduction circuitry. This digital hearing aid is available as a behind-the-ear unit with an open-fit earmold. Ten years ago, 18.8% of all hearing aids sold were behind-the-ear units; in 2007, they were 51% of the hearing-aid market in the United States. The advent of digital circuitry has allowed behind-the-ear units to remain small in size.

The bone-anchored hearing aid (BAHA™) is a surgically implanted system for treatment of such conditions as chronic ear infections, congenital external atresia of the external auditory canal, or "single-sided deafness" resulting from such conditions as acoustic schwannoma. The system was approved by the FDA in 1996 for conductive and mixed hearing loss and in 2002 for unilateral sensorineural hearing loss. It consists of a titanium implant placed into the bone, allowing bone conduction to stimulate the cochlea directly and thus bypass the outer and middle ear. When vibrations through the skull are sent from the sound processor to the external abutment, the titanium implant creates vibrations within the skull and the cochlea, which stimulate the nerve fibers of the inner ear. People with unilateral hearing loss that resulted from removal of an acoustic tumor have significant reductions in self-reported hearing handicap with BAHA. To determine if the BAHA will be useful for them, potential recipients can test it before surgery.

The auditory brain-stem implant is used to restore hearing function in individuals with hearing loss related to bilateral retrocochlear tumors. It is a prosthetic device specifically designed to bypass the cochlea and the auditory nerve, transmitting sound directly to the brain stem. The device is placed directly on the nerve center (cochlear nucleus) at the base of the brain, usually during surgery to remove tumors. According to the House Ear Institute, the auditory brain-stem implant has been used in 500 people worldwide. The device was approved by the FDA in 2000.

References

1. Chisolm T, Johnson C, Danhauer J, et al. A systematic review of health-related quality of life and hearing aids: Final report of the American Academy of Audiology Task Force on the Health Related Quality of Life Benefits of Amplification in Adults. *J Am Acad Audiol.* 2007;18(2):151–183.
2. Leung J, Wang N, Yeagle J, et al. Predictive models for cochlear implantation in elderly individuals. *Arch Otolaryngol Head Neck Surg.* 2005;131(12):1049–1054.

266. An 88-yr-old man comes to you for evaluation after having two previous systolic blood pressure readings >160 mmHg. He is remarkably healthy, with a history only of osteoarthritis, macular degeneration, and multiple basal cell cancers that have been treated successfully. He takes calcium, vitamin D, and acetaminophen as needed.

On examination, blood pressure is 170/88 mmHg and pulse is 70 beats per minute, without postural changes. His physical examination is otherwise unremarkable. His ECG is normal, as are all laboratory tests except for a low-density lipoprotein cholesterol of 128 mg/dL. He eats a healthy diet, exercises regularly, and is not interested in further lifestyle changes.

What is the best approach to treating his blood pressure at this point?

(A) Measure home blood pressure on at least 3 separate occasions.
(B) Begin a thiazide diuretic.
(C) Begin a β-blocker.
(D) Begin an α-blocker.

ANSWER: B

Systolic hypertension in older adults is common and associated with poor outcomes. In several clinical trials (SHEP, Syst-Eur), treatment of systolic hypertension reduced the incidence of stroke, coronary heart disease, and heart failure (versus placebo) (SOE=A). A meta-analysis of eight trials of treatment of systolic hypertension also showed a mortality benefit (SOE=B). Most experts recommend that thiazide diuretics should be the initial agent in the absence of comorbidities that would make other agents preferable (eg, coronary artery disease—β-blockers; diabetes—ACE inhibitors) (SOE=C). However, all four major classes of antihypertensive drugs (diuretics, β-blockers, ACE inhibitors/angiotensin-receptor blockers, and calcium channel blockers) have been shown to reduce cardiovascular events (SOE=A). α-Agonists were found to be inferior to other classes of blood pressure agents in improving clinical outcomes (SOE=A). Recently, some analyses have suggested that β-blockers may be inferior to other agents in older adults (SOE=B). In many cases, combination medication therapy is necessary.

Treatment of systolic hypertension in adults >80–85 yr old has benefits, but optimal agents and the goals of treatment are a topic of continued interest. The recent Hypertension in the Very Elderly Trial (HYVET) showed that treatment of hypertension in patients ≥80 yr old with indapamise with or without perindopril with a target blood pressure of <150/80 mmHg was associated with reduced all-cause mortality, cardiovascular events, stroke-related death, and heart failure. In other studies, hypertensive patients >80 yr old who achieved systolic blood pressures of <140 mmHg appeared to have increased mortality rates, so the ideal blood pressure target in adults >80 yr old is still being debated. Because this patient's systolic blood pressure has been >160 mmHg on three separate occasions, additional home blood pressure recordings before treatment are not indicated. Home blood pressure measurements are most useful when office readings are inconsistent, the diagnosis of hypertension is in question, or when the diagnosis of "white coat" hypertension is being considered (SOE=C).

References

1. Beckett NS, Peters R, Staessen JA, et al. Treatment of hypertension in patients 80 years of age and older (HYVET). *N Engl J Med.* 2008;358(18):1887–1898.
2. Bulpitt CJ, Beckett NS, Cooke J, et al. Results of the pilot study for the Hypertension in the Very Elderly Trial (HYVET). *J Hypertension.* 2003;21(12):2409–2417.
3. Chobanian AV. Clinical Practice. Isolated systolic hypertension in the elderly. *N Engl J Med.* 2007;357(8):789–796.
4. Pickering TG, Hall JE, Appel LJ, et al. Recommendations for blood pressure measurement in humans and experimental animals: part 1: blood pressure measurement in humans: a statement for professionals from the Subcommittee of Professional and Public Education of the American Heart Association Council on High Blood Pressure Research. *Circulation.* 2005;111(5):697–716.

267. An 82-yr-old man, previously independent, comes to the emergency department with 2 days of difficulty swallowing, productive cough, and dyspnea. History includes hypertension and controlled type 2 diabetes mellitus. On examination, he has a low-grade fever and increased blood pressure. Physical examination and chest radiography are consistent with consolidation in the left lower lobe. On bedside testing, he immediately sputters and coughs after drinking a small amount of water from a cup. There are no other neurologic findings. Laboratory testing suggests mild dehydration, and WBC count is slightly increased. MRI reveals a new, small brain-stem infarction and mild generalized cerebral atrophy.

Treatment for aspiration pneumonia is instituted. Seven days after onset of symptoms, swallowing has not improved, and formal evaluation shows aspiration with most consistencies.

Which of the following is the best recommendation?

(A) Careful oral feeding
(B) Gastrostomy feeding
(C) Hospice
(D) Nasogastric feeding
(E) Total parenteral nutrition

ANSWER: B

This patient most likely has pharyngeal-phase dysphagia resulting from brain-stem infarction. He will not be able to obtain adequate nutrition via an oral route at this time. The safest oral feeding may require pureed solids and honey-thick liquids; most people cannot obtain adequate intake with this restrictive diet. Nearly half of patients with dysphagia due to stroke recover effective swallowing within 7 days (SOE=B). Many patients with this type of injury will have significant, if not complete, recovery within 1 yr with rehabilitation (SOE=C). Hospice is not appropriate at this time: given the patient's relatively good premorbid functional status and lack of serious comorbidities, substantial recovery is likely, and he should be encouraged to undergo optimal treatment. Early placement of a gastrostomy tube with appropriate nutritional support and judicious rehabilitation gives this patient the best opportunity to return to his premorbid condition. Many patients can manage their own feeding tube and return to their prior residence (SOE=C).

Nasogastric feeding is a short-term treatment associated with greater need for tube replacement. Nasogastric feeding might be appropriate temporarily if placement of a gastrostomy tube is delayed. Total parenteral nutrition is associated with bacterial and fungal sepsis and makes fluid management more difficult; it also requires central venous access with its associated risks, and thus is not appropriate.

References

1. Dennis MS, Lewis SC, Warlow C; FOOD Trial Collaboration. Effect of timing and method of enteral tube feeding for dysphagic stroke patients (FOOD): a multicentre randomised controlled trial. *Lancet.* 2005;365(9461):764–772.
2. DiBartolo MC. Careful hand feeding: a reasonable alternative to PEG tube placement in individuals with dementia. *J Gerontol Nurs.* 2006;32(5):25–33.
3. Janes SE, Price CS, Khan S. Percutaneous endoscopic gastrostomy: 30-day mortality trends and risk factors. *J Postgrad Med.* 2005;51(1):23–29.
4. McMahon M, Hurley D, Kamath P, et al. Medical and ethical aspects of long-term enteral tube feeding. *Mayo Clinic Proc.* 2005;80(11):1461–1476.
5. Ramsey DJ, Smithard DG, Kalra L. Early assessments of dysphagia and aspiration risk in acute stroke patients. *Stroke.* 2003;34(5):1252–1257.
6. Verhoef MJ, Van Rosendaal GM. Patient outcomes related to percutaneous endoscopic gastrostomy placement. *J Clin Gastroenterol.* 2001;32(1):49–53.

268. A 79-yr-old woman comes to the office to establish care. She reports that she often feels sleepy. History includes osteoporosis, hip fracture, systolic heart failure, hypertension, frequent falls, chronic kidney disease, and post-herpetic neuralgia. Medications include extended-release metoprolol 100 mg/d, gabapentin 600 mg q8h, alendronate 35 mg/wk, vitamin D 800 IU/d, calcium carbonate 500 mg q8h, and aspirin 81 mg/d. Serum creatinine is 1.5 mg/dL, with estimated creatinine clearance of 30 mL/min.

Which of the following would be most likely to relieve this patient's sleepiness?

(A) Reduce gabapentin dosage to 600 mg q12h.
(B) Start lisinopril 2.5 mg/d.
(C) Discontinue alendronate.
(D) Increase vitamin D to 1,200 IU/d.
(E) Switch extended-release metoprolol to metoprolol 50 mg q12h.

ANSWER: A

In patients with chronic kidney disease who take medications that are primarily eliminated by the kidneys, dosage adjustments are often needed to avoid adverse drug events. This patient's lethargy may be related to the excessive gabapentin dosage, particularly in light of her renal impairment. Gabapentin is eliminated by the kidneys unchanged. In patients with creatinine clearance between 30 and 59 mL/min, the total dosage recommendation for gabapentin is 400–1400 mg.

Because this patient has systolic heart failure, an ACE inhibitor may improve survival and reduce morbidity (SOE=A). It may also slow progression of her kidney disease. However, it is unlikely to cause her sleepiness.

Discontinuing alendronate will not reduce the patient's sleepiness. According to the manufacturer, alendronate (and other bisphosphonates) are not recommended for patients with severe renal impairment (creatinine clearance <35 mL/min), because experience in this population is limited. Available evidence suggests that bisphosphonates can be used safely in women with stage 3 chronic kidney disease, such as this patient (SOE=A). There are no comparable data for patients with stage 4 or 5 renal disease.

The recommended vitamin D dosage is 800–1,000 IU/d (SOE=A). Increasing the patient's dosage to 1,200 IU/d will not improve her lethargy. Likewise, changing from extended-release to regular metoprolol will not affect the lethargy.

References

1. Facts & Comparisons. *Drug Facts and Comparisons 2008.* St. Louis, MO; 2008.
2. Jamal SA, Bauer DC, Ensrud KE, et al. Alendronate treatment in women with normal to severely impaired renal function: an analysis of the fracture intervention trial. *J Bone Miner Res.* 2007;22(4):503–508.
3. Miller PD, Roux C, Boonen S, et al. Safety and efficacy of risedronate in patients with age-related reduced renal function as estimated by the Cockcroft and Gault method: a pooled analysis of nine clinical trials. *J Bone Miner Res.* 2005;20(12):2105–2115.

269. An 80-yr-old man comes to the office for routine evaluation. He has a history of osteoarthritis, major depressive disorder, and well-controlled hypertension. Medications include hydrochlorothiazide 12.5 mg/d, escitalopram 20 mg/d, ibuprofen 400 mg q8h, and valsartan 80 mg/d. The patient's blood pressure readings at home average 160/80 mmHg.

Which of the following is the next best step to take in managing his hypertension?

(A) Increase hydrochlorothiazide.
(B) Stop escitalopram.
(C) Stop ibuprofen.
(D) Increase valsartan.
(E) Add amlodipine.

ANSWER: C

There is increasing evidence that hypertension is not age dependent and should be treated in older adults (SOE=A). The evaluation of hypertension in older adults should include a search for exacerbating factors. NSAIDs adversely affect blood pressure, heart failure, and renal function (SOE=B). Medications that may be implicated in worsening blood pressure should be stopped before a new medication is introduced to manage hypertension. Escitalopram does not increase blood pressure. Valsartan or hydrochlorothiazide could be increased if blood pressure remains increased after ibuprofen is discontinued. Amlodipine could be added as a third medication if stopping the ibuprofen and adjusting the dosages of other antihypertensive medications does not successfully lower the patient's blood pressure. For the patient's arthritis, acetaminophen 1 gram q8h may be effective, as well as exercise, heat/cold application, and physical therapy.

References

1. Beckett NS, Peters R, Fletcher AE, et al. Treatment of hypertension in patients 80 years of age or older. *N Engl J Med.* 2008;358(18):1887–1898.
2. Gaziano JM. Nonnarcotic analgesics and hypertension. *Am J Cardiol.* 2006;97(9A):10–16.

270. A 76-yr-old woman comes to the office because she has multiple rough skin lesions on her forehead, temples, cheeks, and forearms. Nasolabial folds are spared. The lesions bleed easily when she picks them off, and then recur. The lesions are scaly, <1 cm in diameter, and feel like sandpaper to touch.

Which of the following is the most appropriate treatment?

(A) Moisturizing cream
(B) Metronidazole gel
(C) Imiquimod 5% cream
(D) Ketoconazole 2% cream
(E) Sunscreen and observation

ANSWER: C

The patient has actinic keratosis. The lesions can be single or multiple, and they are dry, rough, adherent, and scaly. The lesions are on sun-exposed skin, while areas that are less exposed to the sun (eg, nasolabial folds) are spared. The lesions can be skin-colored, brown, or yellow-brown. They are coarse like sandpaper; often they are more easily felt than seen. Prolonged and repeated exposure to the sun in susceptible individuals damages keratinocytes. A moisturizing cream and sunscreen are helpful but insufficient. Actinic keratosis should be treated because of its potential to progress to squamous cell carcinoma (SOE=C). Treatment options include ablative therapies (cryosurgery, curettage) or topical therapies for patients with >15 lesions. Curettage (mechanical scraping) provides tissue for histologic evaluation and is particularly helpful for thick, hyperkeratotic lesions. Topical therapies include various fluorouracil formulations, imiquimod 5% cream, and diclofenac 5% gel. Photodynamic therapy is also effective. It involves application of a topical photosensitizer to the lesions. The skin is then exposed to a light source for photoactivation.

Ketoconazole 2% cream is used to treat facial and trunk seborrheic dermatitis; a mild corticosteroid (eg, hydrocortisone 1%) can also be effective. Lesions associated with seborrheic dermatitis are erythematous patches or plaques with loose, yellowish, greasy scales. They are present in areas where sebaceous glands are most prominent: scalp, eyebrows, nasolabial folds, ears, chest, and intertriginous areas. The etiology of seborrheic dermatitis is thought to be, at least in part, an inflammatory reaction to the yeast *Pityrosporum ovale*.

Metronidazole is used as initial therapy for rosacea, an acneiform disorder with vascular dilation of the central face, including the nose (especially in men), cheek, eyelids, and forehead.

References

1. Chia A, Moreno G, Lim A, Schumack S. Actinic keratoses. *Aust Fam Physician.* 2007;36(7):539–543.
2. Kalisiak MS, Rao J. Photodynamic therapy for actinic keratosis. *Dermatol Clin.* 2007;25(1):15–23.
3. McIntyre WJ, Downs MR, Bedwell SA. Treatment options for actinic keratoses. *Am Fam Physician.* 2007;76(5):667–671.

271. A 76-yr-old man comes to the office because he recently read about the new "shingles shot" and wants to know if he should have it. He had an isolated case of herpes zoster in the past and does not want a recurrence.

Which of the following is true regarding the herpes zoster vaccine Zostavax?

(A) It is recommended for people with acute zoster or ongoing post-herpetic neuralgia.
(B) It is less effective in preventing post-herpetic neuralgia in adults ≥70 yr old than in younger adults.
(C) People with a history of herpes zoster infection were excluded from the stage 3 trial.
(D) Before administration of the vaccine, the patient's history of varicella exposure should be confirmed.

ANSWER: C

Herpes zoster develops in approximately 30% of adults over a lifetime. The risk of herpes zoster increases with age: by age 85, 50% of adults have had herpes zoster. The incidence of post-herpetic neuralgia increases with age. Approximately 40% of adults ≥60 yr older are likely to have neuralgia after an episode of herpes zoster.

The zoster vaccine (Zostavax) was licensed for prevention of herpes zoster after being studied in a large (38,546 participants), double-blind, placebo-controlled trial of adults ≥59 yr old; 90% of participants had more than one underlying chronic medical illness. The average duration of follow-up was 3 yr, and 95% of participants completed the study. The vaccine was more effective in preventing zoster in adults between the ages of 60 and 69 than for those >70 yr old. However, the incidence of post-herpetic neuralgia was lower in the group ≥70 yr old than in adults 60–69 yr old. From this study, 17 persons would need to be vaccinated to prevent 1 case of herpes zoster, and approximately 31 would need to be vaccinated to prevent 1 case of post-herpetic neuralgia (SOE=A).

Adults with a history of zoster were excluded from the trial, possibly because of the risk of recurrent zoster. However, use of the vaccine does not appear to present safety concerns for this group, and patients do not need to be asked about varicella exposure or have a varicella titer determined before receiving the vaccine.

The vaccine is not used to treat people with acute zoster or to treat ongoing post-herpetic neuralgia. It is contraindicated for patients who are immunosuppressed, have a history of tuberculosis, or have recently taken either steroids or chemotherapy for cancer. Typical adverse events of the vaccine are local, varicella-like rash, erythema, pain, swelling, and pruritus at the site of injection.

References

1. Harpaz R, Ortega-Sanchez IR, Seward JF; Advisory Committee on Immunization Practice (ACIP) Centers for Disease Control and Prevention (CDC). Recommendations of the Advisory Committee on Immunization Practices (ACIP). Prevention of herpes zoster. *MMWR Recomm Rep.* 2008;57(RR-5):1–30.
2. Kimberlin D, Whitley R. Varicella-zoster vaccine for the prevention of herpes zoster. *N Engl J Med.* 2007;356(13):1338–1343.

272. An 82-yr-old woman comes to the office for follow-up pain management. She has a history of chronic low-back pain radiating into the buttocks due to spinal stenosis. For 4 yr, the pain had been managed with stable doses of oxycodone plus acetaminophen. The patient usually needed the medication 1 or 2 days each month, and took 4 pills on those days. The patient has reported an increase in pain over the past 3 mo. She has run out of the oxycodone and has requested early refills each month. Last month, she called the office because she lost her prescription and needed a replacement. She would now like a change in the prescription to allow her to take up to 6 pills in 1 day. Her increased usage has coincided with a new living arrangement: the patient's daughter has moved into her apartment to care for her, which has caused the patient substantial stress and anxiety. The patient further reports that her daughter has a drug problem.

There are no new findings on physical examination. Routine laboratory tests, including an erythrocyte sedimentation rate, are unrevealing. MRI of the lumbosacral spine was performed 1 mo before the current visit; it showed stable spinal stenosis (as compared with a scan from a year ago) and no new pathology.

Which of the following is most appropriate?

(A)   Pursue additional radiologic testing to identify the cause of the increase in pain.
(B)   Discontinue oxycodone plus acetaminophen; begin a long-acting opioid medication.
(C)   Defer renewal of the patient's opioid prescription until her daughter undergoes urine drug screening.
(D)   Add a benzodiazepine to the treatment regimen to address pseudoaddiction.
(E)   Schedule an extended appointment for the patient and her daughter to discuss opioid use.

ANSWER: E

Despite limited evidence of long-term efficacy, opioid use for chronic noncancer pain is increasing in the United States. This case raises several red flags for possible opioid misuse or abuse, including an abrupt change in medication requirement, multiple requests for early refills, and report of a lost prescription. These last two situations are frequently used as criteria for establishing opioid misuse or abuse (SOE=C). The most appropriate management strategy would be to express concern about the possibility of misuse or abuse, and to schedule an extended visit with the patient and her daughter to gather more information and to voice concerns with both parties.

A history of substance abuse is a strong and independent predictor of opioid abuse. The daughter may, in fact, be using her mother's medications. However, withholding the medication from the patient would leave her in pain. Many addiction experts advocate urine testing to assess for misuse or abuse, but requiring a urine screen of the daughter is not appropriate, given that she is not the patient. Another possible explanation is that the mother is using the medication to treat her stress and anxiety. Pseudoaddiction is typically defined as drug-seeking behavior that occurs in response to inadequate analgesia; it is sometimes mistaken for addiction. Pseudoaddiction would not be treated successfully by adding a benzodiazepine to the medication regimen.

Further diagnostic imaging is not likely to yield useful information in this case, particularly because the pain has not extended beyond its previous sites, and an MRI scan, obtained after the change in opioid pattern, showed stable spinal stenosis.

Tolerance is defined as the need for an increase in the dosage of a medication to produce the same analgesic effect. While it can occur in patients on long-term opioid therapy, the abruptness and amount of medication requested in this case are not consistent with tolerance.

References
1. Barry LC, Gill TM, Kerns RD, et al. Identification of pain-reduction strategies used by community-living older persons. *J Gerontol A Biol Sci Med Sci.* 2005;60(12):1569–1575.
2. Compton WM, Volkow ND. Major increases in opioid analgesic abuse in the United States: concerns and strategies. *Drug Alcohol Depend.* 2006;81(2):103–107.
3. Ives TJ, Chelminski PR, Hammett-Stabler CA, et al. Predictors of opioid misuse in patients with chronic pain: a prospective cohort study. *BMC Health Serv Res.* 2006;6:46.
4. Katz NP, Sherburne S, Beach M. Behavioral monitoring and urine toxicology testing in patient receiving long-term opioid therapy. *Anesth Analg.* 2003;97(4):1097–1102.

273. A 70-yr-old man who lives in assisted living is admitted to the hospital with several hand fractures related to a fall. The fall was not witnessed, but there are no signs of head trauma. His family notes that he has a 2-yr history of progressive memory impairment.

On examination, the patient is physically agitated and appears anxious. He is verbal but cannot recall where he is or why. His score on the Mini–Mental State Examination is 15/30, and his attention span is normal. He sleeps poorly in the hospital at night and tends to sleep during the day, but he is easily aroused. Physical examination, brain imaging, and laboratory examinations do not identify reversible causes of his impairments.

Which of the following is the most likely cause of this patient's agitation?

(A)   Generalized anxiety disorder
(B)   Alzheimer's disease
(C)   Delirium
(D)   Head trauma
(E)   Major depressive disorder

ANSWER: B

Although each of the options can cause agitation, the most likely cause in this case is dementia related to Alzheimer's disease. Unless they are also delirious, patients with Alzheimer's disease have normal attention but impaired cognition, particularly short-term recall, that has progressed gradually for years. Anxiety can be related to the agitation of dementia, to uncontrolled pain, or to fear of novel settings and people, or it may have no particular trigger beyond the dementia itself.

Unremarkable brain imaging that does not indicate stroke, hematoma, or injury makes head trauma an unlikely cause of this patient's anxiety (SOE=A). The diagnosis of delirium requires an attention deficit.

References

1. Hshieh TT, Fong TG, Marcantonio ER, et al. Cholinergic deficiency hypothesis in delirium: a synthesis of current evidence. *J Gerontol A Biol Sci Med Sci.* 2008;63(7):764–772.
2. Salzman C, Jeste DV, Meyer RE, et al. Elderly patients with dementia-related symptoms of severe agitation and aggression: consensus statement on treatment options, clinical trials methodology, and policy. *J Clin Psychiatry.* 2008;69(6):889–898.

274. A 68-yr-old woman is brought to the office by her daughter, who describes a 2-yr history of reduced attention to personal hygiene and inappropriate behavior. The patient is threatened with eviction because she stopped paying rent. She believes that the landlord is trying to get her to move by infiltrating her apartment with toxic gas through the air vents. She often smells the gas and has several times called the police, but they have not found anything. She believes that the landlord has arranged for her problems to be broadcast each night on the television news, and she hears him in the walls every night, discussing his plans to get rid of her. There is no history of alcohol or substance abuse, or functional decline.

Physical examination, cognitive assessment, laboratory tests, and CT of the head are within normal limits.

Which of the following is the most likely diagnosis?

(A) Alzheimer's disease
(B) Late-onset schizophrenia
(C) Delirium
(D) Major depressive disorder
(E) Delusional disorder

ANSWER: B

This patient has a sustained course of persecutory delusions, ideas of reference, and auditory and olfactory hallucinations. The bizarre nature of her delusions and the prominence of auditory hallucinations point to

schizophrenia rather than to a delusional disorder. An estimated 15%–20% of cases are in patients ≥45 yr old (late-onset schizophrenia). There are no differences between early- and late-onset cases in terms of positive symptoms, family history, brain abnormalities, memory retention, or minor physical abnormalities. Late-onset schizophrenia affects more women than men, whereas there are no gender differences in early-onset disease. Late-onset schizophrenia is more likely to be associated with the paranoid subtype; lower levels of negative symptoms; and less impairment in learning, abstraction, and flexibility. In patients with late-onset disease, premorbid functioning is better with respect to work and marriage.

In very late-onset schizophrenia-like psychosis, symptoms begin after age 60. This disorder has more brain abnormalities and neuropsychologic deficits. Far more women are affected than with early- or late-onset schizophrenia, and there is a greater prevalence of persecutory and partition delusions; higher rates of visual, tactile, and olfactory hallucinations; lower genetic load; more sensory abnormalities; and absent negative symptoms or formal thought disorder such as disorganized thinking. Limited data suggest that older adults with schizophrenia respond to antipsychotic treatment at dosages lower than those required in younger patients (SOE=C).

Late-onset schizophrenia can be differentiated from delirium by its sustained course, lack of visual hallucinations, and absence of an attention deficit. Major depressive disorder can present with psychotic features, although typically these are not bizarre, and reflect depressive themes (mood congruent), such as death and disability. Individuals with major depressive disorder with psychotic features have other symptoms of major depression.

Differentiating late-onset schizophrenia from dementia-related psychosis can be difficult. Sustained systematized delusions and persistent auditory hallucinations are an unlikely presentation of psychosis in Alzheimer's disease. Psychotic symptoms are rare at the onset of dementia in Alzheimer's disease; more typically they emerge after several years (mid-stage) and are typically characterized by simple, repetitive, nonsustained delusions, such as delusions of theft or abandonment, or delusional misidentification of caregivers. Patients with Alzheimer's disease are more likely to have visual than auditory hallucinations.

References

1. Howard R, Rabins PV, Seeman MV, et al. Late-onset schizophrenia and very-late-onset schizophrenia-like psychosis: an international consensus. The International Late-Onset Schizophrenia Group. *Am J Psychiatry*. 2000;157(2):172–178.
2. Manepalli JN, Gebretsadik M, Hook J, et al. Differential diagnosis of the older patient with psychotic symptoms. *Primary Psychiatry*. 2007;14(8):55–62.
3. Mintzer J, Targum SD. Psychosis in elderly patients: classification and pharmacotherapy. *J Geriatr Psychiatry Neurol*. 2003;16(4):199–206.

275. Which of the following statements best describes the use of complementary and alternative medicine in the United States?

(A) Complementary and alternative medicine is replacing the existing healthcare system.
(B) Male gender is the best predictor for use of complementary and alternative medicine.
(C) Use of complementary and alternative medicine is unrelated to age or ethnicity.
(D) Herbal therapy is the most popular form of complementary and alternative medicine.

ANSWER: D

The use of complementary and alternative medicine is common among older adults. Use is significantly influenced by race and ethnicity. In a study of treatment for colds, insomnia, and back pain, Hispanic ethnicity and female gender best predicted use of complementary and alternative medicine. Blacks were more likely than whites to use complementary and alternative medicine. Hispanics were more likely than whites or blacks to choose herbal medications to self-treat colds and insomnia, and more likely than whites to visit practitioners of complementary and alternative medicine for low-back pain. Hispanics were more likely than blacks or whites to treat insomnia with herbal medications rather than with OTC or prescription medications.

Individuals who use complementary and alternative medicine are more likely to use conventional care too. Most people are not using complementary and alternative medicine in place of conventional health care, but as an adjunct to it.

In the United States, the most commonly used complementary and alternative modalities in 2002 were herbal therapy (18.6%, representing >38 million adults), followed by relaxation techniques (14.2%, representing 29 million adults) and chiropractic treatment (7.4%, representing 15 million adults). Among those who used complementary and alternative medicine, 41% used 2 or more types during the previous year. Between 1997 and 2002, the greatest relative increase in use of complementary and alternative medicine was seen for herbal medicine (12.1% versus 18.6%, respectively), while the greatest relative decrease was seen for chiropractic treatment (9.9% versus 7.4%, respectively). The prevalence of complementary and alternative medicine use remained stable from 1997 to 2002.

References

1. Cherniack EP, Ceron-Fuentes J, Florez H, et al. Influence of race and ethnicity on alternative medicine as a self-treatment preference for common medical conditions in a population of multi-ethnic urban elderly. *Complement Ther Clin Pract*. 2008;14(2):116–123.
2. Druss BG, Marcus SC, Olfson M, et al. Trends in care by nonphysician clinicians in the United States. *N Engl J Med*. 2003;348(2):130–137.
3. Grzywacz JG, Quandt SA, Neiberg R, et al. Age-related differences in the conventional health care-complementary and alternative medicine link. *Am J Health Behav*. 2008;32(6):650–663.
4. Tindle HA, Davis RB, Phillips RS, et al. Trends in use of complementary and alternative medicine by US adults. 1997–2002. *Altern Ther Health Med*. 2005;11(1):42–49.

276. A 78-yr-old man is evaluated because he has been unable to take oral nutrition since surgery 3 days earlier after a fall. With encouragement he can take oral medications. Formal speech and language assessment finds mild oral pharyngeal dysphagia.

He lives at home with his wife. History includes Lewy body dementia that has been present at least 6 yr. He has lost approximately 6.8 kg (15 lb) over the last year. He speaks in short, partial sentences and has difficulty following a conversation. At home, he requires assistance with bathing, dressing, grooming, toileting, and set-up for feeding.

Physical examination is unremarkable.

Laboratory results:

Albumin	2.8 g/dL
BUN	28 mg/dL
Creatinine	0.7 mg/dL
Hemoglobin	10.7 g/dL
Total cholesterol	115 mg/dL

Additional laboratory tests are unremarkable.

Which of the following is the most appropriate management?

(A) Arrange for placement of a percutaneous gastrostomy tube.
(B) Determine the patient's goals of medical care and preferences.
(C) Prescribe oral megestrol acetate suspension 400 mg/d.
(D) Prescribe nutritional supplements and multivitamins.
(E) Refer for hospice care.

ANSWER: B

This patient has end-stage dementia; he most likely has adult failure-to-thrive syndrome. The time course is appropriate, and no readily reversible cause of weight loss has been identified. No feeding interventions have consistently been shown to affect prognosis in such cases (SOE=B). There is little harm in a trial of oral supplements, but supplements can be costly. Artificial feeding and hydration via gastrostomy is invasive and has not been shown to improve prognosis or quality of life; careful feeding by hand is preferable and more efficacious. Megestrol acetate suspension is approved for use only in AIDS wasting syndrome; results of one study of megestrol for long-term care patients suggest that the adverse events outweigh the potential small benefit in weight gain. Other medications have not made a substantial difference for most patients in this situation. With weight loss, dependency in ADLs, recurrent illness, and a paucity of speech, the prognosis in dementia is <6 mo. The most appropriate response to this patient's weight loss is to meet with his family to ascertain his goals and preferences in the context of his terminal condition (SOE=C). It is not appropriate to refer him to hospice until a plan of care is agreed on.

References

1. Finucane TE, Christmas C, Travis K. Tube feeding in patients with advanced dementia: a review of the evidence. *JAMA*. 1999;282(14):1365–1370.
2. Golden AG, Daiello LA, Silverman MA, et al. University of Miami Division of Clinical Pharmacology therapeutic rounds: medications used to treat anorexia in the frail elderly. *Am J Ther*. 2003;10(4):292–298.
3. Mitchell SL, Buchanan JL, Littlehale S, et al. Tube-feeding versus hand-feeding nursing home residents with advanced dementia: a cost comparison. *J Am Med Dir Assoc*. 2004;5(2 Suppl):S22–29.
4. Potter JM. Oral supplements in the elderly. *Curr Opin Clin Nutr Metab Care*. 2001;4(1):21–28.
5. White GN, O'Rourke F, Ong BS, et al. Dysphagia: causes, assessment, treatment, and management. *Geriatrics*. 2008;63(5):15–20.

277. Having seen numerous news reports about the "Alzheimer's gene," a middle-aged woman comes to the office to request genetic testing for Alzheimer's disease.

Which of the following statements is correct?

(A) Apolipoprotein E *(APOE)* genetic testing requires physician referral and pre- and post-test counseling by a genetics counselor.
(B) A positive test result causes increased symptoms of anxiety.
(C) The Genetic Information Nondiscrimination Act of 2008 (GINA) does not include protective safeguards for long-term care insurance.
(D) Presence of the ε4 allele of the *APOE* gene is associated with younger age at onset of Alzheimer's disease.

ANSWER: C

The 2008 Genetic Information Nondiscrimination Act (GINA) protects individuals from discrimination by employers and health insurers but does not offer safeguards for life, disability, or long-term care insurance.

The role of the apolipoprotein E *(APOE)* ε4 allele as a susceptibility gene for late-onset Alzheimer's disease has been widely confirmed in multiple studies. The presence of the ε4 allele increases risk of Alzheimer's disease but is neither necessary nor sufficient to cause disease. Testing for the ε4 allele thus differs from predictive genetic testing common to diseases with Mendelian inheritance (eg, Huntington's disease), in which gene markers definitively predict future disease. As such, testing for *APOE* status uses different protocols for risk assessment and counseling, and research is ongoing for such questions as to who is likely to seek testing and how test results will be used. In 2008, a Philadelphia-based company made direct-to-consumer salivary testing for *APOE* commercially available for the first time.

Results from the REVEAL (Risk Evaluation and Education for Alzheimer's Disease) study published in 2005 indicate that 90% of study participants who were informed of their ε4 allele status and its association with Alzheimer's disease had unchanged or reduced levels of anxiety about Alzheimer's disease after their risk was disclosed. A systematic review of the psychologic impact of genetic testing recently reported little or no difference in anxiety symptoms in carriers and noncarriers of predispositional mutations for hereditary breast/ovarian or colon cancers a year after disclosure, indicating that the REVEAL results are not an isolated phenomenon.

The few individuals (1%–2% in population estimates) who are homozygous for *APOE ε4* have a 50% risk of symptomatic Alzheimer's disease by their mid to late 60s, whereas heterozygote status confers a 50% risk of disease by the mid to late 70s. However, if Alzheimer's disease does not develop during these age ranges, the person's risk becomes comparable to that of the general population. In addition, a recent examination of cognitive phenotypes in Alzheimer's disease challenged the idea that presence of an *ε4* allele inevitably lowers age at onset of disease.

Reference

1. Couzin J. Genetics. Once shunned, test for Alzheimer's risk headed to market. *Science.* 2008;319(5866):1022–1023.
2. Heschka JT, Palleschi C, Howley H, et al. A systematic review of perceived risks, psychological and behavioral impacts of genetic testing. *Genet Med.* 2008;10(1):19–32.
3. Hudson KL, Holohan MK, Collins FS. Keeping pace with the times: the Genetic Information Nondiscrimination Act of 2008. *N Eng J Med.* 2008;358(25):2661–2663.
4. Roberts JS, Cupples AL, Relkin NR, et al. Genetic risk assessment for adult children of people with Alzheimer's disease: the risk evaluation and education for Alzheimer's disease (REVEAL) study. *J Geriatr Psychiatry Neurol.* 2005;18(4):250–255.
5. Snowden JS, Stopford CL, Julien CL, et al. Cognitive phenotypes in Alzheimer's disease and genetic risk. *Cortex.* 2007;43(7):835–845.

278. Increased concentrations of interleukin-6 (IL-6) and other inflammatory cytokines have been associated with which of the following conditions?

(A)   Functional decline
(B)   Lewy body dementia
(C)   Mild cognitive impairment
(D)   Alzheimer's disease

ANSWER: D

IL-6 is a potent mediator of inflammatory processes, and levels increase with age. Researchers have proposed that the age-associated increase in IL-6 may account for some of the characteristics typical of advanced age. Age-related changes possibly linked to chronic inflammation include decreased lean body mass, osteopenia, anemia, and decreased serum albumin and cholesterol levels. Increased levels of inflammatory proteins (eg, C-reactive protein), lymphoproliferative disorders, multiple myeloma, osteoporosis, and Alzheimer's disease have all been linked to increased IL-6 expression (SOE=B).

References

1. Ershler WB, Keller ET. Age-associated increased interleukin-6 gene expression, late-life diseases, and frailty. *Annu Rev Med.* 2000;51:245–270.
2. Naugler WE, Karin M. The wolf in sheep's clothing: the role of interleukin-6 in immunity, inflammation and cancer. *Trends Mol Med.* 2008;14(3):109–119.

279. A 66-yr-old man comes to the office because his family has noticed increasing apathy, forgetfulness, and confusion over the past few months. For example, he now gets lost on his way home from familiar places. He and his wife lived in England for 20 yr before her death 10 yr ago. He then moved to the United States and has dated occasionally. He has no significant comorbidities and is on no medications. There is no history of sexually transmitted disease. His family is concerned that he may have early Alzheimer's disease.

Physical examination is normal except for the neurologic exam, which reveals slowing of rapid finger and toe tapping, increased reflexes, short-term memory deficits, and an inability to do relatively simple calculations. He scores 22/30 on the Mini–Mental State Examination. His affect is normal. A cranial CT scan reveals mild to moderate atrophy, but no other changes. There are no metabolic or endocrine abnormalities on laboratory testing.

What is the most likely cause of this patient's dementia?

(A)   Syphilis
(B)   Creutzfeldt-Jakob disease
(C)   Human immunodeficiency virus (HIV) antibody
(D)   Lyme disease

ANSWER: C

One of every 11 new diagnoses of HIV is in an adult >50 yr old. In the United States, older adults are the cohort least likely to practice safe sex; most cases of HIV infection in older adults are acquired through sexual activity. Older adults are more likely than young adults to meet criteria for acquired immune deficiency syndrome (AIDS) at the time of HIV diagnosis, perhaps because nonspecific symptoms such as weight loss, dementia, and failure to thrive are more common in older adults and because, untreated, AIDS progresses faster in older adults. However, once diagnosed, older adults with HIV are as likely to benefit from anti-HIV therapy as young adults, with regard to both survival and immunologic recovery.

HIV-associated dementia can present with many different clinical syndromes. The most common characteristics include fairly rapid decline in memory and concentration, emotional disturbances, and psychomotor slowing. Spasticity, tremor, and ataxia can also be present. This patient's presentation is consistent with HIV-associated dementia, and epidemiologically this is the most prevalent infectious dementia in this age group. Arrest and even reversal of HIV-associated dementia are widely described and expected with combinations of antiretroviral drugs that penetrate the CNS. Although hyperlipidemia, accelerated atherosclerosis, and other metabolic complications are seen in patients on antiretroviral therapies, these effects do not offset the marked benefit of therapy. If treated, this patient can expect marked improvement in his memory and his chance of surviving at least 3 yr is >80%. He should be counseled regarding safe sex and routes of transmission. All his sexual partners within the last 5 yr should be tested for HIV.

Neurosyphilis is a late manifestation of infection with *Treponema pallidum*. Findings include neurocognitive decline and prominent frontal lobe signs. Creutzfeldt-Jakob disease is a rapidly progressive dementia associated with myoclonus, and pyramidal and extrapyramidal signs, which this patient does not exhibit. *Borrelia burgdorferi* is an unusual cause of infectious dementia. Patients can have a history of tick bite, as well as the typical rash of *erythema chronicum migrans*, transient arthritis, cranial nerve palsies, and cardiac conduction disturbances that would precede dementia caused by *B burgdorferi*.

References

1. Duthie EH, Katz PR, Malone ML, ed. *Practice of Geriatrics, 4th ed.* Philadelphia, PA: Saunders Elsevier; 2007.
2. Geschwind MD, Haman A, Miller BL. Rapidly progressive dementia. *Neurol Clin.* 2007;25(3):783–807.
3. Luther VP, Wilkin AM. HIV infection in older adults. *Clin Geriatr Med.* 2007;23(3):567–583.
4. Perez JL, Moore RD. Greater effect of highly active antiretroviral therapy on survival in people aged > or = 50 years compared with younger people in an urban observational cohort. *Clin Infect Dis.* 2003;36(2):212–218.
5. Wellons MF, Sanders L, Edwards LJ, et al. HIV infection: treatment outcomes in older and younger adults. *J Am Geriatr Soc.* 2002;50(4):603–607.

280. A 79-yr-old woman comes to the office for a routine evaluation. Her husband of 58 yr died 6 mo ago. He had dementia and she had taken care of him for 10 yr. During this time, she gradually withdrew from most of her social engagements and activities. History includes hypertension and diabetes, and macular degeneration was recently diagnosed. She finds the prospect of blindness terrifying, and offhandedly mentions that she is certain she could not cope with it.

Which of the following is true of risk factors associated with major depressive disorder in older adults?

(A) Hypertension is a risk factor.
(B) Social isolation is a risk factor if compounded by disability.
(C) Bereavement and caregiver status are risk factors independent of health status.
(D) Diabetes is a risk factor independent of heart disease.
(E) Chronic illness is a risk factor for late-onset major depressive disorder, irrespective of functional limitations.

ANSWER: C

This patient has several risk factors for major depressive disorder: she spent many years as a caregiver, she had a recent loss, she has become socially isolated, she is facing a significant physical disability, she has at least three serious chronic illnesses, and she feels overwhelmed by the stressors she is facing (SOE=B).

Extensive studies support an association between major depressive disorder in older adults and stroke, but not in older adults with hypertension alone. Close to 25% of patients who have had myocardial infarction or stroke, regardless of stroke location, have major depressive disorder. In these patients, the co-occurrence of major depressive disorder is associated with lower adherence to medical recommendations, lower participation in rehabilitation, and overall increase in morbidity and mortality. These findings have prompted studies to determine whether use of antidepressants soon after a cardiovascular event improves overall outcome. Thus far, results are encouraging but not as strong as anticipated.

There is strong evidence for physical disability as a risk factor for development of major depressive disorder in older adults. The association of major depressive disorder with chronic medical conditions (eg, diabetes mellitus, COPD, osteoarthritis, cancer, macular degeneration) is not related to the chronic condition per se, but to the degree of functional limitation and the patient's perceived sense of mastery. Social isolation, caregiver status, and bereavement are each independent risk factors. This patient's multiple risk factors require close monitoring for major depressive disorder and interventions to decrease her social isolation (SOE=C).

References

1. Cole MG, Dendukuri N. Risk factors for depression among elderly community subjects: a systematic review and meta-analysis. *Am J Psychiatry.* 2003;160:1147–1156.
2. Frasure-Smith N, Lespérance F, Talajic M. Depression following myocardial infarction. Impact on 6-month survival. *JAMA.* 1993;270(15):1819–1825.
3. Gallo JJ, Bogner HR, Morales KH, et al. Depression, cardiovascular disease, diabetes and 2-year mortality among older primary care patients. *Am J Geriatr Psychiatry.* 2005;13(9):748–755.
4. Rovner BW, Casten RJ. Preventing late-life depression in age-related macular degeneration. *Am J Geriatr Psychiatry.* 2008;16(6):454–459.

281. A 76-yr-old man has been in a nursing facility for 3 wk since he had a left-hemisphere stroke with right hemiparesis and mild expressive aphasia. His cognitive status was normal before the stroke, and he was living unassisted with his wife in a single-story home. He was initially unable to participate in rehabilitation because of delirium. Currently, he is dependent in transfers and toileting and requires assistance in dressing. His speech is 50% intelligible. His cognitive status has returned to baseline, and the physical therapist reports that he is actively engaged in therapy and follows 3-step commands. Assessments have not been performed for occupational therapy and speech or language pathology.

Which of the following is the most appropriate next step?

(A) Discharge the patient to home with a referral for home-based rehabilitation.
(B) Ask the nursing home to obtain occupational therapy and speech and language pathology consultations.
(C) Instruct the physical therapist to continue therapy at a slower pace.
(D) Refer the patient to an inpatient stroke rehabilitation service.

ANSWER: D

Clinical outcomes are better when patients who have had a stroke receive coordinated, multidisciplinary evaluation and intervention (SOE=A). The intensity of services offered in a stroke rehabilitation unit is associated with better outcomes (SOE=B). Probably the most important factor influencing outcome is a patient's cognitive status (SOE=A). Delirium, a negative risk factor in rehabilitation, appears to have been transient in this case. The patient's level of independence before the stroke is also a predictor of outcome.

Rehabilitation efforts can begin after the patient has been medically stabilized. This patient's ability to follow 3-step commands shows good receptive-speech capability and short-term memory. Generally, expressive speech deficits are not an added risk of poor outcome in stroke rehabilitation. The addition of occupational and speech therapy would allow him to receive up to 3 hour of therapy per day and meet Medicare reimbursement guidelines.

In-home stroke rehabilitation is generally reserved for patients requiring a slower pace of rehabilitation. The presence of a capable caregiver is critical to success. Home rehabilitation is best for patients needing only one type of rehabilitation (eg, physical therapy) (SOE=C).

Stroke rehabilitation provided in a nursing facility can benefit patients needing a slow pace. The number of therapy hours per day is not mandated, as it is with inpatient units. This patient does not appear to have objective reasons for needing a slower pace (SOE=C).

Slowing the pace of therapy would not meet this patient's rehabilitation needs. It could worsen his deconditioning. In addition, he needs occupational therapy to reduce his dependence in ADLs, and speech therapy to improve his aphasia (SOE=D).

References
1. Bates B, Choi JY, Duncan PW, et al. Veterans Affairs/ Department of Defense Clinical Practice Guideline for the Management of Adult Stroke Rehabilitation Care: executive summary. *Stroke*. 2005;36(9):2049–2056.
2. Stroke Unit Trialists' Collaboration. Organized inpatient (stroke unit) care for stroke. *Cochrane Database Syst Rev*. 2002;(1):CD000197.

282. A 77-yr-old man is referred for evaluation and management of multiple myeloma. While travelling in Tibet, he sustained a fracture of the right humerus. Radiography showed a destructive lesion of the right glenoid with intra-articular extension. Bone radiography showed evidence of diffuse osteopenia and a pathologic fracture of the right humerus. Serum protein electrophoresis identified an immunoglobulin Gλ monoclonal protein level of 3.6 g/dL; 24-hour urine protein electrophoresis confirmed a paraprotein level of 200 mg/d.

Laboratory tests are remarkable for hemoglobin of 8.9 g/dL and serum creatinine of 3.8 mg/dL.

Which of the following therapies is most appropriate?

(A) Zoledronic acid
(B) Oral thalidomide and dexamethasone
(C) Bortezomib and dexamethasone
(D) Melphalan and prednisone followed by autologous stem cell transplantation

ANSWER: C

This patient has advanced-stage multiple myeloma characterized by diffuse osteoporosis and a destructive bone lesion, most likely the result of a plasmacytoma. In addition, he has hypercalcemic renal failure, perhaps due to proximal tubule nephropathy from light-chains, or due to one of the many potential causes of renal failure in the setting of multiple myeloma. Although treatment of multiple myeloma has dramatically changed in the last decade, his age and renal insufficiency limit therapy. Bortezomib, a novel proteasome inhibitor, is an effective agent, alone or in combination with other agents, in the treatment of multiple myeloma (SOE=A). It has demonstrated activity in renal failure with an acceptable toxicity profile (SOE=C). The FDA has approved use of bortezomib, without dosage adjustments, in patients with impaired renal function, including those requiring hemodialysis.

In this patient, a bisphosphonate should be part of the treatment regimen, but zoledronic acid is contraindicated in renal failure and should not be administered. Pamidronate, at a dosage adjusted for renal insufficiency, might be safer (SOE=C). An immunomodulatory agent like thalidomide or lenalidomide has distinct advantages over standard alkylator-based chemotherapy, and is better in terms of inducing a response than steroids alone. However, the use of this class of agents in renal insufficiency has not been established. Thalidomide can be associated with significant adverse events (in particular, somnolence) when administered to patients with renal failure. Melphalan and prednisone could be appropriate, but autologous transplantation in older adults, regardless of disease stage, has not been shown to result in a progression-free or overall survival advantage over conventional therapy (SOE=A).

References
1. Moreau P, Hulin C, Facon T. Frontline treatment of multiple myeloma in elderly patients. *Blood Rev*. 2008;22(6):303–309.
2. Palumbo A, Bringhen S, Liberati AM, et al. Oral melphalan, prednisone, and thalidomide in elderly patients with multiple myeloma: updated results of a randomized, controlled trial. *Blood*. 2008;112(8):3107–3114.
3. Tsubokura M, Kami M. Treatment for elderly patients with multiple myeloma. *Lancet*. 2008;371(9617):983.

283. A 48-yr-old woman comes to the office because she is worried that she is likely to develop Alzheimer's disease. She has been the primary caregiver since her mother was diagnosed with Alzheimer's disease 8 yr ago. The daughter asks whether there is anything she can do to minimize her risk.

Which of the following statements is most accurate about modifying risk of Alzheimer's disease?

(A) Long-term use of hormone replacement therapy reduces a woman's risk of Alzheimer's disease.
(B) There is insufficient evidence to recommend use of an NSAID to reduce risk.
(C) Use of high-dose vitamin E supplements is highly effective in reducing risk.
(D) *Ginkgo biloba* extract is both safe and effective in reducing the risk of Alzheimer's disease.

ANSWER: B

Results from randomized, controlled trials of NSAIDs for the prevention of Alzheimer's disease have been inconsistent (SOE=C). Most recently, a randomized, double-blind, placebo-controlled clinical trial designed to investigate the efficacy and safety of celecoxib and naproxen for the primary prevention of Alzheimer's disease found no decrease in disease incidence associated with use of either NSAID. Adults enrolled in this trial were ≥70 yr old, ie, already within the typical age range for onset of Alzheimer's disease. Additional research is needed to determine whether the potentially neuroprotective effects of NSAIDs, as suggested by observational studies, depend on other factors, such as timing or duration of NSAID use.

Evidence on the relationship between hormone replacement therapy and risk of Alzheimer's disease is far from definitive. In a prospective cohort study (Cache County Study), a protective association was found between long-term hormone use and dementia risk, suggesting that there might be a perimenopausal "therapeutic window" during which hormone replacement might reduce later dementia risk. In contrast, initial results from the Women's Health Initiative Memory Study (WHIMS), an ancillary study of the Women's Health Initiative, found that incidences of dementia and Alzheimer's disease on follow-up were higher than expected in women ≥65 yr old who had been randomly assigned to short-term use of either estrogen or estrogen/progestin (SOE=A). In 2008, results from a large, 5-yr prospective cohort study did not support an effect of hormone replacement in prevention of dementia (SOE=B).

The preponderance of evidence from randomized, controlled trials does not support a protective effect on cognition from antioxidant vitamins such as vitamin E. In addition, in meta-analysis of randomized primary and secondary prevention trials, vitamin E increased all-cause mortality regardless of dosage (SOE=A).

The *Ginkgo biloba* extract used in Chinese traditional medicine has become a popular alternative therapy for maintenance or enhancement of cognition. Case reports have suggested a possible causal relationship between use of *Ginkgo biloba* and bleeding, including intracranial hemorrhage (SOE=B). A randomized, placebo-controlled, double-blind trial examined the effect of *Ginkgo biloba* on preventing cognitive impairment in a small group of cognitively intact adults ≥85 yr old. In an intention-to-treat analysis, no significant delay in cognitive decline was found, but a post-hoc analysis controlling for medication compliance showed a protective effect. In this study, there were more incidents of transient ischemic attack and stroke in the treated group (SOE=A). The National Center for Complementary and Alternative Medicine is funding a multicenter, randomized, placebo-controlled, double-blind trial of *Ginkgo biloba* and dementia as its primary outcome.

References
1. ADAPT Research Group. Naproxen and celecoxib do not prevent AD in early results from a randomized controlled trial. *Neurology.* 2007;68(21):1800–1808.
2. Bjelakovic G, Nikolova D, Gluud LL, et al. Mortality in randomized trials of antioxidant supplements for primary and secondary prevention: systematic review and meta-analysis. *JAMA.* 2007;297(8):842–857.
3. Dodge HH, Zitzelberger T, Oken BS, et al. A randomized placebo-controlled trial of *Ginkgo biloba* for the prevention of cognitive decline. *Neurology.* 2008;70(19 Pt 2):1809–1817.
4. Petersen RC, Thomas RG, Grundman M, et al. Vitamin E and donepezil for the treatment of mild cognitive impairment. *N Engl J Med.* 2005;352(23):2379–2388.
5. Petitti DB, Crooks VC, Chiu V, et al. Incidence of dementia in long-term hormone users. *Am J Epidemiol.* 2008;167(6):692–700.
6. Rossouw JE, Prentice RL, Manson JE, et al. Postmenopausal hormone therapy and risk of cardiovascular disease by age and years since menopause. *JAMA.* 2007;297(13):1465–1477.

284. A 70-yr-old retired mailman comes to the office because he now has difficulty climbing 1 flight of stairs. He has dyspnea on exertion that has progressed slowly over 5 yr. He wheezes occasionally. He has had a minimally productive morning cough for many years but no chest pain or discomfort. He has a 50 pack-year cigarette smoking history and still smokes.

On examination, temperature is 36°C (96.8°F), blood pressure is 115/75 mmHg, heart rate is 98 beats per minute, and respiratory rate is 22 breaths per minute. There is no accessory muscle use. Bibasilar crackles are audible. Cardiac and abdominal examinations are normal. There is trace peripheral edema but no cyanosis or clubbing. Chest radiography is normal.

Pulmonary function tests:

FVC	65% of predicted
FEV_1	70% of predicted
FEV_1/FVC ratio	75%

After bronchodilation, FEV_1 increases by 9% and FVC increases by 8%.

Which of the following is the most likely cause of this patient's dyspnea?

(A) Asthma
(B) COPD
(C) Idiopathic pulmonary fibrosis
(D) Pleural effusion
(E) Pulmonary embolism

ANSWER: C

This patient's FEV_1/FVC ratio is ≥70%, which is consistent with either normal spirometry or restrictive disease. Because the FVC is <70% of predicted, the patient's spirometry is consistent with restrictive disease. Spirometry measures the rate of airflow out of the lungs during rapid, forceful, and complete expiration from total lung capacity to residual volume (forced vital capacity maneuver). This test provides an indirect measure of the flow-resistive properties of the lungs. The critical values to interpret are the FEV_1, the FVC, and the FEV_1/FVC ratio. FEV_1 is a measure of airflow, and FVC a measure of volume. The "reversibility" of airflow obstruction is evaluated by repeating spirometry 15 min after administration of a bronchodilator, usually a β_2-agonist such as albuterol. While the presence of "reversibility" indicates that asthma is a component of the disease, it is not pathognomonic for asthma. A reasonable normal range for FEV_1 and FVC is between 80% and 100% of predicted, and ≥70% (actual number, not percent predicted) for the FEV_1/FVC ratio. However, because structural changes occur in the airways with age, some experts recommend using an FEV_1/FVC ratio of ≥65% for adults ≥70 yr old. Significant reversibility is defined as ≥12% increase in either FEV_1 or FVC.

Asthma and COPD cause obstructive, not restrictive, disease. Pulmonary embolism is a pulmonary vascular disease and usually causes neither obstruction nor restriction. Although both pleural effusion and idiopathic pulmonary fibrosis can cause restriction, the absence of

pleural disease on chest radiography makes effusion unlikely. Between 10% and 15% of cases of interstitial lung disease are associated with normal chest radiography. This patient's normal chest radiograph is consistent with idiopathic pulmonary fibrosis (SOE=A).

References

1. Miller MR, Hankinson J, Brusasco V, et al. Standardization of spirometry. *Eur Respir J.* 2005;26(2):319–338.
2. Pellegrino R, Viegi G, Brusasco RO, et al. Interpretative strategy for lung function tests. *Eur Respir J.* 2005;26(5):248–268.

285. For patients recently discharged from the hospital after treatment for an acute ischemic stroke, what is the strongest predictor of return to the emergency department or hospital during the first 30 days after discharge?

(A) Mechanical ventilation during the hospital stay
(B) Female gender
(C) Medicaid enrollment
(D) Discharge from hospital to rehabilitation center

ANSWER: C

A complicated transition (or "bounce back") has been defined as the movement of a patient from a less-intensive to a more-intensive care setting. An example of a complicated transition would be a visit to the emergency department for evaluation of an acute condition by a patient recently discharged from the hospital. A recent study identified predictors of complicated transitions for patients in the 30 days after hospitalization for acute ischemic stroke. Patients who had one or more complicated transitions were more likely to be older, black, and enrolled in Medicaid; have a longer index hospitalization; be initially discharged to a nursing or long-term care facility; and have more chronic diseases (SOE=C).

When compared with patients with one complicated transition, patients with more than one complicated transition were more likely to be male, black, have prior hospitalizations, have fluid and electrolyte disorders, and be discharged to a nursing or long-term care facility. Patients who were initially discharged to a rehabilitation center were less likely to have complicated transitions. The strongest predictor of multiple complicated transitions was black race. Perhaps surprisingly, the need for mechanical ventilation during the hospital stay, a marker of stroke severity, was not a predictor of subsequent complicated transitions.

References
1. Coleman EA, Berenson RA. Lost in transition: challenges and opportunities for improving the quality of transitional care. *Ann Intern Med.* 2004;141(7):533–536.
2. Coleman EA, Min SJ, Chomiak A, et al. Posthospital care transitions: patterns, complications, and risk identification. *Health Serv Res.* 2004;39(5):1449–1465.
3. Kind AJ, Smith MA, Frytak JR, et al. Bouncing back: patterns and predictors of complicated transitions 30 days after hospitalization for acute ischemic stroke. *J Am Geriatr Soc.* 2007;55(3):365–373.

286. An 83-yr-old man comes to the clinic because he recently began having urinary incontinence. Urine leaks when he coughs or bends, and he has painful urgency. He has difficulty with starting to void, stopping and restarting midstream, weak stream, frequency, and urgency, and he awakens several times each night to urinate. He also has abdominal fullness and suprapubic discomfort. He has not been ill and has not started any new medications.

On examination, the lower abdomen is tense; there is dullness on percussion at the midline emanating from the pubic symphysis up to the umbilicus. On palpation of the lower abdomen, the patient feels an intense need to void, yet he is unable to do so.

Portable ultrasonography shows approximately 600 mL of urine in the bladder.

Which of the following is the most appropriate next step?

(A) Give a loading dose of terazosin 10 mg in the clinic, followed by terazosin 10 mg nightly at home.
(B) Start finasteride at 5 mg/d.
(C) Start doxazosin and finasteride.
(D) Insert Foley catheter; if bladder volume is confirmed, leave catheter in and refer for further evaluation.
(E) Give a 500-mL fluid challenge to stimulate voiding.

ANSWER: D

The patient has worsening urinary retention that has not yet progressed to complete retention. This was previously called "overflow" incontinence. The International Continence Society has recommended that this term be replaced by terminology that describes the predominant type of leakage (ie, urge, stress, or mixed urinary incontinence), along with a high postvoid residual volume (SOE=C).

A diagnosis of urinary retention must be considered when there is a midline mass emanating from the suprapubic area that is dull on percussion. These findings are specific but not necessarily sensitive—they can be absent even with postvoid residual volumes of ≥300 mL (SOE=C). The appropriate approach is to confirm retention with catheterization. Inserting a Foley catheter (versus a straight catheter) will avoid a second catheterization if the decision is made to leave the catheter in place. Generally, the catheter remains in place for 1–2 wk to decompress the bladder, after which evaluation may be done to determine the cause of the retention, or a voiding trial may be considered. Patients with large postvoid residuals should be monitored for rapid diuresis in the hours after the bladder is drained.

When symptoms of urinary retention are present, a fluid challenge could exacerbate retention. α-Blockers (eg, terazosin, doxazosin, prazosin, tamsulosin, alfuzosin) and 5-α reductase inhibitors (eg, finasteride, dutasteride) improve symptoms associated with the lower urinary tract, but this patient's symptoms and degree of retention favor bladder drainage (SOE=C). Terazosin should not be given as a loading dose; a 1-mg test dose given at night can identify individuals who are overly sensitive to the medication (SOE=A).

References
1. Kaplan SA, Wein AJ, Staskin DR, et al. Urinary retention and post-void residual in men: separating truth from tradition. *J Urol.* 2008;180(1):47–54.
2. Lepor H, Jones K, Williford W. The mechanism of adverse events associated with terazosin: an analysis of the Veterans Affairs Cooperative Study. *J Urol.* 2000;163(4):1134–1137.
3. Selius BA, Subedi R. Urinary retention in adults: diagnosis and initial management. *Am Fam Physician.* 2008;77(5):643–650.

287. A 79-yr-old man in an assisted-living facility has cough, shortness of breath, and pleuritic chest pain. He has a history of heart failure with bifascicular block and chronic kidney disease with a baseline creatinine of 1.8 mg/dL. His medications are lisinopril, furosemide, and simvastatin. On examination, he is awake and alert. Respiratory rate is 22 breaths per minute, temperature is 39.2°C (102.5°F), heart rate is 90 beats per minute, and blood pressure is 130/80 mmHg. Chest auscultation reveals crackles in the left lower lobe, and a chest radiograph shows an infiltrate. Community-acquired pneumonia is diagnosed, and he is admitted to the hospital. His creatinine is now 3.5 mg/dL, with an estimated creatinine clearance of 20 mL/min. Sputum for Gram stain is not obtainable; a urine for *Streptococcus pneumoniae* and *Legionella* antigen detection is sent.

Which is the most appropriate initial antibiotic choice?

(A) Moxifloxacin 200 mg/d
(B) Ceftriaxone 1 gram/d plus azithromycin 500 mg/d
(C) Levofloxacin 750 mg/d
(D) Aztreonam 2 grams q8h plus vancomycin 1 gram q24h

ANSWER: B

Community-acquired pneumonia in older adults is typically caused by *S pneumoniae*, nontypeable *Haemophilus influenzae, Moraxella cattarhalis, Mycoplasma pneumoniae, Chlamydophila* (previously *Chlamydia*) *pneumoniae, Legionella pneumoniae,* and respiratory viruses. Unless colonization is known, methicillin-resistant *Staphylococcus aureus* (MRSA) pneumonia is uncommon, and gram-negative bacilli (eg, *Pseudomonas, Klebsiella*) are uncommon in the absence of severe COPD (FEV$_1$ <30% predicted). For the most likely organisms, the Infectious Disease Society of America/American Thoracic Society recommend a respiratory fluoroquinolone alone or a β-lactam plus a second-generation macrolide (clarithromycin, azithromycin) for mild or moderate community-acquired pneumonia in older adults (SOE=C). In this patient, aztreonam and vancomycin are not needed for activity against *Pseudomonas* or MRSA, respectively, and are not effective against *M pneumoniae, C pneumoniae,* or *L pneumoniae* (SOE=C). In this patient with heart failure and a bifascicular block, fluoroquinolones are relatively contraindicated because of their effects on the QT interval. In addition, the dosage is too low for moxifloxacin, which does not require dosage adjustment in impaired renal function, and too high for levofloxacin, which does (SOE=D). Neither ceftriaxone nor azithromycin require dosage adjustment depending on renal function, which is likely to fluctuate significantly in this patient over the first few hours of hospitalization. Both medications have minimal effect on the QT interval and together are effective against the most common pathogens, including the "atypical" bacteria.

References

1. Donowitz GR, Cox HL. Bacterial community-acquired pneumonia in older patients. *Clin Geriatr Med.* 2007;23(3):515–534.
2. Mandell LA, Wunderink RG, Anzueto A, et al. Infectious Diseases Society of America/American Thoracic Society Consensus Guidelines on the Management of Community-Acquired Pneumonia in Adults. *Clin Infect Dis.* 2007;44 Suppl 2:S27–72.

288. An 82-yr-old man comes to the office because he is gradually losing erectile function. He reports that his libido is "not what it used to be"; he also reports sleep disturbances, lower energy, and intermittent irritability but no sadness or headache. History includes coronary artery disease, hypertension, dyslipidemia, and obesity. He takes aspirin, simvastatin, lisinopril, metoprolol, and a multivitamin daily.

On examination, he weighs 95 kg (210 lb; body mass index 34 kg/m^2). Blood pressure is 145/86 mmHg and pulse is 80 beats per minute. Cardiovascular and pulmonary examination is normal. Testicular volume is 20 cc bilaterally, and no prostate nodules are palpable.

Fasting morning laboratory results:

Total testosterone	166 ng/dL (5.76 nmol/L) and 142 ng/dL (4.93 nmol/L)
Luteinizing hormone	5 mIU/mL
Follicle-stimulating hormone	7.2 mIU/mL
Total cholesterol	190 mg/dL
High-density lipoprotein	40 mg/dL

Which of the following tests should be ordered next?

(A) Prostate-specific antigen
(B) MRI of the pituitary gland with contrast
(C) Karyotype analysis
(D) Prolactin
(E) Hematocrit

ANSWER: D

Late-onset male hypogonadism is controversial because there is no uniform agreement among endocrinologists as to what constitutes a low testosterone level (SOE=C). The Endocrine Society's clinical practice guideline suggests a threshold between 200 and 300 ng/dL (7 and 10 nmol/L). Others have proposed using an age-adjusted threshold, because testosterone levels decline with aging. Diagnosing late-onset male hypogonadism clinically is challenging because of its many nonspecific signs and symptoms.

The low testosterone levels and normal gonadotropin level suggest that this patient has secondary hypogonadism or hypogonadotropic hypogonadism. The next step is to exclude hyperprolactinemia as a cause of the low testosterone (SOE=C). Treatment of hyperprolactinemia can comprise initiating a dopamine agonist for prolactinoma or discontinuing an offending medication. Occasionally, men need testosterone therapy even after the prolactin level returns to normal.

Levels of prostate-specific antigen and hematocrit should be measured at baseline and 3 mo after starting testosterone therapy, and yearly thereafter. The concern that testosterone promotes prostate cancer is theoretical, not based on clinical evidence (SOE=B). However, before initiating testosterone therapy, secondary causes such as hyperprolactinemia must be excluded.

MRI of the pituitary with contrast is not indicated at this point because there is no clinical suggestion of a tumor, such as headache, visual field deficit, or galactorrhea (SOE=C). If the prolactin level is markedly increased, imaging of the pituitary would be justified.

Karyotype analysis is indicated if gonadotropin levels are high or if there is evidence of hypergonadotropic hypogonadism. Klinefelter's syndrome typically presents after adolescence, when fibrosis causes the testes to become small and hard. Some cases are diagnosed during adulthood, especially mosaic forms, which are typically milder than the classical form. This patient has normal-sized testes and normal gonadotropin levels (SOE=C).

References

1. Bhasin S, Cunningham GR, Hayes FJ, et al. Testosterone therapy in adult men with androgen deficiency syndromes: an endocrine society clinical practice guideline. *J Clin Endocrinol Metab.* 2006;91(6):1995–2010.
2. Marks LS, Mazer NA, Mostaghel E, et al. Effect of testosterone replacement therapy on prostate tissue in men with late-onset hypogonadism. *JAMA.* 2006;296(19):2351–2361.
3. Mohr BA, Guay AT, O'Donnell AB, et al. Normal, bound and nonbound testosterone levels in normally ageing men: results from the Massachusetts Male Ageing Study. *Clin Endocrinol.* 2005;62(1):64–73.
4. Roddam AW, Allen NE, Appleby P, et al. Endogenous sex hormones and prostate cancer: a collaborative analysis of 18 prospective studies. *J Natl Cancer Inst.* 2008;100(3):170–183.

289. Which of the following best characterizes major depressive disorder in later life?

(A) It is a usual part of aging.
(B) Symptoms are most common among adults ≥85 yr old.
(C) The incidence in older adults has increased over the past 10 yr.
(D) The incidence is similar among older white, black, and Hispanic Americans.
(E) Symptoms are more common among older men than among older women.

ANSWER: B

Clinically diagnosed major depressive disorder or a high number of depressive symptoms frequently accompanies physical illness, functional disability, and increased use of healthcare resources. Major depressive disorder is not a normal part of aging; it is a mental illness at any age and should be diagnosed and treated.

The incidence of major depressive disorder increases with age. Adults ≥85 yr old (19%) are more likely to report depressive symptoms than adults 65–74 yr old (13%) or 75–84 yr old (15%). The rate of major depressive disorder in adults >65 yr old has remained relatively stable since 1998. As with other age groups, older women consistently report higher rates of depressive symptoms than do older men: between 1998 and 2004, 11%–12% of men and 17%–19% of women ≥65 yr old reported depressive symptoms. Older men are more likely to commit suicide than women, with the largest difference among men and women ≥85 yr old. In this age range, suicide rates are 45 per 100,000 men and 4 per 100,000 women.

Rates of major depressive disorder in older adults differ across racial and ethnic groups. Rates of documented major depressive disorder are generally lower among black or African Americans and higher among Hispanics of all heritages than among white older adults. However, suicide rates are highest in white older adults.

References

1. Alegria M, Mulvaney-Day N, Torres M, et al. Prevalence of psychiatric disorders across Latino subgroups in the United States. *Am J Pub Health*. 2007;97(1):68–75.
2. Cohen CI, Magai C, Yaffee R, et al. Racial differences in syndrome and subsyndromal depression in an older urban population. *Psychiatric Services*. 2005;56(12):1556–1563.
3. Federal Interagency Forum on Aging-Related Statistics. *Older Americans 2008: Key Indicators of Well-Being*. Federal Interagency Forum on Aging-Related Statistics. Washington, DC: U.S. Government Printing Office; 2008.
4. Wells KB, Stewart A, Hays RD, et al. The functioning and well-being of depressed patients: results from the Medical Outcomes Study. *JAMA*. 1989;262(7):914–919.

290. A 72-yr-old retired bookkeeper is brought to the office by her husband because she has had gradually increasing problems with her memory over the past year. At first he noticed that his wife had trouble remembering the names of new acquaintances. This progressed to difficulty recalling details of books they read together, and more recently she had to telephone him for help because she could not recall where she had parked her car. Last month the husband had to take control of managing the household finances, a job she had performed competently throughout their marriage. Alzheimer's disease is diagnosed after physical examination and evaluation, including laboratory tests and structural neuroimaging. The couple asks you about cholinesterase inhibitor treatment.

Which of the following statements is the most appropriate response?

(A) The most common adverse events are headache and somnolence.
(B) Liver function must be monitored for the first 6 mo of treatment.
(C) Improvement of cognitive symptoms is sustained during the first 5 yr of treatment.
(D) Benefits are likely to be clinically subtle.
(E) Cholinesterase inhibitors differ significantly from one another in their effectiveness.

ANSWER: D

Since their introduction in 1997, cholinesterase inhibitors (eg, donepezil, galantamine, and rivastigmine) have become first-line treatment for Alzheimer's disease. Although their pharmacologic properties differ slightly, they all work by inhibiting acetylcholine esterase, the primary enzyme involved in breaking down the neurotransmitter acetylcholine. A 2006 Cochrane review concluded that all three medications are efficacious for mild to moderate Alzheimer's disease (SOE=B).

The most common adverse events reported with cholinesterase inhibitors are nausea, vomiting, and diarrhea. Because the adverse events are cholinergic and tend to be dose-related, cholinesterase inhibitors require low starting dosages with gradual upward titration. No laboratory monitoring is routinely required.

Most studies have examined treatment response for 1–2 yr, so there is little evidence on duration of effectiveness. Cumulative results to date indicate that use of a cholinesterase inhibitor has a statistically significant positive effect on tests of cognition for 6–12 mo, although the effect is generally modest. Benefits include improved performance on the ADAS-Cog Scale (a global scale of cognition), better ratings of global clinical state by clinicians blinded to other measures, and better ratings on scales of behavior and ADLs. Few studies have reported results in terms of improvements that are likely to be evident to patients and caregivers. Clinically apparent benefits can be subtle or can occur primarily via slowed progression. Patients and caregivers are at risk of therapeutic nihilism in the absence of counseling about treatment expectations.

There have been few comparative trials of different cholinesterase inhibitors. Most have been supported at least in part by pharmaceutical companies and have methodologic weaknesses, such as inadequate study duration. In a 2-yr, double-blind, randomized, multicenter trial from the United Kingdom in which rivastigmine and donepezil were compared, more frequent adverse events were reported for rivastigmine during the titration phase (SOE=A). Although some statistically significant differences between the two medications were reported in subgroup analyses, overall efficacy on cognition and behavior was similar.

References

1. Birks J. Cholinesterase inhibitors for Alzheimer's disease. *Cochrane Database Syst Rev.* 2006;(1):CD005593.
2. Qaseem A, Snow V, Cross JT Jr, et al. Current pharmacologic treatment of dementia: a clinical practice guideline from the American College of Physicians and the American Academy of Family Physicians. *Ann Intern Med.* 2008;148(5):370–378.
3. Raina P, Santaguida P, Ismaila A, et al. Effectiveness of cholinesterase inhibitors and memantine for treating dementia: evidence review for a clinical practice guideline. *Ann Intern Med.* 2008;148(5):379–397.

INDEX

NOTE: References are to question numbers, preceded by Q.

transurethral resection of the prostate for, Q195

Benzodiazepines, Q38, Q203, Q204
  withdrawal from, Q246

Bereavement, Q159, Q280

β_2-Agonists, Q233

β-Blockers
  for hypertension, Q266
  for perioperative management of knee
    replacement, Q1

Biliary stenting, Q27

Biofeedback-assisted pelvic muscle training,
  Q205

Biopsy
  endometrial, Q226
  open muscle, Q196
  prostate, Q133
  temporal artery, Q186

Bipolar disorder, manic type, Q116

Bisphosphonates
  oral, Q148
  -related osteonecrosis of the jaw, Q7, Q164
  for preventing fracture, Q39

Bladder, overactive, Q2, Q179, Q214

Bladder training, Q214

Bleeding
  gastrointestinal, Q135
  vaginal, Q226
  vitreous, Q250

Blood pressure
  ambulatory monitoring, Q188
  orthostatic hypotension, Q199
  postural, Q3

Blood-pressure control. *See also* Hypertension
  dietary management, Q41, Q57

Blood testing, Q77, Q230

Bone-anchored hearing aid (BAHA), Q265

Bone pain, metastatic, Q18, Q74

Bortezomib, Q282

BPH. *See* Benign prostatic hyperplasia

BPPV (benign paroxysmal positional vertigo),
  Q84, Q251

Braden scale, Q177, Q194

Branch retinal artery occlusion, Q190

Breast cancer, Q227
  adjuvant therapy for, Q208
  early, Q191
  pain relief for, Q18
  prevention of recurrence, Q134
  treatment of, Q191

Breast conservation treatment, Q191

Breath, shortness of, Q120

Bromocriptine, Q9

Bronchodilators, Q189

Bruises, Q83

Bullous pemphigoid, Q8

Bupropion, Q260

Burning mouth syndrome, Q178

Buspirone, Q121

Butorphanol, Q106

C

Calcitonin, Q85

Calcium, Q86

Calluses, Q75

Calorie counts, Q248

CAM (Confusion Assessment Method), Q202

Cancer
  advanced, Q47
  breast, Q18, Q134, Q191, Q208, Q227
  cervical, Q104
  colon, Q171
  colorectal, Q92
  oral, Q32
  pancreatic, Q27
  prostate, Q80, Q167

Candidiasis, vaginal, Q104

Canes, Q69

Capsule endoscopy, Q135

Carbamazepine, Q8

Carbidopa/levodopa, Q3, Q9

Cardiac imaging, Q49

Cardiac risk factors, Q198

Cardiovascular disease, Q165

Cardiovascular events, Q228

Care Management Plus, Q185

Caregiver burnout, Q159, Q241

Caregiver status, Q280

Carotid artery stenosis, Q62

Cataracts, Q222, Q250

Causalgia, Q144

Ceftriaxone, Q287

Celecoxib, Q142

Centers for Medicare & Medicaid Services
  (CMS), Q5

Cerebellar infarction, Q84

Cerebrovascular disease, Q123, Q223

Cervical cancer, Q104

Cervical myelopathy, Q237

Cervical spinal stenosis, Q237

Chemotherapy, Q27

Chest pain, Q49, Q120

Cholecalciferol, Q11

Cholecystectomy, emergent, Q31

Cholecystitis, acute, Q11

Cholinesterase inhibitors, Q140, Q290

Chondrocalcinosis, Q66

Chronic athlete's foot, Q259

Chronic obstructive pulmonary disease (COPD),
  Q189

Chronic open-angle glaucoma, Q190

Chronic pain, Q107, Q272

Chronic pelvic pain syndrome, Q14

Cigarette smoking, Q19

Circadian rhythm sleep disorder, Q258

Citalopram, Q73, Q140

Clinical trials, Q136

Clonazepam, Q26

Clopidogrel, Q17, Q82

Clostridium difficile infection, Q94, Q225

CMS (Centers for Medicare & Medicaid
  Services), Q5

Cochlear implants, Q265

Cockcroft-Gault formula, Q149

Codeine
  acetaminophen with, Q174
  for pain relief in osteoarthritis, Q229

Coenzyme Q_{10}, Q41

Cognitive assessment, Q37

Cognitive-behavioral therapy for anxiety attacks,
  Q204

Cognitive impairment, Q176
  mild, Q223

Cognitive testing, Q112

Colchicine, Q10

Colles' fractures, bilateral, Q210

Colon cancer screening, Q171

Colonoscopy, Q92, Q118, Q171

Colorectal cancer, Q92

Communication, Q261
  with hearing aids, Q245
  language interpreters for assistance with, Q44

Community-acquired pneumonia, Q94, Q287

Complementary and alternative medicine, Q275

Complex regional pain syndrome, Q144

Complicated transition, Q285

Comprehensive geriatric assessment, Q129

Comprehensive in-home assessment, Q50

Computed tomography, Q118
  of abdomen and pelvis, Q181
  of head, Q166

Confusion, acute, Q154

Confusion Assessment Method (CAM), Q202

Constipation
  chronic, Q155
  drug-induced, Q102

COPD (chronic obstructive pulmonary disease),
  Q189

Copper deficiency, Q95

Corns and calluses, Q75

Coronary angiography, Q49

Coronavirus, Q131

Corticosteroids
  for COPD, Q189
  for polyarticular gout, Q10

COX-2 inhibitors, Q142

Creatinine, Q198

Crystalline arthritis, Q66

Cubbin-Jackson scale, Q194

Culturally competent care, Q224, Q261

Cyclooxygenase-2 inhibitors (COX-2 inhibitors),
  Q142

Cystocele, Q113

D

25(OH)D, Q231

Dark chocolate, Q41

DASH (Dietary Approaches to Stop
  Hypertension) diet, Q41

Daytime sleepiness, Q249, Q258, Q268

Debridement, sharp, Q46

Obstructive sleep apnea, Q249
25(OH)D, Q231
Ondansetron, Q227
Onychomycosis, Q259
Open-angle glaucoma, Q250
  chronic, Q190
Open muscle biopsy, Q196
Opioids, Q272
  conversion, Q107
Oral bisphosphonates, Q148
Oral cancer, Q32
Oral estrogen therapy, Q239
Oral mucosal pain, Q178
Oral supplements, polymeric, Q23
Orthostasis, Q3
Orthostatic hypotension, Q199
Osteoarthritis
  of hip, Q240
  pain management in, Q229
Osteomyelitis, Q207
Osteonecrosis of the jaw, Q7, Q164, Q182
Osteopenia, Q242
Osteoporosis, Q7, Q148
  preventing fractures with, Q39
  risk factors for, Q175
  screening for, Q62
  treatment of, Q12, Q72, Q85
Ototoxicity, Q122, Q153
Out-of-pocket costs, Q99
Outpatient services, Q99
Overactive bladder, Q2, Q179, Q214
Overflow incontinence, Q286
Overweight, Q17
Oxybutynin
  anticholinergic effects, Q48, Q174
  for urinary incontinence, Q64, Q205, Q239
Oxycodone, Q18, Q229, Q240
Oxygen, Q212

P

PACE (Program of All-inclusive Care of the
  Elderly), Q157
Pacemaker implantation, Q4
Pain
  abdominal, Q181
  chronic, Q107
  chronic pelvic pain syndrome, Q14
  complex regional pain syndrome, Q144
  heel, Q119
  hip, Q180, Q240
  knee, Q66
  low back, Q6, Q74, Q180
  oral mucosal, Q178
  plantar fasciitis, Q119
  shoulder, Q151
Pain relief
  in breast cancer metastatic to bone, Q18
  in chronic pain, Q272
  in diabetic neuropathy, Q106
  multimodality management, Q50
  in osteoarthritis, Q229
Palliative care, Q27

Pamidronate, Q74
Pancreatic cancer, Q27, Q261
Panic attacks, Q204
Pap smear, Q104
Papulopustular rosacea, Q13
Parainfluenza virus, Q131
Parathyroid hormone, Q12, Q85
Parathyroid sestamibi (nuclear scan), Q231
Paratonia, Q71
Parkinson's disease
  assistive devices for, Q69
  falls with, Q3, Q9
  gait of, Q123
  seborrheic dermatitis in, Q209
Paroxetine
  cytochrome P450 interactions, Q229
  impact on mental status, Q174
Paroxysmal positional vertigo, benign, Q251
Patient-centered medical homes, Q184
PCI (percutaneous coronary intervention), Q247
Pelvic muscle training, Q205
Pelvic organ prolapse, Q64
Pelvic pain, Q14
Pemphigus vulgaris, Q8
Percutaneous coronary intervention (PCI), Q247
Percutaneous endoscopic gastrostomy tubes, Q23
Performance status, Q47
Periodontal disease, Q182
Peripheral blood testing for JAK2 mutation, Q77
Peripheral neuropathy, diabetic, Q53
Persantine thallium testing, Q49
Personality changes, Q166, Q221
Personality disorders
  major depressive disorder with, Q244
  narcissistic, Q116
  prevalence of, Q162
Pessaries, Q64
Pharmaceutical industry, Q136
Pharyngeal-phase dysphagia, Q267
Phenobarbital, Q40
Phosphodiesterase inhibitors, Q255
Physical abuse
  bruise characteristics that raise suspicion of,
    Q83
  mistreatment, Q176
Physical activity
  balance-training exercises, Q126
  health promotion in relation to cognition, Q98
  recommendations for, Q65
Physical disability, Q280
Physical therapy
  for complex regional pain syndrome, Q144
  electromechanics-assisted gait training with,
    Q232
  home health care, Q254
  for preventing falls, Q50
Physician house calls (home visits), Q168
Plantar fasciitis, Q119
Plasmapheresis, Q79

Pneumonia
  community-acquired, Q94, Q287
  home health care for, Q51
  organisms that cause, Q131
  postoperative, Q31
Polyarticular gout, Q10
Polymeric oral supplements, Q23
Polymyalgia rheumatica, Q219
Polysomnography, Q249
Positional vertigo, benign paroxysmal, Q251
Positioning maneuvers, Q251
Postoperative pneumonia, Q31
Postprandial hypotension, Q28
Postural hypotension, Q3
Postural instability, Q69
Postvoid residual urine testing, Q172
Potassium supplements, Q145
Prednisolone, Q144
Prednisone, Q10, Q219
Presbycusis, Q122
Pressure Sore Status Tool, Q194
Pressure Ulcer Scale for Healing (PUSH), Q194
Pressure ulcers
  monitoring, Q194
  reducing, in acute-care settings, Q109
  risk assessment of, Q177
  sacral, Q46
  unstageable, Q67
  wound care, Q60
Probenecid, Q10
Program of All-inclusive Care of the Elderly
  (PACE), Q157
Progressive resistance strength training, Q55
Progressive supranuclear palsy, Q183
Prolactin, Q288
Prompted-voiding program, Q179
Propoxyphene, Q106, Q229
Prospective payment, Q51
Prostate biopsy, Q133
Prostate cancer
  localized, Q80
  treatment of, Q167
Prostatectomy, radical, Q80
Proton-pump inhibitors, Q94
Pseudoephedrine, Q205
Psoriasis, Q104
Psychosis
  of Alzheimer's disease, Q71, Q111, Q197
  in dementia, Q197
  late-onset schizophrenia, Q274
  major depressive disorder with, Q30, Q43
Pulmonary disease, chronic obstructive (COPD),
  Q189
Pulmonary fibrosis, idiopathic, Q284
Pulmonary thromboembolism, Q120
PUSH (Pressure Ulcer Scale for Healing), Q194
Pyrazinamide, Q34

Q

Quadriceps muscle weakness, Q65
Quetiapine, Q59, Q102

Thyroidectomy, Q242

Tilt-table testing, Q230

Timed Up and Go test, Q103

Tinnitus, Q235

Tinnitus Handicap Questionnaire, Q158

Tiotropium, Q189

Toes, upgoing, Q6

Tolerance, Q272

Tolterodine, Q2, Q61, Q73, Q172

Tongue, geographic, Q178

Tongue ulcers, Q32

Topiramate, Q40

Total parenteral nutrition, Q267

Toxic epidermal necrolysis, Q8

Toxicity
  aminoglycoside, Q153
  ototoxicity, Q122, Q153
  vitamin A, Q95
  water intoxication, Q100

Training
  balance, Q126
  bladder, Q214
  gait, Q232
  pelvic muscle, Q205
  resistance, Q16, Q55, Q78
  strength, Q55, Q65, Q139

Transdermal fentanyl, Q107

Transrectal ultrasound, Q2

Transurethral resection of the prostate, Q195

Trauma, head, Q166

Trazodone, Q26, Q121

Treadmill stress testing, Q49

Trichophyton rubrum, Q259

Trimethoprim/sulfamethoxazole, Q149

Tuberculin skin test, Q34

Tuberculosis, Q34
  skin test (PPD), Q34

Tumors, thoracic spine, Q6

U

Ulcers
  pressure, Q60, Q67, Q109, Q177, Q194
  risk factors for, Q252
  sacral pressure, Q46
  tongue, Q32

Ultrasonography
  abdominal aorta, Q62
  transrectal, Q2

Undifferentiated somatoform disorder, Q187

Universal precautions, Q94

Urge incontinence, Q48, Q73, Q179, Q239

Urinary frequency, Q14

Urinary incontinence, Q179, Q214
  drug therapy for, Q56
  due to cystocele, Q113

mixed, Q56
  nonpharmacologic interventions for, Q88
  "overflow" incontinence, Q286
  stress, Q205, Q214
  treatment of, Q239
  urge, Q48, Q73, Q179, Q239

Urinary obstruction, Q86

Urinary retention, Q113, Q172, Q286

Urinary tract atrophy, Q152

Urinary urgency, Q2

Urine testing, postvoid residual, Q172

Urodynamic testing, Q239

Urosepsis, Q149

V

Vaccination
  herpes zoster, Q271
  influenza, Q220

Vaginal atrophy, Q104, Q150, Q152, Q216, Q226

Vaginal bleeding, Q226

Vaginal candidiasis, Q104

Vaginal estrogen tablets, Q150

Vaginal pessaries, Q64

Valsartan, Q165, Q269

Vancomycin, Q94, Q225, Q287

Vascular disease, Q58

Vasomotor symptoms, Q216

VDRL (Venereal Disease Research Laboratory) test, Q211

Vegetarian diet, Q134

Venereal Disease Research Laboratory (VDRL) test, Q211

Venlafaxine, Q26

Ventilator care, Q141

Vertigo
  acute onset of, Q84
  benign paroxysmal positional, Q251
  in Ramsay Hunt syndrome, Q235

Vestibular neuritis, Q153

Vibration testing, Q53

Violent behavior, Q201

Viral infections, respiratory, Q131

Vision assessment, Q25, Q63

Vision loss, Q25, Q143
  with diabetic retinopathy, Q250

Vision rehabilitation, Q29

Visual acuity, Q63

Visual hallucinations, Q33, Q173, Q256

Visuospatial cognitive deficits, Q223

Vitamin A toxicity, Q95

Vitamin B_6 deficiency, Q95

Vitamin B_{12}, Q79

Vitamin B_{12} deficiency, Q95, Q124

Vitamin D, Q268, Q283

Vitamin D deficiency, Q231

Vitamin D supplements, Q11, Q16

Vitreous hemorrhage, Q250

Voiding, prompted, Q179

Voiding diary, Q214

Vulvar atrophy, Q35

Vulvar skin changes, Q35

W

Walkers, Q69

Wallenberg's syndrome, Q84

Warfarin therapy, Q4, Q82, Q108

Water intoxication, Q100

Waterlow scale, Q194

Weakness, Q78, Q79, Q124

Weight loss
  in Alzheimer's disease, Q23
  causes of, Q70
  in diabetes mellitus, Q17
  in end-stage dementia, Q276
  intervention for, Q78
  involuntary, Q169
  with macular degeneration, Q29
  significant, Q21

Wet-to-dry dressings, Q46

Whirlpool therapy, Q60

Whisper test, Q158, Q236

White chocolate, Q41

"White-coat" hypertension, Q188

Withholding information, Q261

Women's health
  atrophic vaginitis, Q104, Q150, Q152, Q216, Q226
  hot flushes, Q216
  menopause, Q104, Q257
  myocardial infarction, Q247
  nursing home populations, Q147
  pelvic organ prolapse, Q64
  postmenopausal bleeding, Q226
  screening, Q62
  urinary incontinence, Q214
  vaginal bleeding, Q226
  vasomotor symptoms, Q216
  vulvar skin changes, Q35

Wound care
  for pneumonia, Q51
  with pressure ulcers, Q60

X

Xerosis, Q262

Xerostomia, Q200

Z

Zinc deficiency, Q95

Zoledronic acid, Q7, Q72

Zolpidem, Q59, Q102

Zoster vaccine (Zostavax), Q271